Artificial Intelligence Applications in Dermatology

Emmanouil Karampinis
Efterpi Zafiriou • Dimitrios Mantzaris
Editors

Artificial Intelligence Applications in Dermatology

Dermatology ex Machina: Clinical applications

Springer

Editors
Emmanouil Karampinis
Department of Dermatology
University Hospital of Larissa
Larissa, Larissa, Greece

Efterpi Zafiriou
Department of Dermatology
University Hospital of Larissa
Larissa, Greece

Dimitrios Mantzaris
Computational Intelligence and Health
Informatics Lab, Nursing Department,
School of Health Sciences
University of Thessaly
Larissa, Greece

ISBN 978-3-032-15613-6 ISBN 978-3-032-15614-3 (eBook)
https://doi.org/10.1007/978-3-032-15614-3

This Springer imprint is published by the registered company Springer Nature Switzerland AG
The registered company address is: Gewerbestrasse 11, 6330 Cham, Switzerland

To my mother, Rinio

Foreword

In recent years, the field of dermatology has witnessed a remarkable shift, altering the way dermatologists approach clinical diagnosis, address treatment dilemmas, and monitor skin diseases. The incorporation of AI in dermatology provides innovative tools that function as intelligent assistants, potentially enhancing the customization of diagnosis and treatment for each individual patient. Nevertheless, these assistants are not free of limitations and their suggestions must be approached with caution and consistently assessed for reliability, as the responsibility for diagnosis and treatment decisions ultimately rests with the treating dermatologist.

This book comes at a crucial moment, as dermatologists globally are becoming increasingly aware of this technology and its extensive applications across various fields of dermatology. They are concerned about the legal ramifications of these models, and realize that this technology is accessible not only to specialists but also to patients. Consequently, dermatologists should not withdraw but embrace this new reality. As this AI in dermatology or "Dermatology ex machina" progresses swiftly, our understanding of its capabilities and limitations must also evolve.

This book is a comprehensive guide on the application of AI across various dermatology subjects, ranging from skin cancer, inflammatory dermatoses, and alopecias to cosmetic procedures and laser applications. It provides a foundational resource for dermatologists, both experts and residents, practitioners, medical students, and researchers interested in exploring this domain. Furthermore, readers gain insights into the significance of maintaining a balanced perspective and the benefits derived from the collaboration between dermatologist expertise and machine intelligence.

I congratulate the editors and the authors that have contributed to this book and have provided a high-quality work that in my knowledge is the first book that explores the AI-driven evolution in dermatology.

First Department of Dermatology, Faculty of Health Sciences
Aristotle University
Thessaloniki, Greece

Aimilios Lallas

Preface

The integration of Artificial Intelligence (AI) into our everyday life is undeniable. AI has affected how we manage tasks, how we create texts, and how we make calculations. The world of medicine is not an exception to this change, and particularly Dermatology, which is a specialty based mainly on image patterns and visual assessment. As a result, this book was created to simplify how AI works, to show what AI applications can offer to our specialty, and to provide practical guidance on how AI can perform different tasks on multiple skin entities, ranging from skin cancer (melanoma, non-melanoma skin cancer (NMSC), and skin cancer mimickers) to inflammatory dermatoses (psoriasis, atopic dermatitis, acne, rosacea, and bullous dermatoses) and skin appendage disorders (nail diseases and alopecia). Cosmetic dermatology and laser applications treatments are also explored. This book serves as an invaluable textbook to all dermatologists, who want to know more about AI technology and how this technological swift can affect Dermatology approach and enhance their clinical practice.

The book begins with Part I—which focuses on AI fundamental principles and the social impact of AI-powered Dermatology across various dimensions (Dermatology education, legal framework of AI, the important aspect of ethics, and the patient-dermatologist relationship dynamics that seem to be altered by AI). The reader firstly would encounter the basic concepts of AI technology and would understand how AI operates in a clear manner (principles of machine and deep learning, large language models, etc.) (Chap. 1). This section also explains how AI models can "read" skin images and conclude to a result based on their training. This proves why Dermatology is the ideal field for AI to thrive (Chap. 2). Worth mentioning is that Chap. 1 presents a glossary table, containing terms used in AI technology that readers might need clarification on if they come across them in other parts of the book. Chapter 3 centers on how AI changes the way Dermatology is educated, from learning process to teaching methods within the specialty. Chapter 4 highlights the legal parameters that must be respected as well as the legal boundaries that dermatologists should not exceed when using AI technology in their specialty. Chapter 5 scope is the ethics part that should always be considered, and dermatologists should not forget that machine cannot replace the invaluable human element in patient's care.

Part II examines the AI contribution to skin cancer approach, mainly diagnosis as well as treatment and patient monitoring. Chapter 6 provides practical examples of AI assistance in NMSC patients while Chap. 7 reports a detailed presentation of AI advancements in melanoma diagnosis, with AI models achieving great efficacy in skin cancer detection and AI becoming an invaluable assistant to dermatologists. Chapter 8 presents examples and studies on skin cancer mimickers that stand mainly as control cases and demonstrates the ability of AI models to distinguish between malignant and benign skin lesions. Part III moves to inflammatory dermatoses (psoriasis (Chap. 9), atopic dermatitis (Chap. 10), acne (Chap. 11), rosacea (Chap. 12), and bullous dermatoses (Chap. 13)) with a focus on the AI subjective severity assessment of those diseases. AI differentiation abilities especially in case of challenging cases of inflammatory skin as well as its use in clinical evaluation are also presented. Personalized medicine and AI-tailored dermatology are also topics explained with examples of real-world patients being benefiting from the cooperation of AI and dermatologists.

Part IV steps into the world of cosmetic applications, skin treatment strategies, and the ways that AI can assist in those areas. Chapters 14 and 15 explain how AI models can pre-assess skin quality, identify skin needs, and propose personalized skin-care plan. The area of injection treatments is also benefited as the "Book before you look" concept, with AI-crafted simulations of AI that predicts how the patient would look after a specific treatment or procedure redefines care methods. Chapter 16 underlines the AI integration into laser applications and shows glimpses of the technology revolution of Dermatology that awaits! Part V (Chaps. 17 and 18) presents the AI developments into alopecia and nail disorders approach facilitating patients' care and follow-up. For example, the AI-automated counting of hair follicles saves practitioners substantial amount of time.

Part VI is the final section of the book focusing on the successes (Chap. 19) that AI has achieved so far (great diagnosis accuracy, subjective assessment, personalized approach, and easy-to-reach AI models and chatbots) as well as the limitations (Chap. 20) that AI present in every skin disease and in every aspect of Dermatology practice that dermatologists should be aware of (overdiagnosis, hallucinations, and bias). Toward this direction, Chaps. 21 and 22 present data regarding limitations on the context of age and skin of color parameters and emphasizes the need for more population-specific AI model training. Chapter 23 includes reports of a dermatologist, a bioengineer, a law expert, and an AI chatbot discussing whether AI would replace dermatologists. They conclude that is highly unlikely but dermatologists with AI knowledge and expertise have the potential to replace the ones who do not possess that skill. Only time will tell!

Larissa, Greece Emmanouil Karampinis
Larissa, Greece Efterpi Zafiriou
Larissa, Greece Dimitrios Mantzaris

Acknowledgments

This book is a work that many contributors and colleagues have contributed to its creation. This book comprises the collective efforts of dermatologists, bioengineers, and law experts indicating that AI-integrated Dermatology is a multicomponent topic that need to be evaluated by many aspects. I would like to thank heartfully:

- My co-editors, Prof. Efterpi Zafiriou and Dimitrios Mantzaris, for their invaluable help
- Profs. of Dermatology: Elizabeth Lazaridou, Zoe Apalla, Alexandros Katoulis, Efstratios Vakirlis, Elena Sotiriou, Alexandros Stratigos, Dimitrios Sgouros, Efstathios Rallis, Nkechi Enechukwu, Christian Navarette Duchenne, and Aimilios Lallas, who forwarded the book
- Dermatology Experts: Christophoros Tzermias, Markos Papakonstantis, Ioanna Triantaphylopoulou. Eirini Kyrmanidou, Natalia Rompoti, and Dimitra Koumaki
- Doctors: Olga Toli, Georgia Pappa, Melpomeni Theofili, Vanessa Grech, Maria-Myrto Papadopoulou, Marios Papadakis, Divinefavour Echezona Malachy, Stella-Maria Michelaki, Iasonas Dermitzakis, Christina Zoubourli, and Panagiota Tanga
- Law Experts: Lillian Mitrou, Anna Mavrophorou, Vasso Karzis, and Aikaterini Karampini

The high quality of this book would not have been possible without their contributions.

AI technologies are increasingly shaping academic writing and practices. Authors and editors of the book are in line with Springer AI Authorship Policy and Guidance and they confirm that no AI-generated text was copied or directly incorporated into the content. AI-assisted improvements particularly from LLMs such as ChatGPT included suggestions for better wording and/or formatting changes to the texts. The authors and editors remain fully responsible for the scientific accuracy and integrity of their work.

Emmanouil Karampinis

Contents

Part I

Conceptual and Regulatory Framework of Artificial Intelligence in Dermatology

Artificial Intelligence (AI) Main Concepts: A Glimpse inside "A.I. Black Box"

1

Dimitrios Mantzaris and Emmanouil Karampinis

1.1 Introduction

Artificial intelligence (AI) is a relatively new scientific discipline focused on understanding how the human brain functions and also on creating intelligent systems. AI is a multidisciplinary field that brings together computer scientists, physiologists, and philosophers, encompassing a variety of subfields all centered on the development of machines capable of intelligent behavior.

The term "Artificial Intelligence" was introduced by John McCarthy nearly 70 years ago [1]. Despite its long history, there is still no universally accepted definition of AI. The lack of a clear and universally accepted definition may stem from the ambiguity surrounding the concept of "intelligence," which remains abstract and difficult to measure [2–4]. Many psychologists and experts in knowledge systems argue that intelligence involves the ability to apply the right knowledge in the right context for effective decision-making. Based on this view, AI can be defined as the ability of machines to simulate human intelligence by identifying and utilizing appropriate knowledge at each stage of problem-solving. A system that can plan and execute appropriate actions at the right time is considered to be logically intelligent [5].

Over recent decades, there have been significant advances in AI, machine learning (ML), and deep learning (DL), which have dramatically improved performance

D. Mantzaris (✉)
Computational Intelligence and Health Informatics Lab, Nursing Department, School of Health Sciences, University of Thessaly, Larissa, Greece
e-mail: dmantzar@uth.gr

E. Karampinis
Second Dermatology Department, School of Health Sciences, Aristotle University of Thessaloniki, Thessaloniki, Greece

Department of Dermatology, Faculty of Medicine, School of Health Sciences, University General Hospital of Larissa, University of Thessaly, Larissa, Greece

E. Karampinis et al. (eds.), *Artificial Intelligence Applications in Dermatology*,
https://doi.org/10.1007/978-3-032-15614-3_1

in various domains. These include tasks like visual recognition and language understanding from audio inputs. As a result, AI, ML, and DL have become critical technologies in fields such as engineering, healthcare, and finance, and they play a substantial role in our everyday lives.

In healthcare, AI has demonstrated its usefulness in disease diagnosis. For instance, Esteva and colleagues trained a deep convolutional neural network (CNN) with 129,450 dermatological images and tested it against 21 dermatologists. The AI system matched the diagnostic accuracy of the human specialists in classifying skin lesions [6]. Similarly, ML is effectively used in predicting intraoperative hypotension, detecting anatomical structures via ultrasound, managing postoperative pain, and optimizing drug delivery. The vast data generated in intensive care units (ICUs) makes them ideal environments for AI applications. In this context, deep learning has been used to monitor patient emotions and behaviors to assess conditions like delirium and agitation, using cameras and accelerometers to track facial expressions and movements [7].

This section introduces the foundational concepts of AI, ML, and DL, highlighting their differences and the architectures used in each approach.

1.2 A.I. Principles and Subtypes

Artificial intelligence (AI) is a comprehensive field of research aimed at replicating intelligent behavior in machines without the need for direct human input [8]. John McCarthy, one of the pioneers of the field, defined AI as "the science and engineering of making intelligent machines, particularly intelligent computer programs." He emphasized that while AI is closely linked to efforts to understand human intelligence using computers, it is not limited to methods that mimic biological processes [9].

The roots of AI can be traced back to Alan Turing, who introduced the foundational question, "Can machines think?" through his work on the imitation game [10]. The term "Artificial Intelligence" was later introduced by McCarthy during the 1956 Dartmouth Conference. Although the field initially generated great enthusiasm, it eventually entered a period known as the "AI winter" from the 1970s to the 1990s, when progress was stalled due to technological limitations [11].

In recent years, however, AI has undergone a revival known as the "AI spring," beginning in the 2010s. This resurgence has been driven by rapid technological advancements and has significantly influenced the field of medicine, giving rise to artificial intelligence in medicine (AIM). The widespread digitization of healthcare data has played a critical role in this development, providing the massive datasets required to train intelligent algorithms. For example, Borges do Nascimento and colleagues studied how big data analytics affects health priorities and outcomes defined by the World Health Organization (WHO) in its 2019–2023 General Program of Work and the European Program of Work (EPW). Their findings showed that real-time data analysis can support more accurate diagnosis and prediction, particularly in the management of chronic diseases [12].

1.2.1 AI Subtypes

Artificial intelligence (AI) encompasses several key subfields, including machine learning (ML), deep learning (DL), computer vision (CV), and natural language processing (NLP) (see Fig. 1.1).

Machine Learning (ML) is a branch of AI that enables computer systems to identify patterns in data and make inferences without being explicitly programmed [13]. ML can operate through three main types of learning: supervised, unsupervised, and semi-supervised. In supervised learning, the model is trained using labeled data, where each example is paired with the correct output. The system learns through repeated trial and error. This approach is commonly used in dermatology, such as training models with labeled clinical images [13]. In unsupervised learning, no labeled outputs are provided, and the algorithm independently identifies patterns or groups based on data similarities. Semi-supervised learning combines both approaches, using a mix of labeled and unlabeled data [14].

In ML, input variables (known as covariates) are processed to predict a specific outcome. For instance, in image analysis, the covariates are pixels, and the predicted

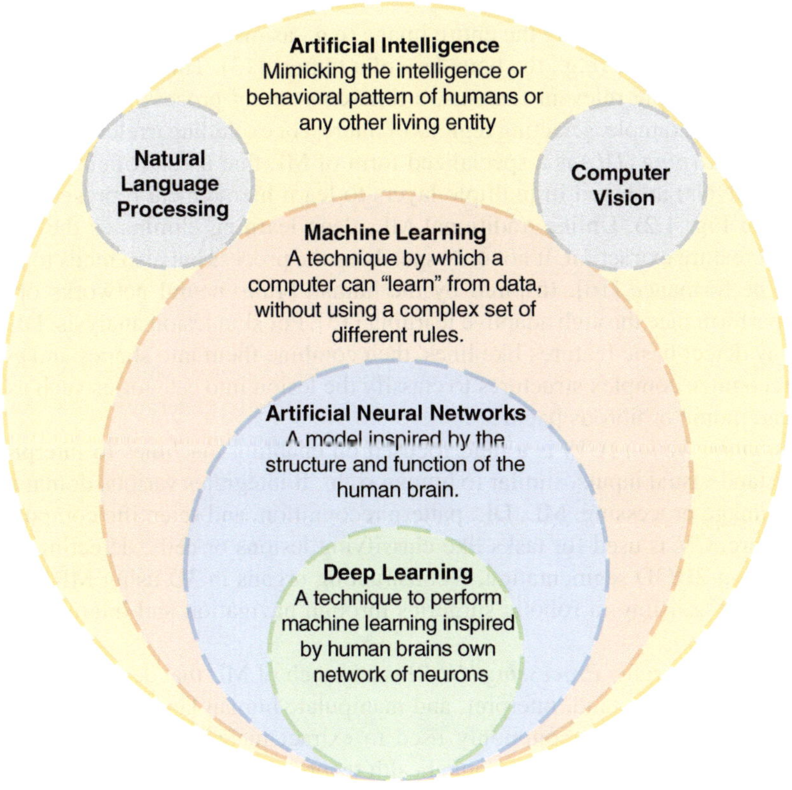

Fig. 1.1 Diagram distinguishing AI-related terms

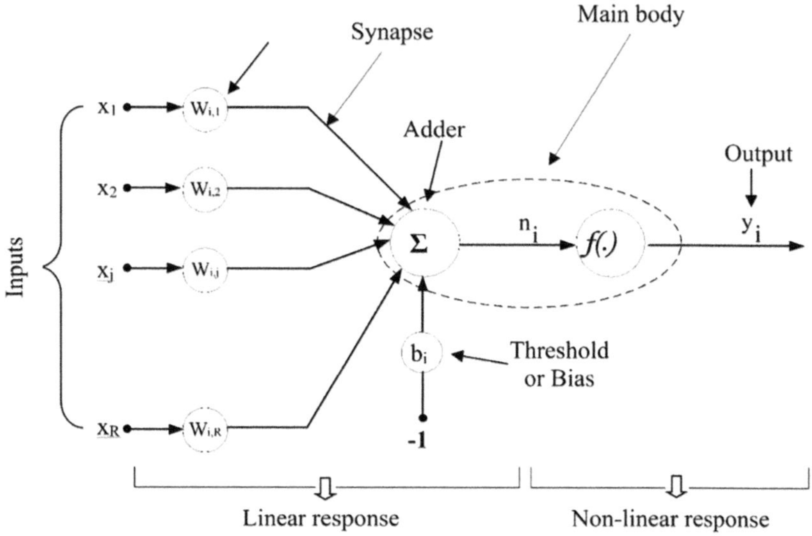

Fig. 1.2 Artificial neuron model

output might be classifying the entire image (e.g., as melanoma or benign) or identifying specific areas (e.g., the boundary of a tumor) [13]. Traditional ML involves manually selecting relevant features, a time-consuming process requiring domain expertise-for example, selecting regions of interest or excluding irrelevant areas [15].

Deep Learning (DL) is a specialized form of ML that uses artificial neural networks (ANNs) arranged in multiple layers to learn hierarchical representations of data (see Fig. 1.2). Unlike traditional ML, deep learning eliminates the need for manual feature extraction. It not only speeds up the process but also tends to achieve better performance [16]. Inspired by the human brain, neural networks optimize their performance through adaptive learning [13]. For skin lesion analysis, DL models may detect basic features like lines, then combine them into shapes and eventually recognize complex structures to classify the lesion into categories such as basal cell carcinoma or fibrous papule.

Computer Vision (CV) is a field focused on enabling machines to interpret and understand visual inputs, similar to human sight. It integrates various domains such as AI, image processing, ML, DL, pattern recognition, and scientific computing. In healthcare, CV is used for tasks like classifying lesions or cells, detecting tumors, performing 2D/3D segmentation, reconstructing organs in 3D using MRI or ultrasound, and assisting in robotic surgeries through navigation and interaction capabilities [17–19].

Natural Language Processing (NLP) is a branch of ML that deals with enabling computers to understand, interpret, and manipulate human language, whether spoken or written. NLP is commonly used to extract meaningful information from unstructured data found in electronic health records (EHRs), such as clinical notes, lab reports, operative summaries, and discharge instructions. Since documentation consumes significant time and contributes to physician burnout, NLP techniques aim to convert free-text into structured, machine-readable data that can be further analyzed using other ML methods [20–22].

1.2.2 Explainable Artificial Intelligence

Despite the impressive progress made in artificial intelligence (AI), including machine learning (ML), deep learning (DL), and natural language processing (NLP), a complete understanding of how deep neural networks function and optimize remains elusive. ML, a core area within AI, focuses on enabling computers to learn from data and improve predictions over time [23]. However, many ML models remain difficult to interpret due to their abstract and nontransparent nature [24]. These models are often criticized for functioning as opaque "black boxes" [25]. Deep learning architectures, such as deep neural networks, typically involve millions of parameters and functions, which are too complex for humans to interpret or analyze. As a result, the inner workings and outcomes of such models can appear mysterious, leading to concerns about their reliability and trustworthiness. Furthermore, there is often no clear way to verify whether the model's outputs are based on flawed, biased, or incorrect reasoning-raising ethical, legal, and financial concerns.

To address these challenges, the field of explainable artificial intelligence (XAI) has emerged. XAI aims to make AI systems more understandable by providing insights into how decisions are made and why certain outcomes are reached. XAI, still an emerging and expansive research area, lacks a universally agreed-upon definition. In [23], it is described as the "science of understanding what a model did or might have done", while [26] defines it as the use of AI to extract meaningful knowledge about data relationships. There are several motivations for making AI models explainable. According to Adadi and Berrada, four key purposes are: justifying decisions, improving user control, refining model performance, and discovering new insights [27].

Furthermore, the researchers are actively developing techniques to make machine learning models more understandable—a field often referred to as explainable machine learning (EML). The goal is to help users intuitively comprehend and trust the models' behavior.

Explainable models can be grouped into three main categories based on their research goals: explainability, interpretability, and transparency. Explainability and interpretability aim to make the model's processes and results comprehensible to humans. Transparency, on the other hand, refers to the degree to which the learning mechanisms of the model are understood. A model is considered transparent if it is inherently self-explanatory [28]. Nowadays, researchers are exploring how neural networks learn, with the goal of making them more transparent [29, 30].

1.2.3 Generative Artificial Intelligence

Generative Artificial Intelligence refers to a branch of AI systems designed to produce new content, such as text, images, audio, and more, by learning patterns from existing datasets [31]. The rise of generative AI began around 2017–2018 with the advent of the first transformer-based models and continued gaining momentum through 2019–2021. Today, the field is experiencing rapid growth and widespread application.

Some of the most significant breakthroughs have occurred in the development of large language models (LLMs), including OpenAI's GPT series (GPT-1 to GPT-4), Meta AI's LLaMA, Google's Gemini models, and Anthropic's Claude models. These LLMs operate using statistical pattern recognition, having been trained on massive textual datasets to identify linguistic structures and probabilistic relationships. When given a prompt, they generate human-like responses based on these learned patterns. However, these models do not understand language the way humans do—they do not possess true semantic comprehension but rather predict the next word or phrase based on probability [32]. Still, the vast amount of data used in training makes them capable of producing outputs that closely resemble those of human experts in various fields [33]. Despite their relatively recent emergence, LLMs already provide substantial value to businesses by assisting with translation, summarization, and question-answering tasks [34].

Generative AI also plays a major role in image creation. Using deep generative neural networks and diffusion models, tools like stable diffusion, midjourney, and DALL·E can generate high-quality images from text-based prompts [35].

In the realm of software development, tools like GitHub Copilot can understand and generate code in widely used programming languages such as Python, JavaScript, and C [36]. There have also been notable advances in AI-driven audio generation [37], and research is ongoing in the area of video generation [38].

A particularly promising frontier is *multimodal generative AI*, which integrates multiple data types—such as text, images, and video—into a single system [39]. These multimodal models are expected to enable more complex and adaptive applications by processing and generating diverse forms of content simultaneously.

1.3 Deep Learning—Artificial Neural Networks

Artificial neural networks (ANNs) are a subset of machine learning, based on algorithms that are designed to recognize patterns that are inspired by the human brain's neural network [40].

Research on neural networks started quite a long time ago, and it has become a broad and interdisciplinary research field today. Though neural networks have various definitions across disciplines, this book uses a widely adopted one: "Artificial neural networks are massively parallel interconnected networks of simple (usually adaptive) elements and their hierarchical organizations which are intended to interact with the objects of the real world in the same way as biological nervous systems do" [41]. In the context of machine learning, neural networks refer to "neural networks learning", or in other words, the intersection of machine learning research and neural networks research.

The basic element of neural networks is neuron, which is the "simple element" in the above definition. In biological neural networks, the neurons, when "excited", send neurotransmitters to interconnected neurons to change their electric potential (see Fig. 1.2). When the electric potential exceeds a threshold, the neuron is activated (i.e., "excited"), and it will send neurotransmitters to other neurons.

An artificial neural network is structured as one input layer of neurons, one or more "hidden layers" and one output layer (see Fig. 1.3a). The input data is processed through a large number of highly interconnected elements, which are called neurons or nodes [42]. Deep learning (DL) is a subset of artificial neural network with stacked neural networks composed of one input and one output layer, and more than one hidden layer (see Fig. 1.3b). Deep learning algorithms require advanced computation and very large data [20, 40].

Feed-forward neural networks were the earliest implementations within deep learning. These networks are called feed-forward because the information within them moves only in one direction (forward)—that is, from the input nodes (units) toward the output units.

The term back propagation refers to the path followed by the transmission of the error during the training of the neural network. Specifically, the error between the actual value and the computed value of the ANN is transmitted from the output layer to the input layer, to modify the network's weighting coefficients.

The implementation of deep learning based on deep neural networks (DNNs). Deep neural networks can be divided into normal (one-dimensional) or convoluted (two or three-dimensional). Convolutional neural networks have gained importance in medical image analysis for extracting patterns from images. One of the advantages of deep learning over other types of ML is its scalable behavior. Namely, the performance of deep learning models gets better as the amount of data used to train the model increases, and features are automatically extracted by the network. The structure of DNNs consists of anything from several layers to millions of layers, which makes their mathematical explanation intractable. This nature of neural networks is thus somewhat "black box" in character [43].

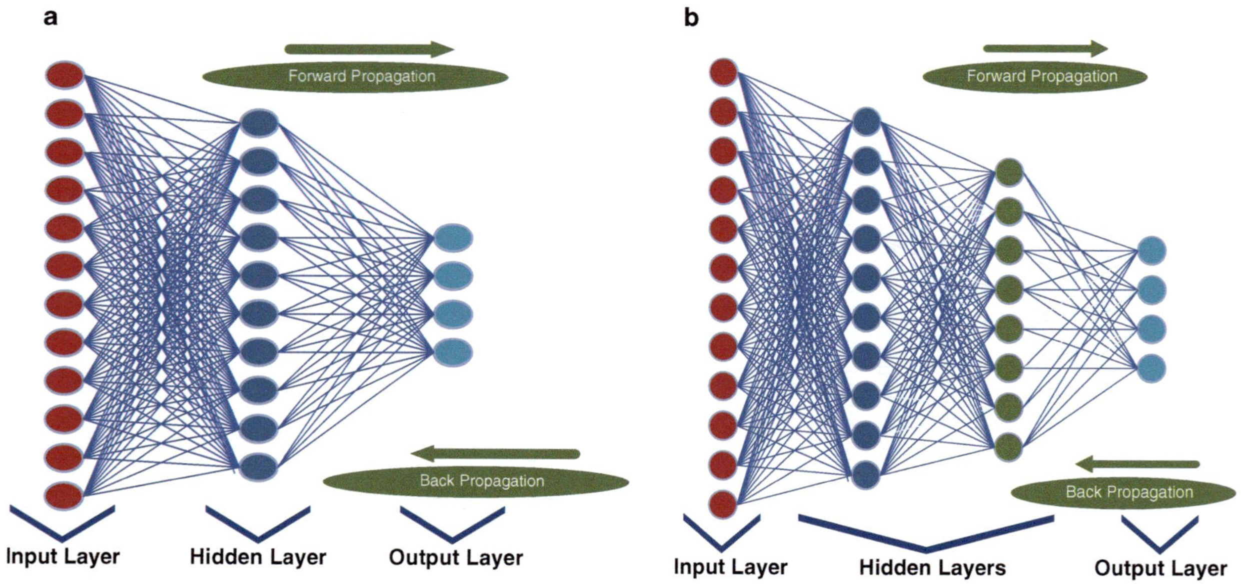

Fig. 1.3 (**a**) Artificial neural network (ANN). The ANNS consists of one hidden layer. (**b**) Deep neural network (DNN). This DNN consists of two hidden layers

1.4 Convolutional Neural Networks—How the AI Brains Constructed and Learn?

Convolutional neural networks (CNNs) are among the most extensively used models in deep learning, drawing inspiration from the animal visual cortex [44, 45]. CNNs have significantly advanced the field of computer vision, enabling breakthroughs in tasks once considered unattainable. Specifically, CNNs have demonstrated remarkable success in image recognition, consistently achieving leading performance on various benchmarks. This success stems from their ability to learn and represent spatial hierarchies in visual data through multiple layers of convolutions, each capturing features at different levels of detail [46, 47].

CNNs have been widely adopted across multiple domains, delivering state-of-the-art results in numerous applications, including image classification, object detection, object tracking, pose estimation, text detection and recognition, action recognition, scene labeling, and speech and natural language processing [48, 49].

1.4.1 Convolutional Neural Network Architecture

A convolutional neural network (CNN) is a type of feedforward neural network designed to automatically extract features from data using convolutional structures. Unlike traditional feature extraction techniques [50, 51], CNNs eliminate the need for manual feature engineering. Their design is inspired by the human visual system [52], where artificial neurons mimic biological neurons, convolutional kernels act like receptors that detect various features, and activation functions simulate the process where only signals surpassing a certain threshold are passed on to subsequent neurons.

A CNN is typically composed of three primary types of layers: convolutional layers, pooling (or aggregation) layers, and fully connected layers. Together, these layers form the core architecture of a CNN. A basic example of this architecture, used for image classification, includes two convolutional layers followed by four fully connected layers, as shown in Fig. 1.4 [53, 54]. Each layer contributes a specific role within the network, enabling the hierarchical extraction and processing of features.

Convolutional Layer: This is the fundamental component of a CNN [55], responsible for applying convolution operations to the input using a set of trainable filters. These filters (also known as kernels) are small matrices that move across the input image, computing dot products with localized regions at each step. The result is a series of feature maps that highlight various characteristics of the input image.

Pooling Layer: Pooling layers are used to downsample the feature maps generated by convolutional layers, reducing their spatial dimensions [56]. Each feature map is processed independently, with operations like max pooling or average pooling applied to nonoverlapping regions. This not only lowers computational load but also enhances the network's ability to generalize by making it more resilient to small shifts in the input.

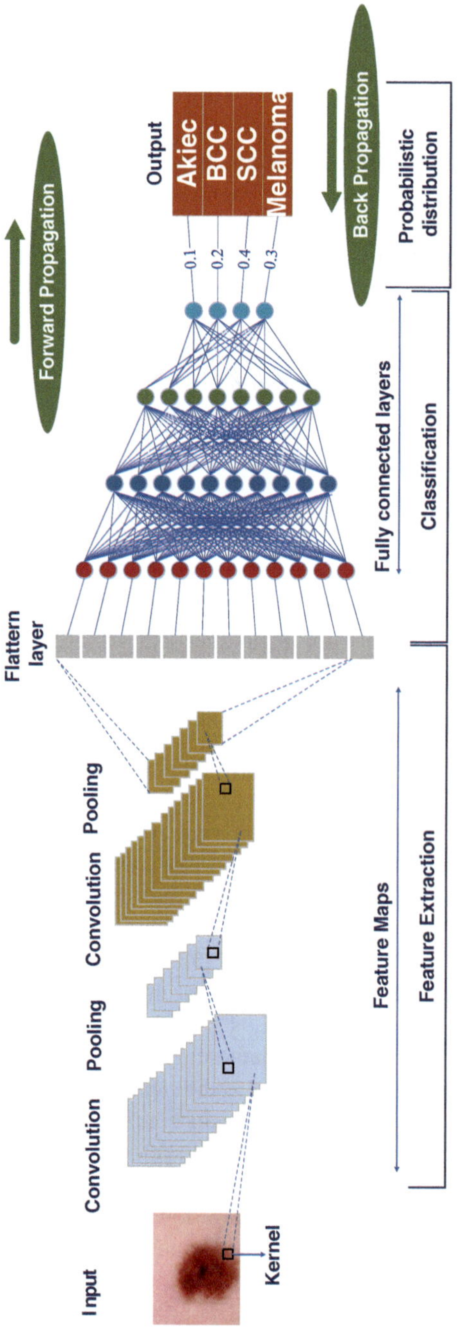

Fig. 1.4 Convolution neural network architecture

Activation Layer: This layer introduces nonlinearity into the network by applying a nonlinear activation function to the outputs of the preceding layer [57, 58]. This is crucial for enabling the CNN to model complex patterns and relationships in the data.

Batch Normalization Layer: Batch normalization standardizes the output of the previous layer by adjusting it based on the batch's mean and standard deviation [59]. This helps to stabilize and speed up training by reducing internal covariate shifts.

Dropout Layer: During training, the dropout layer randomly disables a fraction of neurons from the previous layer [60]. This acts as a regularization technique, reducing the risk of overfitting and promoting the learning of more generalized features.

Fully Connected Layer: This layer connects each neuron to every neuron in the previous layer, functioning like a traditional neural network layer [60]. It is typically positioned at the end of the CNN and is responsible for producing the final classification or prediction output.

In summary, each type of layer in a CNN plays a specific and complementary role in extracting and learning features from input data. By understanding how these layers function together, practitioners can design more efficient and effective CNN architectures tailored to various computer vision applications [61, 62].

CNN Training: Fig. 1.4 presents a CNN architecture for image classification using dermatological lesion images. The input image is first processed by the input layer, then passed through a series of hidden layers where convolutional filters extract hierarchical features from low-level edges and textures to high-level abstract patterns. The final output layer produces a probability distribution over three classes (car, bus, and plane), and the class with the highest probability is selected.

Training involves optimizing convolutional kernels and fully connected layer weights to minimize prediction error, typically using backpropagation. This process updates parameters by computing loss during forward propagation and adjusting weights based on gradients via gradient descent.

1.4.2 Convolution Operation

Convolution is a fundamental mathematical operation widely used in fields such as signal processing, image analysis, and computer vision [63, 64]. It involves combining two functions or signals to generate a third function that expresses how one signal modifies or influences the other, shaped by the form of the second signal. In the context of computer vision, convolution is a key technique used in CNNs to extract meaningful features from images.

In deep learning, the terms convolution and cross-correlation are often used interchangeably, both in academic literature and practical implementations. Mathematically, for a given input I(t) and a kernel $K(\alpha)$, the convolution operation is represented mathematically by the symbol * and the operation: $(I*K)(t)$. The essence of the operation is that the kernel is a much shorter set of data points compared to the input, and the output of the convolution operation is higher when the input is similar to the kernel.

The mathematical definition of the convolution operation for given an input $I(t)$ and a kernel $K(\alpha)$ is:

The convolution operation can be extended to two dimensions, in which case the input $I(m, n)$ and a kernel $K(a, b)$.

In the case of image processing, the image itself is the two-dimensional signal that the CNN will process. Fig. 1.5a presents a two-dimensional signal (image) and a one-dimensional kernel. In case the kernel is two-dimensional, the principle function is illustrated in Fig. 1.5b. The convolution operation is applied to each channel of the input image separately, and the resulting feature maps are combined to form the output.

1.4.3 Feature Maps

In CNNs, a feature map plays a vital role as it represents the output generated by a convolutional layer [65]. It is a two-dimensional matrix that indicates how well various local regions of the input image align with the filters applied. Each value in the feature map corresponds to the activation of a neuron, capturing specific visual characteristics from the input.

The creation of a feature map involves applying a set of filters (kernels) to the input image through convolution. Each filter produces its own single-channel feature map, emphasizing a distinct feature or pattern within the image. By combining the outputs from multiple filters in the same layer, a multichannel feature map is formed, providing a richer and more comprehensive representation of the image's content. In essence, feature maps are fundamental to CNNs, enabling the network to detect and learn relevant visual features from input data. This ability underpins the effectiveness of CNNs in a wide variety of image recognition and classification tasks.

1.4.4 CNN Architectures

Since the groundbreaking introduction of AlexNet [66], the development of CNN architectures has rapidly evolved. Researchers have progressively designed models that are deeper, wider, or more efficient. Each of these architectures has significantly advanced the fields of computer vision and deep learning (DL). This section briefly reviews several key CNN architectures, emphasizing their unique innovations, characteristics, and performance contributions.

LeNet: Was introduced by Yann LeCun and colleagues in 1990 [65] and later refined in 1998 [67]. It was primarily designed for digit recognition and was applied to tasks like reading handwritten ZIP codes. LeNet consists of two convolutional

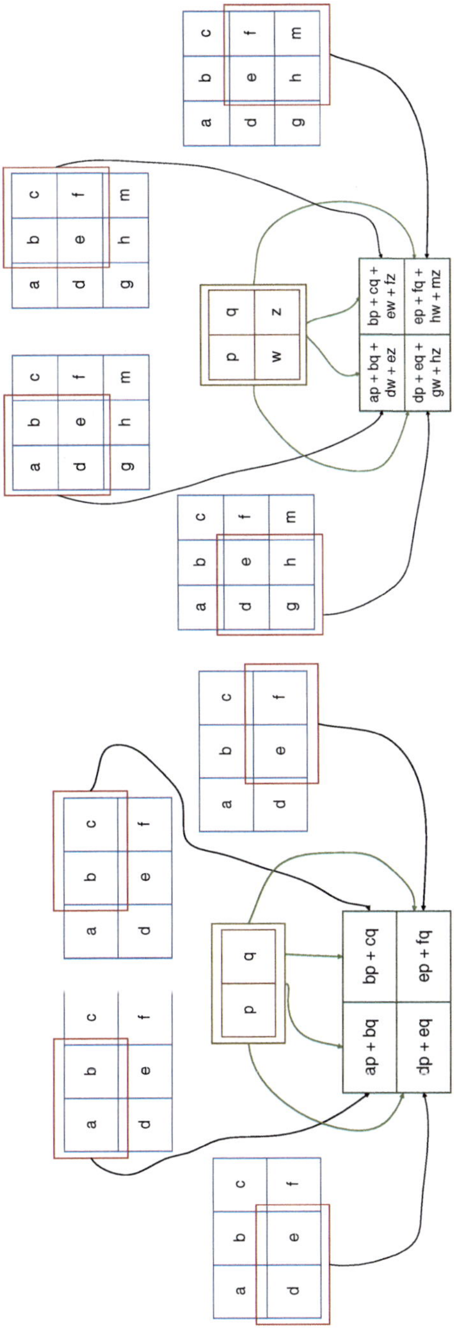

Fig. 1.5 (**a**) Convolution operation: Two-dimensional image and one-dimensional kernel. (**b**) Convolution operation: Two-dimensional image and two-dimensional kernel

layers followed by two fully connected layers [68]. The convolutional layers use small filters combined with pooling layers to extract features, while the fully connected layers produce class probabilities. The network has around 60,000 trainable parameters.

AlexNet: Developed by Alex Krizhevsky et al. in 2012, AlexNet marked a major breakthrough by winning the 2012 ImageNet large-scale visual recognition challenge (ILSVRC) [69]. While structurally similar to LeNet, AlexNet differs in that it stacks all convolutional layers together without alternating with pooling layers. The architecture includes five convolutional layers, three fully connected layers, and approximately 60 million parameters. Notable enhancements include the use of larger filters, local response normalization, and overlapping pooling, making it much deeper and more powerful than LeNet.

VGGNet: Developed by the visual geometry group (VGG) at the University of Oxford, Karen Simonyan and Andrew Zisserman in 2014, VGGNet, a convolutional neural network (CNN) architecture, earned recognition as the runner-up in the ILSVRC 2014 competition while still achieving state-of-the-art results [70]. The architecture builds upon AlexNet, significantly increasing the depth and feature extraction capabilities. VGG-16, one of the most commonly used variants, consists of 16 convolutional layers grouped into blocks: three blocks with two 3×3 convolutions followed by 2×2 max pooling, and two blocks with three 3×3 convolutions followed by 2×2 max pooling. This is followed by two fully connected layers with 4096 neurons each. With roughly 138 million parameters, VGG offers improved accuracy by using smaller convolution filters in series, which reduces the number of parameters while maintaining a large receptive field [70].

GoogLeNet/InceptionNet: Introduced by Christian Szegedy et al. in 2014, GoogLeNet won the ILSVRC 2014 competition by proposing a novel "inception module" that allows efficient computation [71]. Each inception module includes multiple convolution filters of varying sizes along with pooling layers. The outputs of these parallel operations are concatenated to form a composite feature map. GoogLeNet includes auxiliary classifiers to help with gradient flow during training and reduce overfitting. The model is 22 layers deep yet remarkably efficient, requiring only about five million parameters-much fewer than VGGNet's 138 million.

Inception v4: In 2015, Szegedy and colleagues further improved upon GoogLeNet by integrating residual connections, inspired by He et al.'s ResNet architecture [72]. This hybrid design enhanced training efficiency and performance. Inception v4 demonstrated superior accuracy and played a crucial role in winning the 2015 ILSVRC competition.

ResNet (Residual Network): Introduced by Kaiming He et al. in 2015, ResNet revolutionized deep learning by addressing the vanishing gradient problem, which plagued very deep networks [73]. It achieved an unprecedented milestone by surpassing human-level performance on ImageNet. The core innovation of ResNet is the residual (or skip) connection, which bypasses one or more convolutional layers and adds the input directly to the output of a block. This allows for very deep networks-ResNet-152, for instance—without the degradation in performance often observed in deeper architectures. The model contains around 65 million parameters. Some residual blocks include bottlenecks, using 1 × 1 convolutions at the start and end to reduce computation. Batch normalization is also applied after each convolution. While ResNet performs exceptionally well, its evaluation can be computationally expensive due to the large number of parameters, though removing the initial fully connected layer can significantly reduce this burden without impacting accuracy.

DenseNet: In 2017, Huang et al. [74] proposed DenseNet, a CNN with a densely connected structure. It has the characteristics of feature sharing and arbitrary interlayer interconnection. The advantages of DenseNet are feature map reuse through dense connections, reducing interdependence between layers by reusing feature maps from different layers, providing compact and differentiated input features by shortcut connections of different lengths, and effectively reducing the gradient disappearance problem that is difficult to optimize in deep networks. The final prediction is to use features from all layers to obtain better performance and model robustness on a standard dataset with a smaller model size and computational effort.

U-Net: The U-net is a neural network architecture, which utilized fully CNNs, developed primarily for image segmentation [75]. It features a fundamental two-path design (see Fig. 1.6). The initial segment is the contracting path, also known as the encoder or analysis path. This part functions like a conventional CNN, extracting features and providing classification data. Each block within this path sequentially applies two 3 × 3 convolutions, followed by a rectified linear unit (ReLU) activation, and then a max-pooling layer. This sequence is repeated multiple times. *The U-net's innovation lies in its second component: the expansion path, also known as the decoder or synthesis path*

There are various U-net architectures: *3D U-net, attention U-net, inception U-net, residual U-Net, dense U-net, U-net++, adversarial U-net, cascaded arrangement, and parallel arrangement.*

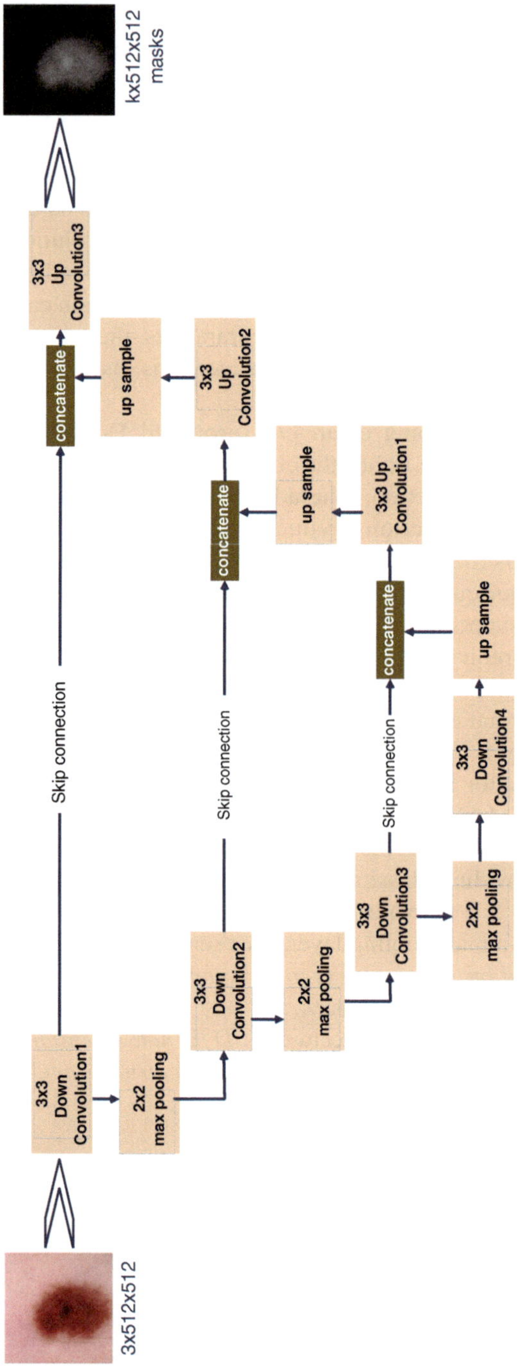

Fig. 1.6 Basic U-net architecture

1.5 Vision Transformer

Transformers [76] were initially developed for natural language processing (NLP), bringing a significant shift to deep learning through their architecture based on self-attention mechanisms [77]. Models like BERT [78] and RoBERTa [79] demonstrated remarkable performance, which inspired researchers to explore the use of transformers in computer vision (CV) tasks as well. Traditionally, CNNs served as the backbone for visual recognition, using convolutional and pooling operations to effectively extract hierarchical features from images [80]. While transformers were first integrated with CNNs [81], vision transformers (ViTs) have since evolved into standalone models, fully replacing convolutional layers with self-attention mechanisms.

A standard transformer model consists of L layers, each comprising two main components: a multi-head self-attention (MSA) layer, which applies attention across different projections of the input tokens, and a multi-layer perceptron (MLP). Both components are preceded by layer normalization (LN) and followed by residual (skip) connections [82]. Originally used for processing 1D sequences in NLP [83, 84], the attention mechanism has now been extended to work with 2D image data and even 3D video [85].The core elements of a transformer include MSA, MLP, and layer normalization [86]. GELU (Gaussian error linear unit), introduced in [87], is widely used as a high-performing activation function. Unlike batch normalization, which is not ideal for recurrent networks, layer normalization [88] normalizes across individual training cases, stabilizing dynamics in recurrent models and significantly improving training speed.

In the vision domain, transformer-based approaches fall into two main categories. The first involves pure attention-based models, aiming to replace convolution entirely. The second combines self-attention with convolutional layers [89]. These self-attention architectures have already transformed NLP and are now driving rapid progress in image analysis tasks like classification and object detection [90, 91].

Transformers can be used either alongside or in place of CNNs in vision applications. Remarkably, CNNs are no longer essential, as pure transformers can effectively classify images by directly processing sequences of image patches. Unlike traditional transformers that accept sequences of words, Dosovitskiy et al. [92] adapted the architecture to process images with minimal changes, giving rise to the vision transformer (ViT). As shown in Fig. 1.7, ViT divides an image into a grid of square patches. Each patch is flattened into a vector and then linearly projected to match the model's input dimensions. Since transformers lack inherent spatial structure, learnable positional embeddings are added to help the model understand the spatial relationships between patches. The sequence is then fed into a transformer encoder, pre-trained in a supervised manner on a large dataset and fine-tuned on specific downstream tasks such as image classification.

The Image GPT (iGPT) approach [93] extends the GPT-2 model [94] to image pixels, using unsupervised generative pretraining to develop robust visual representations. iGPT demonstrated that even without convolutional structures, transformers

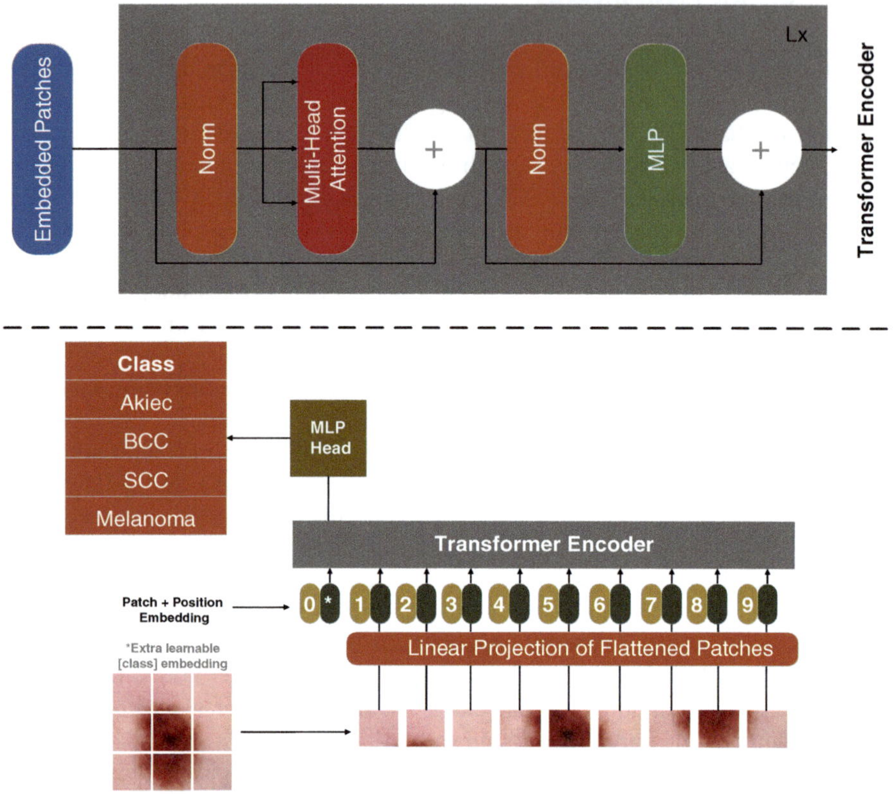

Fig. 1.7 Vision transformer architecture

could achieve impressive results on visual tasks like image generation and completion.

To reduce dependency on massive labeled datasets, data-efficient Image transformers (DeiT) [95] adopt a student–teacher training setup, along with strong data augmentation and regularization strategies such as stochastic depth [96] and repeated augmentation [97]. In this framework, the teacher network guides the student, introducing a convolutional inductive bias to improve performance without the need for large datasets [98].

LeViT, inspired by ViT and trained using the DeiT method, achieves a favorable speed-to-accuracy trade-off, significantly outperforming both CNNs and vision transformers in terms of efficiency [99]. On CPUs, LeViT runs five times faster than EfficientNet at comparable accuracy levels.

To further enhance image classification, CrossViT [100] was proposed by Chen et al. [101]. This architecture uses a dual-branch transformer design to learn multi-scale features, with one branch processing small patches and the other handling larger patches.

Lastly, transformer-in-transformer (TNT) [102] introduces a hierarchical approach that models both patch-level and pixel-level relationships. It consists of an outer transformer block that processes patch embeddings and an inner transformer block that captures interactions between individual pixel embeddings, offering a richer and more detailed representation of image data.

1.6 Large Language Models—Are they Really AI?

Language plays a crucial role in human communication and self-expression, as well as in our interactions with machines. The need for generalized models has grown due to the increasing demand for machines to perform complex language tasks like translation, summarization, information retrieval, and conversational interactions. Recently, significant advancements in language models have been driven by transformers [103], enhanced computational power, and the availability of large-scale training datasets. These developments have led to the creation of large language models (LLMs), which are capable of achieving near-human performance across a wide range of tasks [104, 105]. An LLM involves data preprocessing, tokenization, parameter tuning, activation function, attention mechanism, and normalization layer. A visualization of MLLs is provided in Fig. 1.8.

LLMs represent a significant leap forward in artificial intelligence research [106], capable of performing a broad spectrum of natural language processing (NLP) tasks. These models have greatly improved machines' ability to understand and generate human-like language [104] and have been successfully applied in various fields, such as content and text generation, text analysis, translation, sentiment analysis, question answering, communication, knowledge dissemination, and similar functions.

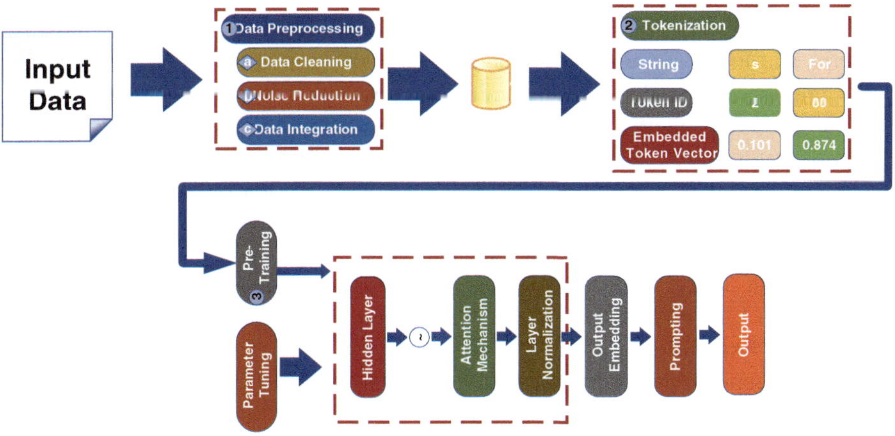

Fig. 1.8 Large language model principles

1.6.1 Large Language Models' Operation

At their core, large language models (LLMs) are a form of artificial intelligence that replicates human-like intelligence. They achieve this by utilizing advanced statistical models and deep learning techniques to process vast amounts of text data [107]. By identifying complex patterns and relationships within this data, LLMs can generate content that mirrors the style and characteristics of specific authors or genres [108].

The process begins with pre-training, where the model is exposed to a large corpus of text from various sources such as books, articles, and websites. Through unsupervised learning, the model learns to predict the next word in a sentence based on the context of the preceding words, allowing it to understand grammar, syntax, and semantics [109]. The pre-training pipeline begins with the collection of a vast amount of text data, divided into two categories: general and specialized data. Once gathered, the data must be preprocessed, which includes removing noisy, redundant, unnecessary, or harmful content [110, 111].

The second step involves quality filtering, where low-quality or irrelevant data is removed using techniques such as language filtering, statistical filtering, and keyword filtering [110]. The third step is deduplication, which addresses the issue of duplicate data that can reduce the diversity of the training corpus and negatively impact model performance [112]. The fourth step is privacy reduction, ensuring that personal or sensitive information, such as personally identifiable information (PII), is removed from the dataset to avoid privacy breaches [113]. The final preprocessing step is tokenization, where raw text is divided into individual tokens for input into the LLM.

After pre-training, the LLM undergoes fine-tuning, which tailors the model to a specific task or domain. During this phase, the model is trained on labeled examples, allowing it to generate more accurate and contextually appropriate responses for specific applications, such as language translation, question-answering, or text generation [109]. Fine-tuning enables LLMs to specialize in a range of tasks.

The success of LLMs is largely attributed to their ability to capture the statistical patterns and linguistic nuances of the data they are trained on [114]. By analyzing large amounts of text, these models gain a deep understanding of language, enabling them to produce coherent, contextually relevant responses. In the inference stage, when a user interacts with an LLM, they provide a prompt or query, which the model processes to generate a response based on its learned knowledge. This response is created using probabilistic methods that consider the likelihood of various words or phrases, given the input context.

LLMs can be classified into two categories: pre-trained and fine-tuned models. Pre-trained LLMs have significantly enhanced natural language understanding and generation. Examples of notable pre-trained models include [115]: GPT-3, T5, mT15, PanGau-a, CPM-2, ERNIE 3.0, Jurassic-1, HyperCLOVA, Yuan 1.0, Gopher and many others. Fine-tuned models, on the other hand, have been further trained for specific tasks or applications, including T0, mT0, Tk-Instruct, GopherCite, WebGPT, and Sparrow, among others [115].

In more specialized applications, LLMs are used in fields such as dermatology. For example, First Derm [116, 117] is a teledermoscopy application that allows dermatologists to remotely assess skin conditions, and Pahola [118] is a chatbot designed to provide guidance on alcohol consumption.

1.6.2 Perspective

Large language models (LLMs) are expected to have a profound impact on clinical healthcare, research, and medical education. However, it is essential to recognize and address their limitations. LLMs are known to replicate existing biases and are prone to generating inaccurate information, commonly referred to as "hallucinations", which can lead to the spread of misinformation [28]. In educational settings, including both medical and nonmedical fields, students may be misled by this misinformation, potentially hindering the development of essential critical thinking skills. Currently, there are no reliable systems in place to verify the accuracy of an LLM's output. This limitation significantly restricts the use of LLMs in clinical environments, where errors or false information could have life-threatening consequences. The lack of accountability for LLM-generated content further complicates this issue. On the other hand, safety measures designed to mitigate risks in LLMs may inadvertently introduce their own issues, such as bias prevention strategies that overlook gender differences in symptom presentation. Despite these challenges, newer models specifically trained with medical data show encouraging signs of progress in the healthcare sector [2, 5]. Nevertheless, fundamental concerns related to safety, accuracy, and ethical considerations must be fully addressed before LLMs can be widely implemented in medicine.

1.7 Dictionary of AI Terms

Terms	Terminology/Explanation
AlexNet	A groundbreaking convolutional neural network (CNN) architecture that revolutionized the field of deep learning and computer vision. Introduced in 2012 by Alex Krizhevsky, Ilya Sutskever, and Geoffrey Hinton
CAM	Class activation map: The original technique that generates a heatmap to visualize the important regions in an image that a convolutional neural network (CNN) used to make a specific class prediction
Grand CAM	A more generalized and widely applicable successor to CAM. It uses gradients of the target class score with respect to feature maps to produce the heatmap, making it applicable to virtually any CNN architecture without modifications
Chatbot	A computer program that simulates and processes human conversation (written or spoken). Chatbot is powered by various levels of AI, from simple rule-based systems to advanced generative AI models (like ChatGPT, Gemini, etc.) that use natural language processing (NLP) to understand and respond to user queries They are widely used in customer service, information retrieval, content generation, and many other applications

Terms	Terminology/Explanation
CNN	Specialized type of deep learning neural network, automatically extracting features from data using convolutional structures
Data augmentation	A set of techniques used in machine learning, particularly in deep learning, to increase the amount and diversity of training data by creating modified versions of existing data
DeepLab	A powerful family of deep learning models developed by Google research, specifically designed for semantic image segmentation
DenseNet	Type of convolutional neural network where every layer is directly connected to every other layer in a feed-forward fashion within a "dense block". These connections are a most distinguishing feature, named dense connections
DenseNet201	A specific version of DenseNet architecture. The "201" indicates the 201 layers in its deep structure
EfficientNet	A family of convolutional neural networks incorporating compound scaling method that uniformly scales all three dimensions (width, depth, and resolution) with a fixed ratio
ESRGANs	Enhanced super-resolution generative adversarial networks designed to produce high-quality image super-resolution. It leverages deep learning techniques to enhance image details, making it a preferred choice for applications requiring precise image clarity
Explainable AI (XAI)	The development of AI systems that provide clear, understandable explanations for their decisions and actions, making them more transparent and trustworthy to users
Faster R-CNN	Fast region-based convolutional network: An object detection algorithm that significantly improved upon its predecessor, R-CNN, by addressing its computational inefficiencies. Fast R-CNN made object detection faster and more accurate
Feature pyramid network (FPN)	A top–down architecture with lateral connections for building high-level semantic feature maps at all scales. The FPN operates by constructing the feature pyramid within a deep convolutional neural network
GANs	Generative adversarial network: A deep learning framework that uses two neural networks, a generator and a discriminator, in a competitive learning process The generator produces new data instances that resemble the training data The discriminator tries to distinguish between real data and the generator's output The generator and discriminator are trained simultaneously in a competitive manner, allowing the generator to learn to create highly realistic data
Heatmap	Refers to the visual output of CAM or grad-CAM. It's an overlay on the original image where warmer colors (e.g., red and yellow) indicate regions of higher importance or activation for a specific class prediction, while cooler colors (e.g., blue and green) indicate lower importance
Inception (such as inception-v3)	A family of convolutional neural network for computer vision, particularly image recognition, introduced by researchers at Google as GoogLeNet and later renamed inception-v1) The series was historically important as an early CNN that separates the stem (data ingest), body (data processing), and head (prediction), an architectural design that persists in all modern CNN Inception v3 is an improved version of inception v2 (added batch normalization and removed dropout) by using factorized convolutions

Terms	Terminology/Explanation
Internet of things (IoT)	Describes devices with sensor processing ability, software, and other technologies that connect and exchange data with other devices and systems over the internet or other communication networks
LightGBM	Light gradient-boosting machine: A breakthrough tree-based ensemble learning approach to overcome the efficiency and scalability difficulties of XGBoost in high-dimensional input feature and massive dataset contexts
LIME	Local interpretable model-agnostic explanations: A technique that approximates any black box machine learning model with a local, interpretable model to explain each individual prediction
LLM	Large language model: A type of machine learning model designed for natural language processing (NLP) tasks. LLMs are language models with many parameters and are trained with self-supervised learning on a vast amount of text
Overfitting	A behavior that occurs when the ML model gives accurate predictions for training data but not for new data
Random forest	A machine learning algorithm that uses an ensemble of decision trees to make predictions. It's a popular choice for both classification and regression tasks because it often outperforms individual decision trees due to its ability to reduce overfitting and improve accuracy
Region proposal network (RPN)	A fully convolutional network that efficiently generates potential bounding boxes (region proposals) within an image where objects are likely to be located
ResNet (such as ResNet-152)	Residual neural network: A deep learning architecture addressing the degradation problem and extracting more information from the original data The ResNet-152 has the ability to learn rich feature representations through its 152-layered network, which is particularly beneficial in differentiating subtle features of human faces with and without masks
Semantic image segmentation	A computer vision task where the goal is to assign a class label (e.g., "road", "person", and "lesion") to every single pixel in an image, effectively partitioning the image into meaningful regions
Single-shot detector (SSD)	A type of object detection algorithm is used in computer vision and machine learning. SSD algorithm is based on a deep convolutional neural network that takes an image as input and procedures a set of bounding boxes and class predictions for all objects in the image
Support vector machine (SVM)	A supervised machine learning algorithm used for both classification and regression tasks. It is well-known for its effectiveness in classification, especially with complex, high-dimensional datasets
Swin transformer	Swin transformer capably serves as a general-purpose backbone for computer vision. The swin transformer builds hierarchical feature maps by merging image patches in deeper layers and has linear computation complexity to the input image size due to the computation of self-attention only within each local window
Transfer learning	A technique in machine learning in which knowledge learned from a task is reused in order to boost performance on a related task
Tuning	The processing of optimizing a model's parameters to improve its performance on a specific task Fine-tuning is a specific type of tuning where a pre-trained model is further trained on a new, smaller dataset to specialize it for a particular use case
UNet	A powerful convolutional neural network architecture primarily used for image segmentation tasks in AI, particularly in computer vision. It is known for its U-shaped design, consisting of an encoder and a decoder

Terms	Terminology/Explanation
Underfitting	A behavior that occurs when the ML cannot adequately capture the underlying structure of the data
VGG-16	A pre-trained specific type of convolutional neural network architecture that was proposed by the visual geometry group (VGG). It is characterized by its depth, consisting of 16 layers, including 13 convolutional layers and three fully connected layers
Vision transformer (ViT)	A model for image classification that employs a transformer-like architecture over patches of the image. The idea behind vision transformer (ViT) is to break down an image into small blocks, treat each patch like a token and then feed these tokens into a transformer model
YOLO (such as YOLOv3)	A real-time object detection algorithm based on convolutional neural networks YOLOv3, introduced in 2018, includes the use of a more complex backbone network, multiple scales for detection, and a more sophisticated loss function, in contrast to the YOLOv1 and YOLOv2

1.8 Conclusions

The development in the field of artificial intelligence is rapid. This is due to computers and their rapid rate of development, which have increased human expectations of finding answers to the nature and functioning of the human brain. In this chapter, the concepts regarding artificial intelligence, the different technologies that have been implemented and their mode of operation have been presented in detail. In addition, the differentiations of AI technologies were clarified, and applications in the health sector were presented, with particular emphasis on dermatological imaging.

References

1. McCarthy J, Minsky ML, Rochester N, Shannon CE. A proposal for the dartmouth summer research project on Artificial Intelligence, August 31, 1955.
2. Haugeland E. Artificial intelligence: the very idea. Cambridge: MIT Press; 1985.
3. Kurzweil R. The age of intelligent machines. Cambridge: MIT Press; 1990.
4. Newell A, Simon A. Human Problem Solving. Englewood Cliffs: Prentice-Hall; 1972.
5. Russel S., and Norvig P., "Artificial intelligence: a modern approach" Prentice-Hall, Englewood Cliffs, 1995.
6. Kulikowski CA. Beginnings of artificial intelligence in medicine (AIM): computational artifice assisting scientific inquiry and clinical art-with reflections on present AIM challenges. Yearb Med Inform. 2019;28:249–56.
7. Isgut M, Gloster L, Choi K, Venugopalan J, Wang MD. Systematic review of advanced AI methods for improving healthcare data quality in post COVID-19 era. IEEE Rev Biomed Eng. 2023;16:53–69.
8. Hamet P, Tremblay J. Artificial intelligence in medicine. Metabolism. 2017;69:S36–40.
9. McCarthy J. What is artificial intelligence. 2004. Accessible on: http://www-formal.stanford.edu/jmc/whatisai.html.
10. Amisha MP, Pathania M, Rathaur VK. Overview of artificial intelligence in medicine. J Family Med Prim Care. 2019;8(7):2328–31. https://doi.org/10.4103/jfmpc.jfmpc_440_19.

11. Kaul V, Enslin S, Gross SA. History of artificial intelligence in medicine. Gastrointest Endosc. 2020 Oct;92(4):807–12. https://doi.org/10.1016/j.gie.2020.06.040.
12. Borges do Nascimento IJ, Marcolino MS, Abdulazeem HM, et al. Impact of big data analytics on people's health: overview of systematic reviews and recommendations for future studies. J Med Internet Res. 2021;23(4):e27275. https://doi.org/10.2196/27275.
13. Murphree DH, Puri P, Shamim H, Bezalel SA, Drage LA, Wang M, Pittelkow MR, Carter RE, Davis MDP, Bridges AG, Mangold AR, Yiannias JA, Tollefson MM, Lehman JS, Meves A, Otley CC, Sokumbi O, Hall MR, Comfere N. Deep learning for dermatologists: part I fundamental concepts. J Am Acad Dermatol. 2020;87:1343.
14. Hogarty DT, Su JC, Phan K, Attia M, Hossny M, Nahavandi S, Lenane P, Moloney FJ, Yazdabadi A. Artificial intelligence in dermatology-where we are and the way to the future: a review. Am J Clin Dermatol. 2020;21(1):41–7. https://doi.org/10.1007/s40257-019-00462-6.
15. Brinker TJ, Hekler A, Utikal JS, Grabe N, Schadendorf D, Klode J, Berking C, Steeb T, Enk AH, von Kalle C. Skin cancer classification using convolutional neural networks: systematic review. J Med Internet Res. 2018;20(10):e11936. https://doi.org/10.2196/11936.
16. Marka A, Carter JB, Toto E, Hassanpour S. Automated detection of nonmelanoma skin cancer using digital images: a systematic review. BMC Med Imaging. 2019;19(1):21. https://doi.org/10.1186/s12880-019-0307-7.
17. Shapiro L, Stockman G. Computer vision. Prentice-Hall; 2001. p. 13.
18. Chen CH. An introduction to computer vision in medical imaging. In: Chen CH, editor. Computer vision in medical imaging. Singapore: World Scientific Publishing; 2014. p. 1–17.
19. Pun T, Gerig G, Ratib O. Image analysis and computer vision in medicine. Comput Med Imaging Graph. 1994;18:85–96.
20. Esteva A, Kuprel B, Novoa RA, Ko J, Swetter SM, Blau HM, et al. Dermatologist-level classification of skin cancer with deep neural networks. Nature. 2017;542:115–8.
21. Craft JA 3rd. Artificial intelligence and the softer side of medicine. Mo Med. 2018;115:406–9.
22. Shanafelt TD, Dyrbye LN, Sinsky C, Hasan O, Satele D, Sloan J, et al. Relationship between clerical burden and characteristics of the electronic environment with physician burnout and professional satisfaction. Mayo Clin Proc. 2016;91:836–48.
23. Gilpin LH, Bau D, Yuan BZ, Bajwa A, Specter M, Kagal L. Explaining explanations: an overview of interpretability of machine learning. In: Proceedings of the 2018 IEEE 5th International Conference on Data Science and Advanced Analytics (DSAA), Turin, Italy, 1–3 October 2018; 2018. p. 80–9.
24. Gunning D, Aha DW. DARPA'S explainable artificial intelligence program. AI Mag. 2019;40:44–58.
25. Alain G, Bengio Y. Understanding intermediate layers using linear classifier probes. 2018. Available online: https://arxiv.org/abs/1610.01644v4. Accessed 1 Sept 2020.
26. Murdoch WJ, Singh C, Kumbier K, Abbasi-Asl R, Yu B. Definitions, methods, and applications in interpretable machine learning. Proc Natl Acad Sci USA. 2019;116:22071–80.
27. Adadi A, Berrada M. Peeking inside the black-box: a survey on explainable artificial intelligence (XAI). IEEE Access. 2018;6:52138–60.
28. Shi X, De-Silva V, Aslan Y, Ekmekcioglu E, Kondoz A. Evaluating the learning procedure of CNNs through a sequence of prognostic tests Utilising information theorctical measures. Entropy. 2022;24:67. https://doi.org/10.3390/e24010067.
29. Cheng H, Lian D, Gao S, Geng Y. Utilizing information bottleneck to evaluate the capability of deep neural networks for image classification. Entropy. 2019;21:456.
30. Yu S, Wickstrom K, Jenssen R, Príncipe JC. Understanding convolutional neural networks with information theory: an initial exploration. IEEE Trans Neural Netw Learn Syst. 2020;32:435–42.
31. Goodfellow I, Bengio Y, Courville A. Deep learning. The MIT Press; 2016.
32. Janik RA. Aspects of human memory and large language models. arXiv:2311.03839. 2023; https://doi.org/10.48550/arXiv.2311.03839.
33. Wang Z, Valdez J, Basu Mallick D, Baraniuk RG. Towards human-like educational question generation with large language models. In: Rodrigo MM, Matsuda N, Cristea AI, Dimitrova

V, editors. Artificial Intelligence in Education. Springer International Publishing; 2022. p. 153–66. https://doi.org/10.1007/978-3-031-11644-5_13.
34. Brown TB, Mann B, Ryder N, Subbiah M, Kaplan J, Dhariwal P, Neelakantan A, Shyam P, Sastry G, Askell A, Agarwal S, Herbert-Voss A, Krueger G, Henighan T, Child R, Ramesh A, Ziegler DM, Wu J, Winter C, et al. Language models are few-shot learners. arXiv:2005.14165. 2020; https://doi.org/10.48550/arXiv.2005.14165.
35. Chang Z, Koulieris GA, Shum HPH. On the design fundamentals of diffusion models: a survey. arXiv:2306.04542. 2023; https://doi.org/10.48550/arXiv.2306.04542.
36. Yetistiren B, Ozsoy I, Tuzun E. Assessing the quality of GitHub copilot's code generation. In: Proceedings of the 18th international conference on predictive models and data analytics in software engineering; 2022. p. 62–71. https://doi.org/10.1145/3558489.3559072.
37. Borsos Z, Marinier R, Vincent D, Kharitonov E, Pietquin O, Sharifi M, Roblek D, Teboul O, Grangier D, Tagliasacchi M, Zeghidour N. AudioLM: a language modeling approach to audio generation. IEEE/ACM Trans Audio Speech Lang Process. 2023;31:2523–33.
38. Li Y, Yu Y, Li H, Chen Z, Khashanah K. TradingGPT: multi-agent system with layered memory and distinct characters for enhanced financial trading performance. arXiv:2309.03736. 2023; https://doi.org/10.48550/arXiv.2309.03736.
39. Suzuki M, Matsuo Y. A survey of multimodal deep generative models. Adv Robot. 2022;36(5–6):261–78. https://doi.org/10.1080/01691864.2022.2035253.
40. A Beginner's Guide to Neural Networks and Deep Learning. Available from: https://pathmind.com/wiki/neural-network. Last accessed on 30 Apr 30 2025.
41. Kohonen T. An introduction to neural computing. Neural Netw. 1988;1(1):3–16.
42. Choy G, Khalilzadeh O, Michalski M, Do S, Samir AE, Pianykh OS, et al. Current applications and future impact of machine learning in radiology. Radiology. 2018;288:318–28.
43. Castelvecchi D. Can we open the black box of AI? Nature. 2016;538:20–3.
44. Ramachandran R, Rajeev DC, Krishnan SG, Subathra P. Deep learning an overview. IJAER. 2015;10(10):25433–48.
45. Hubel DH, Wiesel TN. Receptive fields and functional architecture of monkey striate cortex. J Physiol. 1968;195:215.
46. Chen Y, Jiang H, Li C, Jia X, Ghamisi P. Deep feature extraction and classification of hyperspectral images based on convolutional neural networks. IEEE Trans Geosci Remote Sens. 2016;54:6232–51.
47. Tu F, Yin S, Ouyang P, Tang S, Liu L, Wei S. Deep convolutional neural network architecture with reconfigurable computation patterns. IEEE Trans Very Large Scale Integr (VLSI) Syst. 2017;25:2220–33.
48. Dua S, Kumar SS, Albagory Y, Ramalingam R, Dumka A, Singh R, Rashid M, Gehlot A, Alshamrani SS, AlGhamdi AS. Developing a speech recognition system for recognizing tonal speech signals using a convolutional neural network. Appl Sci. 2022;12:6223.
49. Donahue J, Hendricks LA, Guadarrama S, Rohrbach M, Venugopalan S, Saenko K, Darrell T. Long-term recurrent convolutional networks for visual recognition and description. IEEE Trans Pattern Anal Mach Intell (PAMI). 2017;39(4):677–91.
50. Lindeberg T. Scale invariant feature transform. Scholarpedia. 2012;7(5):10491.
51. Ahonen T, Hadid A, Pietikainen M. Face description with local binary patterns: application to face recognition. IEEE Trans Pattern Anal Mach Intell. 2006;28(12):2037–41.
52. Hubel DH, Wiesel TN. Receptive fields, binocular interaction and functional architecture in the cat's visual cortex. J Physiol. 1962;160(1):106–54.
53. Szegedy C, et al. Going deeper with convolutions. In: Proceedings of the IEEE conference on computer vision and pattern Recognition (CVPR); 2015. p. 1–9.
54. Ioffe S, Szegedy C. Batch normalization: accelerating deep network training by reducing internal covariate shift. In: Proceedings of the international conference on machine learning; 2015. p. 448–56.
55. Pandian JA, Kanchanadevi K, Kumar VD, Jasinska E, Gono R, Leonowicz Z, Jasinski M. A five convolutional layer deep convolutional neural network for plant leaf disease detection. Electronics. 2022;11:1266.

56. Galanis NI, Vafiadis P, Mirzaev KG, Papakostas GA. Convolutional neural networks: a roundup and benchmark of their pooling layer variants. Algorithms. 2022;15:391.
57. Ouyang W, Xu B, Hou J, Yuan X. Fabric defect detection using activation layer embedded convolutional neural network. IEEE Access. 2019;7:70130–40.
58. Khan ID, Farooq O, Khan YU. Automatic seizure detection using modified CNN architecture and activation layer. J Phys Conf Ser. 2022;2318:012013.
59. Wang SH, Hong J, Yang M. Sensorineural hearing loss identification via nine-layer convolutional neural network with batch normalization and dropout. Multimed Tools Appl. 2020;79:15135–50.
60. Setiawan W. Character recognition using adjustment convolutional network with dropout layer. IOP Conf Ser Mater Sci Eng. 2021;1125:012049.
61. Liu H, Zhang C, Deng Y, Xie B, Liu T, Zhang Z, Li YF. TransIFC: invariant cues-aware feature concentration learning for efficient fine-grained bird image classification. IEEE Trans Multimed. 2023:1–14. https://doi.org/10.1109/TMM.2023.3238548.
62. Liu T, Liu H, Yang B, Zhang Z. LDCNet: limb direction cues-aware network for flexible human pose estimation in industrial behavioral biometrics systems. IEEE Trans Ind Inform. 2023:1–11. https://doi.org/10.1109/TII.2023.3266366.
63. Ma Y, Cao Y, Vrudhula S, Seo JS. Optimizing the convolution operation to accelerate deep neural networks on FPGA. IEEE Trans Very Large Scale Integr Syst. 2018;26:1354–67.
64. Zhao B, Hua X, Yu K, Tao W, He X, Feng S, Tian P. Evaluation of convolution operation based on the interpretation of deep learning on 3-D point cloud. IEEE J Sel Top Appl Earth Obs Remote Sens. 2020;13:5088–101.
65. Jiang P, Xue Y, Neri F. Convolutional neural network pruning based on multi-objective feature map selection for image classification. Appl Soft Comput. 2023;139:110229.
66. Krizhevsky A, Sutskever I, Hinton GE. ImageNet classification with deep convolutional neural networks. In: Proceedings of the advances in neural information processing systems, vol. 25; 2012. p. 1097–105.
67. LeCun Y, Bottou L, Bengio Y, Haffner P. Gradient-based learningapplied to document recognition. Proc IEEE. 1998;86:2278.
68. Wei G, Li G, Zhao J, He A. Development of a LeNet-5 gas identification CNN structure for electronic noses. Sensors. 2019;19:217.
69. Chen HC, Widodo AM, Wisnujati A, Rahaman M, Lin JCW, Chen L, Weng CE. AlexNet convolutional neural network for disease detection and classification of tomato leaf. Electronics. 2022;11:951.
70. Zhu Y, Su H, Tang S, Zhang S, Zhou T, Wang J. A novel fault diagnosis method based on SWT and VGG-LSTM model for hydraulic axial piston pump. J Mar Sci Eng. 2023;11:594.
71. Wang Y, Jing C, Huang W, Jin S, Lv X. Adaptive spatiotemporal InceptionNet for traffic flow forecasting. IEEE Trans Intell Transp Syst. 2023;24:3882–907.
72. Szegedy C, Ioffe S, Vanhoucke V. Inception-v4, inception-resnet and the impact of residual connections on learning. arXiv:1602.07261. 2016;
73. Liu K, Qin S, Ning J, Xin P, Wang Q, Chen Y, Zhao W, Zhang E, Lang N. Prediction of primary tumor sites in spinal metastases using a ResNet-50 convolutional neural network based on MRI. Cancer. 2023;15:2974.
74. Huang G, Liu Z, Der Maaten V, Weinberger KQ. Densely connected convolutional networks. arXiv:1608.06993. 2016. https://arxiv.org/abs/1608.06993.
75. Ronneberger O, Fischer P, Brox T. U-net: Convolutional networks for biomedical image segmentation. In: Medical Image Computing and Computer-Assisted Intervention – MICCAI 2015. Springer; 2015. p. 234–41.
76. Vaswani A, Shazeer N, Parmar N, Uszkoreit J, Jones L, Gomez AN, Kaiser L, Polosukhin I. Attention is all you need. arXiv:1706.03762. 2017;
77. Vaswani A, Shazeer N, Parmar N, Uszkoreit J, Jones L, Gomez AN, Kaiser Ł, Polosukhin I. Attention is all you need. Adv Neural Inf Process Syst. 2017;30 https://doi.org/10.48550/arXiv.1706.03762.

78. Devlin J, Chang MW, Lee K, Toutanova K. Bert: Pre-training of deep bidirectional transformers for language understanding. arXiv. 2018:arXiv:1810.04805.
79. Liu Y, Ott M, Goyal N, Du J, Joshi M, Chen D, Levy O, Lewis M, Zettlemoyer L, Stoyanov V. Roberta: a robustly optimized bert pretraining approach. arXiv:1907.11692. 2019;
80. Tan M, Le Q. Efficientnet: rethinking model scaling for convolutional neural networks. In: Proceedings of the international conference on machine learning, Long Beach, CA, USA, 9–15 June 2019; 2019. p. 6105–14.
81. Bello I, Zoph B, Vaswani A, Shlens J, Le QV. Attention augmented convolutional networks. In: Proceedings of the IEEE/CVF International Conference on Computer Vision, Seoul, Republic of Korea, 27 October–2 November 2019; 2019. p. 3286–95.
82. Thickstun J. The transformer model equations. 2019; pp. 1–5. Available: https://homes.cs.washington.edu/thick-stn/docs/transformers.pdf.
83. Bahdanau D, Cho K, Bengio Y. Neural machine translation by jointly learning to align and translate. In: 3rd International Conference on Learning Representations, ICLR 2015; 2015. p. 1–15.
84. Luong M, Pham H, Manning C. Effective approaches to attention-based neural machine translation. In: Proceedings of the 2015 conference on empirical methods in natural language processing; 2015. p. 1412–21.
85. Wang X, Girshick R, Gupta A, He K. Non-local neural networks. In: Proceedings of the IEEE conference on computer vision and pattern recognition; 2018. p. 7794–803.
86. Vaswani A. Attention is all you need. In: Advances in neural information processing systems 30: annual conference on neural information processing systems; 2017. p. 5999–6009.
87. Hendrycks D, Gimpel K. Gaussian error linear units (GELUs), 2016; pp. 1–9 [Online]. Available: http://arxiv.org/abs/1606.08415.
88. Ba J, Kiros J, Hinton G. Layer normalization. 2016. Available: http://arxiv.org/abs/1607.06450.
89. Chen Z, Xie L, Niu J, Liu X, Wei L, Tian Q. Visformer: The vision-friendly transformer. 2021. Available: http://arxiv.org/abs/2104.12533.
90. Srinivas A, Lin T.-Y, Parmar N, Shlens J, Abbeel P, Vaswani. Bottleneck transformers for visual recognition. 2021. Available: http://arxiv.org/abs/2101.11605.
91. Zhao H, Jiang L, Jia J, Torr P, Koltun V. Point transformer. 2020. Available: http://arxiv.org/abs/2012.09164.
92. Dosovitskiy A. An image is worth 16x16 words: Transformers for image recognition at scale. 2020. Available: http://arxiv.org/abs/2010.11929.
93. Chen M. Generative pretraining from pixels. In: The 37th International Conference on Machine Learning (ICML 2020), vol. PartF16814; 2020. p. 1669–81.
94. Radford A, Wu J, Child R, Luan D, Amodei D, Sutskever I. Language models are unsupervised multitask learners. 2019. Available: http://arxiv.org/abs/2007.07582.
95. Ramachandran P, Bello I, Parmar N, Levskaya A, Vaswani A, Shlens J. Stand-alone self-attention in vision models. Adv Neural Inf Process Syst. 2019;32 https://doi.org/10.48550/arXiv.1906.05909.
96. Huang G, Sun Y, Liu Z, Sedra D, Weinberger K. Deep networks with stochastic depth. LNCS. 2016;9908:646–61.
97. Hoffer E, Ben-Nun T, Hubara I, Giladi N, Hoefler T, Soudry D. Augment your batch: better training with larger batches. 2019. Available: http://arxiv.org/abs/1901.09335.
98. Touvron H, Cord M, Douze M, Massa F, Sablayrolles A, Jegou. Training data- efficient image transformers distillation through attention; 2020. pp. 1–22. Available: http://arxiv.org/abs/2012.12877.
99. Graham B. Levit: a vision transformer in convnet's clothing for faster inference. 2021. Available: http://arxiv.org/abs/2104.01136.
100. Chen C.-F, Fan Q, Panda R. Crossvit: cross-attention multi-scale vision transformer for image classification. 2021. Available: http://arxiv.org/abs/2103.14899.
101. Liu Y. Roberta: A robustly optimized bert pretraining approach. 2019. Available: http://arxiv.org/abs/1907.11692.

102. Han K, Xiao A, Wu E, Guo J, Xu C, Wang Y. Transformer in transformer; 2021. pp. 1–12. Available: http://arxiv.org/abs/2103.00112.
103. Chernyavskiy A, Ilvovsky D, Nakov P. Transformers: "the end of history" for natural language processing? In: Machine learning and knowledge discovery in databases. Research Track: European Conference, ECML PKDD 2021, Bilbao, Spain, September 13–17, 2021, Proceedings, Part III 21. Springer; 2021. p. 677–93.
104. Wang A, Pruksachatkun Y, Nangia N, Singh A, Michael J, Hill F, Levy O, Bowman S. SuperGLUE: a stickier benchmark for generalpurpose language understanding systems. Adv Neural Inf Process Syst. 2019;32:26–9.
105. Adiwardana D, Luong M-T, So DR, Hall J, Fiedel N, Thoppilan R, Yang Z, Kulshreshtha A, Nemade G, Lu Y, et al. Towards a humanlike open-domain chatbot. arXiv preprint arXiv:2001.09977. 2020;
106. Pinker S. The language instinct: how the mind creates language. London: Penguin; 2003.
107. Dergaa I, Chamari K, Zmijewski P, Saad HB. From human writing to artificial intelligence generated text: examining the prospects and potential threats of chatgpt in academic writing. Biol Sport. 2023;40(2):615–22.
108. Hoffmann J, Borgeaud S, Mensch A, Buchatskaya E, Cai T, Rutherford E, Casas D d L, Hendricks LA, Welbl J, Clark A, et al. Training compute-optimal large language model. arXiv preprint arXiv:2203.15556. 2022;
109. Keskar NS, McCann B, Varshney LR, Xiong C, Socher R. CTRL: a conditional transformer language model for controllable generation. arXiv preprint arXiv:1909.05858. 2019;
110. Chowdhery A, Narang S, Devlin J, Bosma M, Mishra G, Roberts A, Barham P, Chung HW, Sutton C, Gehrmann S, et al. Palm: scaling language modeling with pathways. arXiv preprint arXiv:2204.02311. 2022;
111. Rae JW, Borgeaud S, Cai T, Millican K, Hoffmann J, Song F, Aslanides J, Henderson S, Ring R, Young S, et al. Scaling language models: Methods, analysis & insights from training gopher. arXiv preprint arXiv:2112.11446. 2021;
112. Hernandez D, Brown T, Conerly T, DasSarma N, Drain D, El- Showk S, Elhage N, Hatfield-Dodds Z, Henighan T, Hume T, et al. Scaling laws and interpretability of learning from repeated data. arXiv preprint arXiv:2205.10487. 2022;
113. Carlini N, Ippolito D, Jagielski M, Lee K, Tramer F, Zhang C. Quantifying memorization across neural language models. arXiv preprint arXiv:2202.07646. 2022;
114. Li P, Zhang M, Lin P, Wan J, Jiang M. Conditional embedding pre-training language model for image captioning. Neural Process Lett. 2022;54(6):4987–5003.
115. Naveed H, Khan AU, Qiu S, Saqib M, Anwar S, Usman M, Akhtar N. A comprehensive overview of large language models. arXiv:2307.06435v10 [cs.CL]. 2024;
116. Börve A, Molina-Martinez R. A pilot study of a medical information service using mobile phones in Sweden. J Telemed Telecare. 2009;15:421–2.
117. Börve A, et al. Smartphone teledermoscopy referrals: a novel process for improved triage of skin cancer patients. Acta Derm Venereol. 2015;95:186–90.
118. Monteiro MG, Pantani D, Pinsky I, Hernandes Rocha TA. The development of the Pan American Health Organization digital health specialist on alcohol use. Front Digit Health. 2022;4:948187.

Dermatology: The Ideal Field for A.I. to Thrive

2

Dimitrios Mantzaris and Emmanouil Karampinis

2.1 Introduction

Skin diseases have become increasingly prevalent in recent decades and represent a major chronic health issue worldwide [1]. These conditions range from common skin conditions such as eczema, chickenpox, measles, warts, and acne, to more severe and life-threatening cases like skin cancers [2, 3]. Among the latter, melanoma and squamous cell carcinoma are particularly life-threatening if not diagnosed and treated promptly. Due to the significant global burden posed by skin-related conditions, early detection is essential. This underscores the importance of fully automated diagnostic systems, especially in developed countries, where they can alleviate the workload of dermatologists and reduce patient wait times [1]. Traditional diagnostic methods remain limited in frequency and are often expensive, restricting access for large segments of the population. However, advances in machine learning and image analysis have made automated detection and classification of skin diseases more feasible and efficient. Deep learning, a powerful branch of machine learning, leverages complex algorithms to analyze medical images and classify skin conditions based on various visual features.

In the study of Abbas et al., for example, several CNN-based architectures—specifically a sequential CNN, DenseNet-121, and ResNet-50—were used for feature

D. Mantzaris (✉)
Computational Intelligence and Health Informatics Lab, Nursing Department, School of Health Sciences, University of Thessaly, Larissa, Greece
e-mail: dmantzar@uth.gr

E. Karampinis
Second Dermatology Department, School of Health Sciences, Aristotle University of Thessaloniki, Thessaloniki, Greece

Department of Dermatology, Faculty of Medicine, School of Health Sciences, University General Hospital of Larissa, University of Thessaly, Larissa, Greece

E. Karampinis et al. (eds.), *Artificial Intelligence Applications in Dermatology*,
https://doi.org/10.1007/978-3-032-15614-3_2

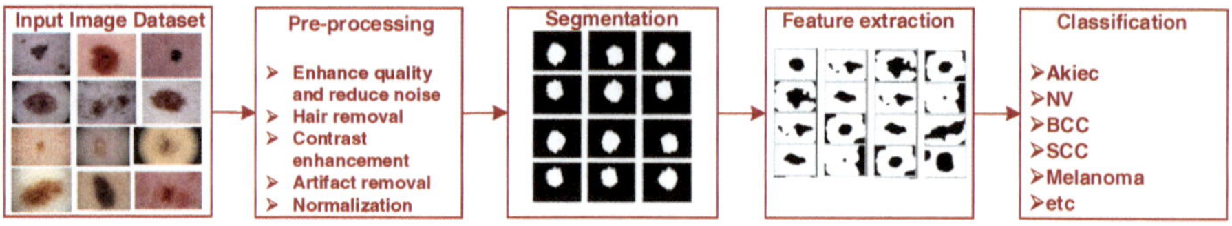

Fig. 2.1 Flowchart of a typical AI model classifying dermatological images. The training images are labeled with their diagnosis, and this labeling can be binary (benign/malignant) or multi-label (BCC, SCC, melanoma, nevi, etc). Following the preprocessing stage, removing hair, or irrelevant details and noise. Segmentation usually occurs right after preprocessing, as a step to clean and isolate region of interest (ROI) before features is extracted for classifier training. The next step is feature extraction can be done with machine learning or deep learning using CNNs to automatically learn features. Then, there is the AI architecture and algorithm selection in the classification stage. Data images are usually split into training, validation, and testing groups. Validation and tuning occur during or following training classifier, to maximize performance. It is essential to outline that each flowchart in each study that involves the implementation of an AI model can differ

extraction. These models were trained and evaluated using the HAM10000 and ISIC dermoscopic image datasets [4].

The diagnostic workflow is structured into four main phases: (1) image preprocessing, (2) segmentation, (3) feature extraction via CNN models, and (4) classification of skin disease types using a variety of machine learning (ML) and deep learning (DL) classifiers (Fig. 2.1). To address the issue of class imbalance in the datasets, data augmentation techniques were employed, enhancing the robustness and generalizability of the classification models [4].

CNNs, especially when combined with transfer learning, play a vital role in the analysis, segmentation, and classification of dermatological images, significantly improving diagnostic accuracy. Nonetheless, ongoing challenges must be addressed to further refine the performance and reliability of these advanced technologies in clinical dermatology.

2.2 Image Acquisition

Traditionally, dermatological diagnosis depends heavily on clinical examination, often supported by histopathological analysis. However, clinical evaluation alone may not always yield accurate results, and while skin biopsies are valuable, they carry a risk of morbidity. As medical technologies continue to advance, a variety of innovative imaging techniques have emerged to assist dermatologists in diagnosing and managing skin diseases [5].

2.2.1 Digital Photographic Imaging

Medical photography plays a key role in dermatology, particularly for tracking patient progress over time and assessing treatment effectiveness. It uses principles of reflectance, and back-scattered light-reflectance enhances surface detail, while back-scattering reveals subsurface structures. Polarizing filters help distinguish these by enabling parallel-polarized photography to highlight skin texture and scale, and cross-polarized photography to accentuate vascular and pigmentary features. Total-body digital photography (TBDP) captures the entire skin surface in a single session and is especially useful for monitoring patients with multiple moles or melanocytic lesions. It supports early detection of changes or new lesions and improves biopsy targeting. Commercial systems now offer standardized lighting and positioning, and often include dermoscopic overlays and algorithms for improved lesion recognition. However, 2D photography may distort lesion size due to angle variations-an issue that 3D imaging helps resolve [6].Three-dimensional imaging provides a full 360° body scan with rapid acquisition, reducing motion artifacts, and improving consistency. It allows dermoscopic close-ups to be overlaid on body maps. Additionally, smartphone applications allow patients to store TBDP images, promoting self-monitoring and enhancing patient engagement [6, 7]. Despite its benefits, TBDP faces limitations such as variability in positioning and lighting, difficulty imaging hair with 3D systems, large physical space requirements, high costs for equipment upgrades, limited insurance coverage, and time-consuming image capture [6].

2.2.2 Dermoscopy

Dermoscopy, also known as epiluminescence microscopy, uses a handheld device to magnify skin up to 10x, enabling visualization of the epidermis and superficial dermis. Polarizing filters enhance image quality by reducing light interference. Contact dermoscopy—using a liquid interface like gel or alcohol—improves clarity by minimizing refraction differences, although noncontact models are also available. Modern dermatoscopes often include both polarized and non-polarized light options [7]. This technique is particularly valuable for skin cancer diagnosis, improving sensitivity, and allowing better biopsy selection. It is especially effective in detecting early or thin melanomas that might go unnoticed during standard clinical exams. Several diagnostic algorithms, such as the ABCD rule and 7-point checklist, assist clinicians in identifying suspicious lesions [8, 9]. Despite its high sensitivity (around 90%), dermoscopy's specificity is lower (approximately 59%), and requires significant training for accurate interpretation. Unfortunately, formal training resources remain limited [8].

2.2.3 Confocal Microscopy

Confocal microscopy enables high-resolution imaging at the cellular level by using an 830-nm laser that exploits differences in the refractive indices of skin components such as melanin, keratin, and collagen. This laser interacts with the skin, and a pinhole filter ensures that only light from a specific focal plane is captured, producing clear, horizontally oriented images that are parallel to the skin surface-offering a more detailed view than conventional histopathology [8–10]. There are two main types of confocal microscopy: reflectance confocal microscopy (RCM) and fluorescence confocal microscopy (FCM). RCM leverages the natural reflective properties of skin cells to generate detailed images, making it particularly useful for diagnosing skin cancers like basal cell carcinoma (BCC), squamous cell carcinoma (SCC), and melanoma. It also plays a role in assessing tumor boundaries and monitoring treatment effectiveness. FCM, which uses fluorescent dyes to enhance contrast, is especially effective in identifying nonmelanoma skin cancers and is often used during margin assessment in procedures like Mohs surgery [10, 11]. Despite its high resolution and sensitivity, confocal microscopy has some drawbacks. Its imaging depth is limited to approximately 200–300 mm, potentially missing deeper lesions. The relatively narrow field of view can make it difficult to visualize larger tumors, and interpreting the images requires specialized training. Additionally, the equipment is expensive. Nonetheless, confocal microscopy remains a valuable tool in the diagnosis and treatment of skin cancers [11].

2.3 Dermatological Image Datasets

According to the Oxford dictionary [12], a dataset is defined as a collection of data that a computer processes as a single unit. Datasets serve as the core element of any artificial intelligence (AI) system and are crucial for the success and scalability of machine learning (ML) applications. They allow for diverse data types to be processed together as a unified whole, helping algorithms learn and detect consistent patterns across the entire dataset. In fact, the availability of large, high-quality datasets is one of the key drivers behind the rapid adoption of machine learning technologies. With sufficient data volume, patterns can be uncovered, trends identified, and data-driven decisions effectively made [13].

Before being used to train ML models, datasets typically undergo preprocessing and are then split into separate subsets: training, validation, and testing. This division is critical for assessing a model's accuracy and robustness. The test set remains isolated during training to ensure an unbiased evaluation of the model's generalization performance. The validation set helps minimize bias, ensuring that the model does not become too dependent on one data distribution. While a large dataset is often necessary for successful training, excessive training can lead to overfitting, where the model performs well on the training data but poorly on unseen data [14].

Advancements in dermatological imaging have made it possible to visualize the skin surface with greater detail, enabling the creation of specialized datasets. Widely used datasets in dermatology include HAM10000, ISIC (International Skin Imaging Collaboration), DermQuest, DermIS, and MED-NODE [15–18].

The *HAM10000* dataset (Fig. 2.2) has been extensively used for skin cancer detection, classification of common pigmented lesions, and melanoma diagnosis through deep learning models [18, 19]. Techniques applied to this dataset include convolutional neural networks (CNNs), DenseNet, Inception ResNet v2, Mask

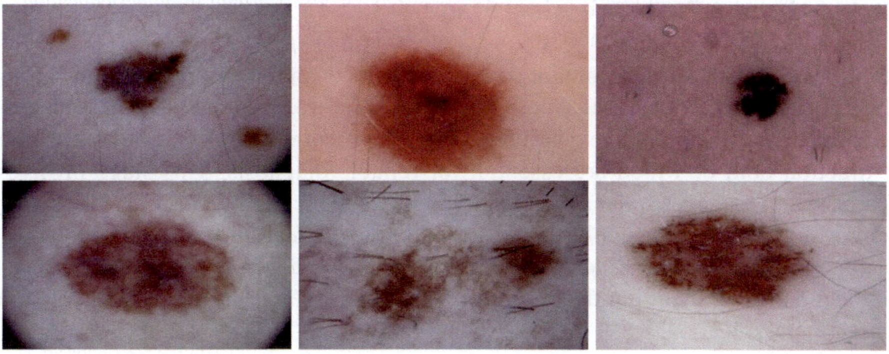

Fig. 2.2 Presents images from HAMA10000. (Dermatological images found in https://dataverse.harvard.edu/dataset.xhtml?persistentId=doi:10.7910/DVN/DBW86T)

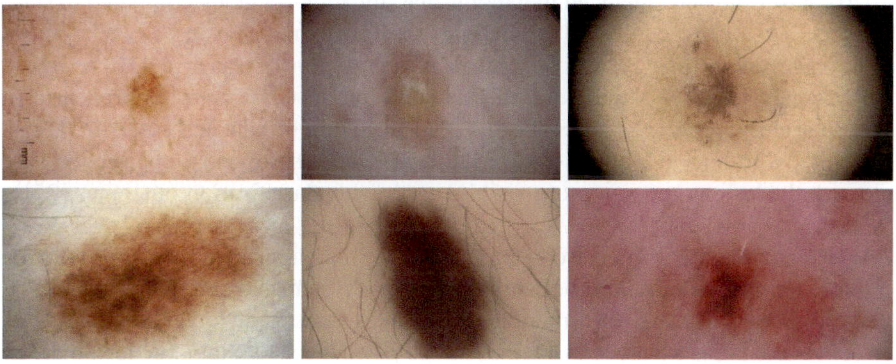

Fig. 2.3 ISIC2020 testing dataset. (Dermatological images [17])

R-CNN, and ResNet15 for tasks such as skin cancer classification and skin condition identification [19].

The *ISIC* dataset (Fig. 2.3) supports a range of deep learning implementations, including deep CNNs for classifying skin lesions and melanoma. It has also been utilized in segmentation tasks, incorporating techniques to predict and correct errors, and applying hybrid CNN models and fine-tuned deep features for more accurate skin lesion classification [20, 21].

The DermQuest, DermIs, and MED-NNODE datasets have provided the input data for classification of skin lesions using AlexNet, a convolutional neural network architecture developed for image classification tasks [22].

The *PH2* dataset includes 200 dermoscopic images of skin lesions, collected at the Dermatology Department of Pedro Hispano Hospital in Matosinhos, Portugal. It was designed to support research in the segmentation and classification of malignant skin regions. As noted in [23], this dataset was randomly split into two equal subsets of 100 images—one for training and the other for evaluation.

2.4 Image Preprocessing Stage

Skin lesion images often contain unwanted artifacts and noise, such as hair or air bubbles, which can obscure critical features. Therefore, preprocessing plays a crucial role in enhancing image quality and ensuring accurate segmentation and feature extraction both of which are essential for reliable diagnosis. This stage involves preparing raw images for analysis by AI models, and includes several key steps: hair removal, image resizing, color normalization, transfer learning, data augmentation, and normalization. The effectiveness of these methods depends heavily on the quality and nature of the input data used for training machine learning models for skin disease classification.

Hair Removal In dermoscopy, removing hair is important to prevent occlusion of the lesion area. Hair often introduces visual noise, complicating the analysis. Kim and Hong [24] utilized CycleGAN for hair removal, and their results on the ISIC 2020 dataset showed enhanced melanoma classification accuracy compared to standard methods. Zhao et al. [25] applied inpainting techniques using a black top-hat filter on grayscale images to replace pixels in hairy regions. Attia et al. [26] reviewed various hair detection strategies and evaluated hybrid CNN-based approaches. In deep learning models, activation maps tend to highlight hair and ruler markings, which aids in their identification and removal. Once these visual obstructions are cleared, the lesions become more visible, improving classification outcomes [25].

Image Resizing Resizing is frequently applied to match image dimensions with the input requirements of neural networks or display systems. When done correctly, it preserves critical visual information and enables consistent image analysis. One effective technique involves extracting image patches that contain key lesion areas. A widely used resizing method is bicubic interpolation, which evaluates a 4x4 grid of neighboring pixels and computes new pixel values using a weighted average-helping to maintain image sharpness and detail [27, 28].

Color Normalization To reduce variability caused by lighting differences or camera inconsistencies, color normalization techniques are applied. These adjust the color distribution across images, making them more uniform. This ensures that the model focuses on relevant lesion features rather than lighting artifacts [29].

Transfer Learning Transfer learning involves reusing knowledge from a previously trained model on a new, but related task. Transfer learning offers a more efficient approach for differentiating between such visually similar conditions, making it a preferred strategy in dermatological image analysis [30].

The ImageNet dataset, containing around 1.2 million images, is widely utilized for developing powerful model architectures due to its extensive size and diversity. Models trained on ImageNet have shown strong generalization when applied to unrelated tasks, making them particularly valuable for transfer learning. There are three main strategies for fine-tuning pretrained models: (a) feature extraction, which involves using the model to extract relevant features and replacing only the final output layer; (b) architecture reuse, where the model's structure is retained but all weights are reinitialized and retrained from the beginning on the new dataset; and (c) selective training, which freezes certain layers while fine-tuning others.

Commonly used pre-trained convolutional neural networks (CNNs) for these strategies include AlexNet, SqueezeNet, MobileNet, Google Inception, ResNet, Xception, VGGNet, and DenseNet.

Data Augmentation Deep learning models require large volumes of labeled data to generalize well. Since annotated medical images are often limited, data augmentation is widely used to expand training datasets and reduce overfitting. This involves applying transformations such as flipping, rotating, cropping, and color adjustments to existing images [31]. Perez et al. [32] evaluated 13 augmentation methods across CNN architectures, while Kato et al. [33] improved diagnostic accuracy by applying flipping operations. Several commonly used data augmentation strategies include geometrical transformation, color jitter, noise addition, multisample technique, generative adversarial networks, and autoaugment.

Geometrical Transformations These techniques involve altering the spatial orientation or dimensions of images through operations such as random reflection, rotation, translation, shearing, zooming, scaling, and resizing [34].

Color Jitter Color jittering techniques commonly involve modifying brightness, contrast, saturation, and hue–value–saturation (HVS) components. These adjustments alter the balance between color channels or apply varying intensity levels. Oukil et al. [35] effectively utilized color features in dermoscopic images, achieving promising results.

Noise Addition Noise addition involves introducing random values from various noise distributions—such as Gaussian, Poisson, and Salt & Pepper—while maintaining the essential features of the image. This technique helps prevent overfitting, especially when the neural network focuses on irrelevant high-frequency details. It is commonly used in conjunction with GANs, where informative noise aids in preventing mode collapse and accelerates convergence [36].

Multisample Technique The synthetic minority over-sampling technique (SMOTE) [37] generates new samples for underrepresented classes through interpolation, effectively addressing class imbalance and enhancing classifier performance. Another method, sample pairing [38], creates new training samples by randomly selecting two images, applying basic augmentations (e.g., random flips), and averaging their pixel values, with one of the original labels assigned to the new sample. The third approach, mixup [39], blends images and labels to produce synthetic data. Lee and Chin [40] extended this by implementing various mixing strategies, such as vertical, horizontal, diagonal-quadrant, four-quadrant, four-column, and region of interest (ROI) mixing. These techniques aim to enrich the training set and better approximate the true data distribution.

Generative Adversarial Networks (GANs) GANs [41] offer advanced data augmentation techniques and solutions for tasks requiring generative models. In recent years, GANs have gained rapid development and have been applied to skin lesion classification [25, 42, 43]. For instance, Abdelhalim et al. [43] used GANs to generate high-quality 256x256 skin lesion images, improving CNN-based melanoma detection with a 5.6% increase in sensitivity. Zhao et al. [25] employed a style-based GAN and DenseNet201 for skin lesion classification, achieving a balanced multiclass accuracy of 93.64% on the ISIC 2019 dataset. Pollastri et al. [42] demonstrated that Laplacian GANs (LAPGAN) can boost accuracy by the equivalent of adding 138% more real annotated images when the dataset exceeds 500 images.

AutoAugment AutoAugment [44] leverages reinforcement learning to identify the most effective image transformation strategies directly from the data, tailoring augmentation techniques to specific tasks.

The GANs and the AutoAugment methods are commonly applied for unsupervised data augmentation.

Data Normalization This is a standard preprocessing step for neural networks, as it facilitates the smooth operation of the optimization algorithm during training. It also helps prevent the model from settling into suboptimal solutions and promotes faster convergence [29].

2.5 Feature Extraction Stage

Feature extraction is a key step in analyzing dermoscopic images, aimed at isolating relevant information that can distinguish between benign and malignant skin lesions. In computer-aided diagnosis (CAD) systems, this process focuses on identifying patterns and features within skin lesion images to support early detection and classification. A widely used approach for this task in earlier detection systems is based on the ABCD rule due to its simplicity, accuracy, and ease of implementation.

Feature extraction directly influences the effectiveness of classification algorithms used in CAD systems. One of the most popular traditional methods is the ABCD dermoscopy rule [45], which assesses four key characteristics of skin lesions: asymmetry, border irregularity, color variation, and diameter. Another reputable diagnostic framework is the 7-point checklist, introduced by Johr in 2002 [46], which identifies dermoscopic features commonly associated with malignancy.

Recently, deep learning (DL) approaches have gained prominence for feature extraction and classification in dermoscopic image analysis [19]. Within these frameworks, convolutional neural networks (CNNs) serve as automated feature extractors, learning complex and abstract representations from raw image data.

Unlike handcrafted features, which are designed manually by experts, CNNs automatically learn useful features during the training phase, often outperforming traditional techniques. For instance, features extracted from deep CNN layers can function similarly to well-known descriptors like scale-invariant feature transform (SIFT) [47].

Despite their advantages, CNN-based methods come with certain challenges. Their performance typically depends on the availability of large, well-annotated datasets and requires substantial computational resources.

Overall, modern research in automated skin lesion detection can be broadly classified into three categories based on the feature extraction strategy: (i) handcrafted features, (ii) deep learning-based features, and (iii) hybrid approaches that combine handcrafted and deep learning features.

2.5.1 Handcrafted Feature Techniques

Handcrafted (HC) features—including texture, color, shape, and border characteristics, or combinations of these—have long been utilized in the classification of dermoscopic images, particularly for distinguishing between melanoma and non-melanoma lesions.

In one study, Bakheet (2017) proposed a melanoma detection framework using support vector machines (SVMs) based on an optimized set of histogram of oriented gradients (HOG) features. This method involves calculating orientation histograms of local gradients across the lesion area, normalizing them at the block level, and compiling them into a comprehensive feature vector [48].

Khan et al. (2019) designed a computer-aided diagnostic tool that begins with noise suppression using a Gaussian filter during preprocessing. K-means clustering is then applied for image segmentation, followed by the extraction of both global and local texture features, as well as RGB-based color descriptors, to identify melanoma [49].

Warsi et al. (2019) introduced a multidirectional 3D color-texture feature (CTF) extraction technique specifically for dermoscopic images. These features are then fed into a multilayer neural network (NN) utilizing backpropagation for classification purposes [50].

2.5.2 Deep Learning-Based Feature Techniques

Deep learning machines (DLMs) have gained significant recognition in the field of medical imaging, especially for their ability to function as both feature extractors and classifiers. Salido and Ruiz (2018) implemented a preprocessing step to remove hair artifacts from dermoscopic images in the PH2 dataset and used AlexNet for both feature extraction and classification [51]. Similarly, Dorj et al. (2018) employed a pre-trained AlexNet alongside an error-correcting output codes support vector machine (ECOC-SVM) to classify four types of skin cancer [52].

Shahin et al. (2018) introduced an ensemble method that combined ResNet-50 and Inception v3 for classifying images in the ISIC 2018 dataset [53]. In a unique approach by Dascalu and David (2019), deep learning models were integrated with audio analysis techniques for skin cancer detection [54]. Pham et al. (2019) applied U-net, U-net with a VGG16 encoder, and an ensemble of U-net models to segment images from the ISIC 2017 dataset [55]. These segmented images were then classified using deep CNNs, including Inception-v4, ResNet-152, and DenseNet-161, achieving the highest classification accuracies of 86.3% for melanoma and 88.7% for seborrheic keratosis using DenseNet-161.

In a study by Brinker et al. (2019), the performance of a CNN model trained on publicly available images was compared to dermatologists with varying levels of expertise. The results showed that CNN models outperformed dermatologists, highlighting their potential to assist clinicians in accurately detecting melanoma [56]. Carcagnì et al. (2019) used a DenseNet architecture combined with an SVM classifier on the HAM10000 dataset [57]. This method applied specialized network architectures and multilevel fine-tuning to improve feature discriminability and classification accuracy.

Naeem et al. (2020) provided a comprehensive review of DLM-based binary classification systems for detecting malignant melanoma [58]. Kumar et al. (2021) utilized deep learning to assess carcinoma severity levels [59]. Ali et al. (2021) proposed a deep CNN for skin cancer classification, incorporating preprocessing steps to remove noise, air bubbles, and other artifacts from the HAM10000 dataset [58]. Sevli (2021) developed a CNN model capable of classifying seven distinct types of skin lesions within the same dataset [60].

2.5.3 Fusion of Handcrafted and Deep Learning Techniques

Li et al. (2018) proposed a two-stage classification approach for dermoscopic images in the ISIC 2018 dataset, which combines DL features with HC features based on clinical criteria [61]. A modified U-net model is used for generating lesion masks, while DenseNet201 and ResNet50v2 are employed to extract global DL features. The HC features include color, texture, and morphological characteristics. These features are fused and optimized using LightGBM to select the best ensemble parameters [61].

Khan et al. (2019) introduced a hybrid approach that utilizes an optimized color feature (OCF) derived from lesion segmentation combined with a Deep Convolutional Neural Network (DCNN) for skin lesion classification. This method was validated on the ISBI 2016, ISBI 2017, and ISBI 2018 datasets [62].

Jayapriya and Jacob (2020) introduced a two-stage framework for segmentation and classification of skin lesions, focusing on melanoma detection [63]. VGG16 and GoogLeNet are used for lesion segmentation, while the final classification integrates features from a deep residual network with traditional HC techniques. This method was evaluated on the ISBI 2016 and ISIC 2017 datasets [63].

Tiwari et al. (2021) presented a hybrid classification model that combines a neural network (NN) and a convolutional neural network (CNN) [64]. Features are extracted using higher-order standardized moment induced-local binary patterns (HOSMI-LBP) and fed into an NN for classification, while the CNN directly classifies images. The final prediction is made by averaging the outputs of both networks. A key enhancement in their method is the inclusion of a preprocessing step that removes hair artifacts from dermoscopic images, which can obscure essential lesion features like texture, shape, and boundary. This step improves the quality of feature extraction and enhances classification accuracy compared to existing state-of-the-art hybrid melanoma detection methods [64].

2.6 Image Segmentation Stage

Segmentation plays a crucial role in image processing, particularly in medical imaging, where it is used to divide an image into distinct regions. This process helps separate areas of interest, such as diseased regions, from stable ones. Accurately identifying the region-of-interest (ROI) is essential for effective feature segmentation and image analysis [65]. Proper segmentation is vital because it supports subsequent processing steps and enables precise spatial statistics by quantitatively capturing the shapes of objects within the image [66, 67]. In medical image analysis, effective segmentation is necessary for accurate and efficient processing. There are various segmentation techniques, and choosing the right one is crucial for obtaining the correct results. Below are some of the most commonly used image segmentation methods:

Edge-Based Segmentation This technique detects variations in pixel intensity across a segmented image by analyzing the gradient strength, helping to identify edges within the region of interest (ROI). Common edge detection methods include the Prewitt, Sobel, Roberts, Laplacian, and Canny operators. The advantage of this method is its simplicity, as edges are key in separating regions. However, edge detection algorithms may sometimes detect nonexistent boundaries, generate redundant edges, and are prone to image noise [68]

Region-Based Segmentation This method segments the image into regions or groups of related pixels based on specific image properties. Common approaches include region growing [69], splitting and merging [70], and the Mumford–Shah method [71]. Regions provide more information for analysis since they consist of more pixels than edges. However, the presence of texture and edges can complicate region detection. The main drawback of this technique is that noise can affect the results, leading to false edge detection and inaccurate segmentation [72].

Threshold-Based Segmentation This technique uses characteristics of the image, such as histograms, to segment the image through point- or pixel-based methods.

Examples of threshold-based methods include Otsu's method, adaptive thresholding and Renyi's entropy [73].

Intelligence-Based Segmentation Two main intelligent approaches are used for segmentation: (i) ANN models genetic algorithms Fuzzy C-means (FCM) and (ii) deep learning: fully convolutional neural network (FCNN) U-net deep residual—SegNet. The first technique represents some of the most widely used approaches in automated dermatological analysis [74]. Key advantages of this approach include robust fault tolerance, high adaptability, efficient computational speed during the inference stage, and superior overall performance [72]. The second approach, based on deep learning, is capable of automatically learning optimal hierarchical features directly from raw images, eliminating the need for manually designed, hand-crafted features by the network developer [75].

Fusion-Based Segmentation This method combines two or more segmentation techniques to create a more sophisticated approach. By integrating multiple thresholding methods, for example, it is possible to find the optimal threshold value, benefiting from the strengths of each technique for more accurate segmentation. However, this approach tends to be more complex and requires higher computational resources [72].

2.7 Image Segmentation Challenges

Accurately segmenting skin lesions is a complex challenge due to the significant variability in lesion characteristics, such as structure, size, color, texture, and location within medical images. Below are some of the key challenges that arise during the segmentation process:

Indistinct Boundaries In many cases, the borders of skin lesions are not clearly defined, making it difficult for segmentation algorithms to accurately detect and delineate the lesion.

Variations in Illumination Lighting conditions can vary widely across different imaging environments. The appearance of a lesion may change depending on the lighting setup, affecting color and contrast. In clinical settings, consistent lighting with appropriate intensity and color balance is essential for reliable imaging.

Artifacts and Unwanted Elements The presence of irrelevant features such as hair, moles, skin burns, bubbles, blood vessels, or wrinkles can obscure lesion boundaries. These artifacts can interfere with segmentation accuracy and may lead to false or misleading lesion detection.

Imaging Equipment and Resolution The type of camera and its resolution play a critical role in image quality. Variations in imaging hardware can significantly affect the clarity and detail of skin lesion images, impacting segmentation performance.

Age-Related Skin Changes As individuals age, their skin undergoes various changes such as the development of wrinkles, stretch marks, and altered pigmentation. These changes can influence skin texture and appearance, complicating the segmentation process.

Background Complexity Clean, uniform backgrounds help facilitate lesion segmentation and feature extraction. In contrast, complex or cluttered backgrounds can introduce noise and hinder accurate analysis.

Ethnicity and Geographic Factors Skin color is influenced by ethnic background and environmental exposure. For example, individuals in colder climates often have lighter skin tones and may receive earlier diagnoses of melanoma compared to those in warmer, tropical regions.

This section also introduces various segmentation techniques frequently employed in the literature for skin lesion segmentation, such as edge-based, region-based, and thresholding methods, as well as those utilizing artificial intelligence (AI).

Deep learning models are capable of extracting and representing data through multiple levels of abstraction, enabling them to recognize complex patterns in large datasets. These versatile methods include not only traditional neural networks but also hierarchical probabilistic models and various supervised and unsupervised feature learning techniques.

This section provides an overview of several deep learning approaches that have been used for image segmentation tasks, particularly in skin lesion analysis. Various deep learning models have been introduced by researchers, achieving excellent performance in segmenting skin lesions [76]. Each of these architectures has its strengths and weaknesses, contributing to their unique performance in segmentation tasks.

2.8 Image Segmentation AI Applications

Mirikharaji et al. (2021) presented D-LEMA, a novel deep ensemble learning framework designed to address inter-annotator variability in skin lesion segmentation. This architecture comprises an ensemble of five Bayesian encoder–decoder CNNs with residual and skip connections. The model was trained on 2223 ISIC Archive images, each annotated by two to five experts. Evaluation was performed on the ISIC, PH2, and DermoFit datasets (2000; 200; 1300 images, respectively). The ensemble achieved Jaccard indices of 72.1% (ISIC), 85.2% (PH2), and 74.3%

(DermoFit), outperforming the baseline. The authors concluded that leveraging multiple annotations through deep ensembles enhances both segmentation accuracy and uncertainty estimation in medical imaging [77].

Akyel and Arici (2022) introduced LinkNet-B7, a new model for noise removal and skin cancer image segmentation. The architecture is based on LinkNet, with EfficientNetB7 as the encoder. They also created a new noise dataset containing 2500 images and masks that include artifacts like hair, rulers, ink spots, and other noise elements. This dataset fills a gap in existing literature, as no such dataset was previously available. The dataset includes images from the ISIC and PH2 datasets. To minimize pixel value loss, images were divided into 16 slices. The authors noted that if input data resolutions fall below certain thresholds, data loss is inevitable. LinkNet-B7 outperformed LinkNet by 6%, achieving a training accuracy of 95.72% for noise removal and 97.80% for lesion segmentation. The authors highlighted that their method addresses inaccuracies in cancer diagnosis caused by ineffective noise removal and segmentation, a common issue with existing automated methods [78].

Alahmadi (2022) proposed the multi-scale attention U-net (MSAU-Net) for skin lesion segmentation, improving upon the standard U-net by incorporating an attention mechanism at the bottleneck. This module captures hierarchical representations by aggregating multi-level features and uses a Bidirectional Convolutional Long Short-Term Memory (BDC-LSTM) to emphasize important features. The model was tested on three publicly available skin lesion datasets: ISIC 2017, ISIC 2018, and PH2, with 2000 images in ISIC 2017, 2594 in ISIC 2018, and 200 in PH2. The results showed that the MSAU-net performed well for skin lesion segmentation, showing enhanced results in this challenging task [79].

Zhao et al. (2022) introduced an improved U-net++ model for skin lesion segmentation, addressing issues such as parameter redundancy and gradient disappearance in fully convolutional networks (FCNs) and U-net. The enhanced U-net++ integrates deep supervision and transfer learning. The model was pre-trained on the Data Science Bowl 2018 dataset and fine-tuned on the ISIC2018 Task I skin lesion dataset. The results showed that the improved model achieved a Jaccard index of 84.73% on the ISIC2018 Task I dataset, demonstrating improved performance in skin lesion image segmentation. The authors suggested that their model could assist dermatologists in diagnoses [80].

Mohammed et al. (2022) presented the deep residual fully convolutional neural network (ResFCNET) for skin lesion segmentation. This model combines residual learning with a fully convolutional network (FCN) to enhance the semantic segmentation of skin lesions. The model addresses challenges in melanoma detection, such as varied lesion sizes, fuzzy boundaries, irregular shapes, and low contrast with surrounding skin. The model was evaluated using the ISBI 2016 and ISBI 2017 datasets. The results demonstrated that ResFCNET achieved high-precision classification with a Jaccard index of 0.866, accuracy of 0.971, sensitivity of 0.925, and specificity of 0.989. The authors proposed ResFCNET as a novel approach providing valuable insights for dermatological image segmentation [81].

2.9 Image Classification Stage

Skin disease classification has become a prominent area of research, driven by the rapid advancements in deep learning and machine learning technologies [4]. The image classification process follows the feature extraction stage, where skin images are classified by inputting the extracted feature values into an AI algorithm for training. This section explores the potential of AI, ML, and DL in the classification of skin lesions. It highlights recent developments in skin disease detection using skin image data and discusses the challenges AI systems face in solving this problem.

2.9.1 Machine Learning Image Classification Techniques

Before the rise of DL methods, image analysis primarily relied on manually extracting and selecting features such as texture patterns, shape descriptors, and grayscale histograms. Once these features were identified, traditional ML algorithms like support vector machines (SVMs), logistic regression, and random forests were commonly used for classification tasks. In dermatological image analysis, classifiers such as SVM, K-nearest neighbor (KNN), and Naive Bayes were often applied [82, 83]. Several studies have explored the use of ML for skin lesion classification, comparing the effectiveness of different classifiers and segmentation methods.

Between 2018 and 2020, several studies focused on enhancing computer-aided diagnostic (CAD) systems for classifying skin images using combinations of different machine learning techniques. In 2018, a CAD system was proposed that classified images into multiple categories using five different classifiers: decision trees, KNN, SVM with various kernels, and artificial neural networks [84]. In 2019, Murugan et al. developed a method based on watershed segmentation that incorporated shape descriptors, the ABCD rule (a common guideline for mole assessment), and GLCM (a texture analysis method). Their approach, which used SVM for classification, outperformed random forest and KNN in terms of both accuracy and generalization to new data [85]. In 2020, Balaji et al. introduced a dynamic graph-cut segmentation method combined with a Naive Bayes classifier. This system classified images efficiently into multiple categories, providing quick predictions and being relatively simple to implement. Although traditional machine learning methods have their uses, they rely heavily on the manual identification and extraction of features from isolated skin lesions, whereas DL techniques have shown greater success by automatically identifying important features and achieving higher classification accuracy.

Swamy and colleagues introduced a new approach to classifying skin diseases using machine learning techniques, which are becoming increasingly common in medical diagnoses. These ML algorithms identify key features in images and use them for classification. Their method includes three main stages: feature identification, model training, and performance testing. The model learns from various skin images using well-established ML techniques. In skin image classification, color, texture, and shape are typically the most important distinguishing features, either individually or together. This particular study focuses on classifying skin conditions based on color and texture, noting that healthy skin has different color properties compared to diseased skin. Texture details, such as smoothness or roughness, provide valuable information for accurate diagnosis. These extracted features are then used to build deep learning-based classification models, including support vector machines (SVMs) and decision trees (DTs). In the decision tree method, entropy is used for the initial splits in the tree, and further changes are applied at later levels to refine the final structure. Additionally, the maximum histogram value from the hue–saturation–value (HSV) system aids in separating different parts of the image during tree-based classification [86].

2.9.2 Deep Learning Image Classification Techniques

Deep learning (DL), a subset of machine learning (ML), has emerged as a powerful approach, especially in medical image classification, surpassing traditional ML techniques. Deep convolutional neural networks (DCNNs) are now the preferred choice for automatic feature extraction and classification of dermatological images. A significant advancement came from Nasiri et al., who proposed a CNN-based classification model for skin lesions. This model, using 16 layers of convolution and pooling, was tested on 1796 dermoscopic images and showed significant improvements in image categorization. However, its application is mostly limited to melanoma detection [87]. Ahmad et al. introduced a hybrid framework that combines a DCNN with a stacked bidirectional long short-term memory (BLSTM) network. By leveraging the strengths of both, this hybrid model improved classification accuracy, particularly in differentiating between similar benign and malignant lesions, achieving an average accuracy of 91.73% on dermatological datasets [88].

While complex DL systems offer impressive performance, they often require substantial computational resources and time for training. To address this issue, a new model, Eff2Net, was introduced in 2022. By replacing the traditional squeeze-and-excitation (SE) module in the EfficientNetV2 architecture with the efficient channel attention (ECA) mechanism, this model reduced the number of parameters without compromising performance. The model delivered excellent classification results with low computational complexity [89].

In a study by Zia Ur Rehman et al., enhanced CNNs like MobileNetV2 and DenseNet201 were used for better skin cancer detection, achieving 95.5% accuracy by adding more convolutional layers and using Grad-CAM for model interpretability [90].

Ahmad et al. introduced an innovative approach to skin lesion classification by integrating ResNet152 and InceptionResNet-V2 models with a triplet loss function. This technique, which was the first of its kind in dermatological images, improved accuracy by embedding input images into Euclidean space and calculating L2 distances to extract discriminative features [91]. Wu et al. applied transfer learning to CNNs, using pre-trained models such as ResNet-50, Inception-v3, and DenseNet121 to achieve outstanding performance across six facial skin classification tasks, further proving the effectiveness of transfer learning in dermatological image classification [92].

Recent studies have introduced cutting-edge deep learning models for skin lesion diagnosis. A notable model, residual deep convolutional neural network (RDCNN), demonstrated superior feature extraction and classification on limited datasets, excelling in binary classification tasks [93]. Another efficient model, InSiNet, achieved 94.59% accuracy on the ISIC 2018 dataset by reducing noise and processing images quickly for benign/malignant distinction [94]. A new multimodal transformer algorithm, introduced by Gan et al., fused image data and clinical metadata using two encoders and a mutual attention decoder, significantly outperforming previous models in dermatological diagnosis [95].

While DL techniques are highly successful in classifying neoplastic and inflammatory skin conditions, their application to pigmented skin diseases, such as vitiligo, remains underexplored. In 2019, a pioneering method for vitiligo detection used three distinct CNN models (ResNet50, VGG16, and Inception v2) trained on a vitiligo dataset, employing various color space representations. This integration of complementary color information resulted in a significant improvement in detection performance [96]. Building on this, in 2020, a vitiligo diagnosis system used images generated under a wood lamp via CycleGAN and advanced super-resolution techniques for enhanced image clarity, followed by classification with ResNet50, leading to improved accuracy [97]. In 2022, Guo et al. introduced a hybrid DL model for vitiligo lesion detection, integrating YOLO v3 for lesion localization and U-net++ for segmentation, which was particularly useful for detecting small lesions.

Sadic et al. proposed a skin disease classification approach using CNN, MobileNet, and Xception architectures, achieving high accuracy rates, with Xception reaching 97.0% after transfer learning. Their study utilized several DL models, including DenseNet and ResNet50, to classify skin conditions from five distinct categories, demonstrating the effectiveness of the approach in skin disease identification [98]. Similarly, Magdy et al. explored both deep learning and traditional machine learning techniques for skin cancer classification, including CNNs and pre-trained models like VGG-16 and AlexNet, as well as KNN and SVM for comparative analysis [99].

Lastly, Cai et al. introduced a multimodal transformer model for skin disease identification, integrating both image data and medical metadata to enhance diagnostic performance. This model included a vision transformer (ViT) for image feature extraction and a soft tag encoder (SLE) for embedding clinical information, resulting in improved classification accuracy by optimizing the integration of image and metadata features [95].

2.10 Deep Learning Challenges in Dermatological Imaging

Although deep learning (DL) has shown promising results in dermatological diagnosis, several issues still need to be addressed before DL can be widely used in clinical settings [100].

Limitations of Datasets The core issue is that DL models need vast amounts of labeled data for effective training. Moreover, dataset imbalances, where rare conditions or minority populations are underrepresented, can introduce biases into the algorithms, leading to poor performance, especially in multi-class classification tasks [101].

The Interpretability of Deep Learning Algorithms Techniques A significant barrier to the adoption of DL in medical applications is the "black box" nature of these models. Because it's difficult to understand how DL models arrive at their decisions, their trustworthiness is undermined, especially in critical areas like disease diagnosis. For DL models to be widely adopted in clinical settings, improving their transparency and interpretability is crucial, as both doctors and patients need to understand the reasoning behind a diagnosis [100].

Uniformity in Research Efforts Dermatological image classification and segmentation predominantly target common, high-risk skin cancers like melanoma, often relying on dermoscopic images. However, less-studied but equally important conditions, such as vitiligo, require more focused research for accurate diagnosis. While smartphone photography offers a promising avenue for skin lesion assessment, these images must meet rigorous clinical quality standards to be useful in healthcare settings. This highlights a need for broader research focus and quality control in non-dermoscopic imaging [100, 102].

More Sophisticated Algorithms Justification The limitations of current DL approaches in dermatological diagnosis are clear. Most models rely on widely used architectures with minimal advancements, often applying the same models across different skin diseases without tailoring them to specific diagnostic tasks. Additionally, these models often work with unimodal data, limiting the depth and accuracy of their diagnostic capabilities. To improve classification and diagnosis, it is essential to use multimodal data, which combines various types of information to provide a more comprehensive understanding of the disease [102].

2.11 Conclusions

Recent years have seen significant strides in the application of machine learning (ML) and deep learning (DL) techniques to dermatological diagnosis, with growing interest from researchers. While both ML and DL have proven to be highly effective in this field, the increasing complexity of diagnostic tasks and the expanding volume of data are driving DL to become the leading method with greater potential. Studies have shown that DL approaches can achieve diagnostic performance on par with that of experienced dermatologists. This section has highlighted key aspects such as image acquisition, dermatological image datasets, preprocessing methods, feature extraction techniques, and the segmentation and classification algorithms used for skin lesion analysis with ML and DL. Additionally, the main challenges facing DL in dermatological diagnosis have been addressed. Looking ahead, further progress in dermatological image processing will require the development of more standardized datasets, enhanced visualization tools, innovations in model architectures, and the integration of various techniques.

References

1. Pezzolo E, Naldi L. Epidemiology of major chronic inflammatory immune-related skin diseases in 2019. Expert Rev Clin Immunol. 2020;16:155–66.
2. Tizek L, Schielein M, Seifert F, Biedermann T, Böhner A, Zink A. Skin diseases are more common than we think: screening results of an unreferred population at the Munich Oktoberfest. J Eur Acad Dermatol Venereol. 2019;33:1421–8.
3. Han WH, Yong SS, Tan LL, Toh YF, Chew MF, Pailoor J, Kwan Z. Characteristics of skin cancers among adult patients in an urban Malaysian population. Australas J Dermatol. 2019;60:e327–9.
4. Abbas M, Arslan M, Bhatty RA, Yousa F, Khan AA, Rafay A. Enhanced skin disease diagnosis through convolutional neural networks and data augmentation techniques. J Comput Biomed Info. 2024;07(01)
5. Schneider S, Kohli I, Hamzavi I, Council MC, Rossi A, Ozog D. Emerging imaging technologies in dermatology, published in final edited form as. J Am Acad Dermatol. 2019;80(4):1114–20.
6. de Menezes M, Rosati R, Ferrario VF, Sforza C. Accuracy and reproducibility of a 3-dimensional stereophotogrammetric imaging system. J Oral Maxillofac Surg. 2010;68(9):2129–35.
7. Hibler BP, Qi Q, Rossi AM. Current state of imaging in dermatology. Semin Cutan Med Surg. 2016;35(1):2–8.
8. Chuah SY, Attia AB, Long V, et al. Structural and functional 3D mapping of skin tumours with non-invasive multispectral optoacoustic tomography. Skin Res Technol. 2017;23(2):221–6.
9. Que SK, Fraga-Braghiroli N, Grant-Kels JM, Rabinovitz HS, Oliviero M, Scope A. Through the looking glass: basics and principles of reflectance confocal microscopy. J Am Acad Dermatol. 2015;73(2):276–84.
10. Hibler BP, Yelamos O, Cordova M, et al. Handheld reflectance confocal microscopy to aid in the management of complex facial lentigo maligna. Cutis. 2017;99(5):346–52.
11. Verdoes M, Edgington LE, Scheeren FA, et al. A nonpeptidic cathepsin S activity-based probe for noninvasive optical imaging of tumor-associated macrophages. Chem Biol. 2012;19(5):619–28.
12. Nersisson R, Iyer TJ, Joseph Raj AN, Rajangam V. A dermoscopic skin lesion classification technique using YOLO-CNN and traditional fea-ture model. Arab J Sci Eng. 2021;46:9797–808.
13. Strzelecki M, Kociołek M, Strakowska M, Kozłowski M, Grzybowski A, Szczypinski P. Artificial intelligence in the detection of skin cancer: state of the art. Clin Dermatol. 2024;42:280–95.
14. What is a Dataset in Machine Learning: The Complete Guide. 2021. https://labelyourdata.com/articles/what-is-datasetin-machine-learning. Accessed 15 Jan 2022
15. Tschandl P, Rosendahl C, Kittler H. The HAM10000 dataset, a large collection of multi-source dermatoscopic images of common pigmented skin lesions. Sci Data. 2018;5:1–9.
16. ISIC Challenge. https://challenge.isic-archive.com/data/. Accessed 10 May 2025
17. DermIS. https://www.dermis.net/dermisroot/en/home/index.htm. Accessed 8 May 2025
18. Le DNT, Le HX, Ngo LT, Ngo HT. Transfer learning with class-weighted and focal loss function for automatic skin cancer classification. Ithaca, New York: Cornell University. p. 1–7.

19. Acosta MFJ, Tovar LYC, Garcia-Zapirain MB, Percybrooks W. Melanoma diagnosis using deep learning techniques on dermatoscopic images. BMC Med Imaging. 2021;21
20. Mahbod A, Schaefer G, Ellinger I, Ecker R, Pitiot A, Wang C. Fusing fine-tuned deep features for skin lesion classification. Comput Med Imaging Graph. 2019;71:19–29.
21. Hasan M, Elahi ME, Alam MA. Dermoexpert: skin lesion classification using a hybrid convolutional neural network through segmentation, transfer learning, and augmentation. Inf Med Unlocked. 2021;28
22. Hosny K, Kassem M, Fouad M. Classification of skin lesions using transfer learning and augmentation with alex-net. PLoS One. 2019;14:e0217293.
23. Asadi-Aghbolaghi M, Azad R, Fathy M, Escalera S. Multi-level context gating of embedded collective knowledge for medical image segmentation. arXiv. 2020:2003.05056.
24. Kim D, Hong B-W. Unsupervised feature elimination via generative adversarial networks: application to hair removal in melanoma classification. IEEE Access. 2021;9:42610.
25. Zhao C, Shuai R, Ma L, Liu W, Hu D, Wu M. Dermoscopy image classification based on StyleGAN and DenseNet201. IEEE Access. 2021;9:8659–79.
26. Attia M, Hossny M, Zhou H, Nahavandi S, Asadi H, Yazdabadi A. Digital hair segmentation using hybrid convolutional and recurent neural networks architecture. Comput Methods Programs Biomed. 2019;177:17–30.
27. Seung-Hun N, Wonhyuk A, Seung-Min M, Jinseok P, Dongkyu K, In-Jae Y, et al. Content-aware image resizing detection using deep neural network. In: 2019 IEEE International Conference on Image Processing; 2019. p. 106–10.
28. Pran DB, Mrutyunjay B, Abhranta P, Manish O. CNN based image resizing detection and resize factor classification for forensic applications. In: 2nd International Conference on Range Technology; 2021. p. 1–6.
29. Ghosh H, Rahat I, Mohanty S, Ravindra J, Sobur A. A study on the application of machine learning and Deep learning techniques for skin cancer detection. WASET. 2024;18(1)
30. Jain S, Singhania U, Tripathy B, Nasr EA, Aboudaif MK, Kamrani AK. Deep learning-based transfer learning for classification of skin cancer. Sensors. 2021;21(23):8142.
31. Esteva A, Kuprel B, Novoa RA, Ko J, Swetter SM, Blau HM, Thrun S. Dermatologist-level classification of skin cancer with deep neural networks. Nature. 2017;542(7639):115–8.
32. Perez F, Vasconcelos C, Avila S, Valle E. Data augmentation for skin lesion analysis. In: "OR 2.0 Context-Aware Operating Theaters, Computer Assisted Robotic Endoscopy", clinical image-based procedures, and skin image analysis. Cham: Springer; 2018. p. 303–311.1864.
33. Kato K, Nemoto M, Kimura Y, Kiyohara Y, Koga H, Yamazaki N, Christensen G, Ingvar C, Nielsen K, Nakamura A, Sota T, Nagaoka T. Performance improvement of automated melanoma diagnosis system by data augmentation. Adv Biomed Eng. 2020;9:62–70.
34. Liu Y, Jain A, Eng C, Way DH, Lee K, Bui P, Kanada K, de Oliveira Marinho G, Gallegos J, Gabriele S, Gupta V. A deep learning system for differential diagnosis of skin diseases. Nat Med. 2020;26(6):900–8.
35. Oukil S, Kasmi R, Mokrani K, García-Zapirain B. Automatic segmentation and melanoma detection based on color and texture features in dermoscopic images. Skin Res Technol. 2022;28(2):203–11.
36. Ahmad B, Jun S, Palade V, You Q, Mao L, Zhongjie M. Improving skin cancer classification using heavy-tailed student T-distribution in generative adversarial networks (TED-GAN). Diagnostics. 2021;11(11):2147.
37. Chawla NV, Bowyer KW, Hall LO, Kegelmeyer WP. SMOTE: synthetic minority over-sampling technique. J Artif Intell Res. 2002;16(1):321–57.
38. Inoue H. Data augmentation by pairing samples for images classification. arXiv. 2018:1801.02929.
39. Zhang H, Cisse M, Dauphin YN, Lopez-Paz D. Mixup: beyond empirical risk minimization. arXiv. 2017:1710.09412.
40. Lee KW, Chin RKY. The effectiveness of data augmentation for melanoma skin cancer prediction using convolutional neural networks. In Proc. IEEE 2nd Int. Conf. Artif. Intell. Eng. Technol. (IICAIET); 2020. p. 1–6.

41. Goodfellow I, Pouget-Abadie J, Mirza M, Xu B, Warde-Farley D, Ozair S, Courville A, Bengio Y. Generative adversarial nets. Proc Adv Neural Inf Process Syst. 2014;27:1–9.
42. Pollastri F, Bolelli F, Paredes R, Grana C. Augmenting data with GANs to segment melanoma skin lesions. Multimed Tools Appl. 2020;79(21–22):15575–92.
43. Abdelhalim ISA, Mohamed MF, Mahdy YB. Data augmentation for skin lesion using self-attention based progressive generative adversarial network. Expert Syst Appl. 2021;165:113922.
44. Cubuk ED, Zoph B, Mane D, Vasudevan V, Le QV. AutoAugment: Learning augmentation policies from data. arXiv. 2018:1805.09501.
45. Nachbar F, Stolz W, Merkle T, Cognetta AB, Vogt T, Landthaler M, Plewig G. The ABCD rule of dermatoscopy: high prospective value in the diagnosis of doubtful melanocytic skin lesions. J Am Acad Dermatol. 1994;30(4):551–9.
46. Johr RH. Dermoscopy: alternative melanocytic algorithms—the ABCD rule of dermatoscopy, menzies scoring method, and 7-point checklist. Clin Dermatol. 2002;20(3):240–7.
47. Nanni L, Ghidoni S, Brahnam S. Handcrafted vs. non-handcrafted features for computer vision classification. Pattern Recogn. 2017;71:158–72.
48. Bakheet S. An SVM framework for malignant melanoma detection based on optimized hog features. Computation. 2017;5(1):4.
49. Khan MQ, Hussain A, Rehman SU, Khan U, Maqsood M, Mehmood K, Khan MA. Classification of melanoma and nevus in digital images for diagnosis of skin cancer. IEEE Access. 2019;7:90132–44.
50. Warsi F, Khanam R, Kamya S, Su'arez-Araujo CP. An efficient 3D color-texture feature and neural network technique for melanoma detection. Inf Med Unlocked. 2019;17
51. Salido JAA, Ruiz C. Using deep learning to detect melanoma in dermoscopy images. Int J Mach Learn Comput. 2018;8(1):61–8.
52. Dorj UO, Lee KK, Choi JY, Lee M. The skin cancer classification using deep convolutional neural network. Multimed Tools Appl. 2018;77(8):9909–24.
53. Shahin AH, Kamal A, Elattar MA. Deep ensemble learning for skin lesion classification from dermoscopic images. In: In 9th Cairo International Biomedical Engineering Conference (CIBEC). IEEE; 2018. p. 150–3.
54. Dascalu A, David EO. Skin cancer detection by deep learning and sound analysis algorithms: a prospective clinical study of an elementary dermoscope. EBioMedicine. 2019;43:107–11.
55. Pham HN, Koay CY, Chakraborty T, Gupta S, Tan BL, Wu H, Nguy QH. Lesion segmentation and automated melanoma detection using deep convolutional neural networks and XGBoost. In: International Conference on System Science and Engineering. IEEE; 2019. p. 142–7.
56. Brinker TJ, Hekler A, Enk AH, Berking C, Haferkamp S, Hauschild A, Weichenthal M, Klode J, Schadendorf D, Holland-Letz T, von Kalle C, Frohling S, Schilling B, Utikal JS. Deep neural networks are superior to dermatologists in melanoma image classification. Eur J Cancer. 2019;119:11–7.
57. Carcagni P, Leo M, Cuna A, Mazzeo PL, Spagnolo P, Celeste G, Distante C. Classification of skin lesions by combining multilevel learnings in a densenet architecture. In: International Conference on Image Analysis and Processing. Springer; 2019. p. 335–44.
58. Ali MS, Miah MS, Haque J, Rahman MM, Islam MK. An enhanced technique of skin cancer classification using deep convolutional neural network with transfer learning models. Mach Learn Appl. 2021;5:100036.
59. Kumar M, Alshehri M, AlGhamdi R, Sharma P, Deep VV. A DE-ANN inspired skin cancer detection approach using fuzzy C-means clustering. Mobile Network Appl. 2020;25:1319–29.
60. Sevli O. A deep convolutional neural network-based pigmented skin lesion classification application and experts evaluation. Neural Comput Applic. 2021;33:12039–50.
61. Li X, Wu J, Jiang H, Chen EZ, Dong X, Rong R. Skin lesion classification via combining deep learning features and clinical criteria representations. bioRxiv. 2018:382010.
62. Khan MA, Sharif MI, Raza M, Anjum A, Saba T, Shad SA. Skin lesion segmentation and classification: a unified framework of deep neural network features fusion and selection. Expert Syst. 2019;

63. Jayapriya K, Jacob IJ. Hybrid fully convolutional network based skin lesion segmentation and melanoma detection using deep feature. Int J Imaging Syst Technol. 2020;30(2):348–57.
64. Tiwari AK, Mishra MK, Panda AR, Panda B. Hosmi-lbp-based feature extraction for melanoma detection using hybrid deep learning models. J Mech Med Biol. 2021;21(03):2150029.
65. Qureshi I, Yan J, Abbas Q, Shaheed K, Riaz A, Wahid A, Waseem M, Khan J, Szczuko p. Medical image segmentation using deep semantic-based methods: a review of techniques, applications and emerging trends. Inf Fusion. 2023;90:316–52.
66. Jiang F, Grigorev A, Rho S, Tian Z, Fu YS, Jifara W, Adil K. Medical image semantic segmentation based on deep learning. Neural Comput & Applic. 2018;29(5):1257–65.
67. Taghanaki SA, Abhishek K, Cohen JP, Adad JC, Hamarneh G. Deep semantic segmentation of natural and medical images: a review. Artif Intell Rev. 2021;54(1):137–78.
68. Adeyinka AA, Viriri S. Skin lesion images segmentation: a survey of the state-of-the-art. In: Proc. Mining Intell. Knowl. Explor., 6th Int. Conf. (MIKE). Cluj-Napoca; 2018. p. 321–30.
69. Guo Y, Ashour A, Smarandache F. A novel skin lesion detection approach using neutrosophic clustering and adaptive region growing in dermoscopy images. Symmetry. 2018;10(4):119.
70. Oliveira RB, Filho ME, Ma Z, Papa JP, Pereira AS, Tavares JMRS. Computational methods for the image segmentation of pigmented skin lesions: a review. Comput Methods Prog Biomed. 2016;131:127–41.
71. Nezhadian FK, Rashidi S. Melanoma skin cancer detection using color and new texture features. In: Proc. Artif. Intell. Signal Process. Conf. AISP; 2017. p. 1–5.
72. Hosny K, Elshoura D, Mohamed E, Vrochidou E, Papakostas G. Deep learning and optimization-based methods for skin lesions segmentation: a review. IEEE Access. 2023;11:85467.
73. Razmjooy N, Ashourian M, Karimifard M, Estrela VV, Loschi HJ, Nascimento DD. Computer-aided diagnosis of skin cancer: a review. Current Med Imag. 2020;16(7):93–781.
74. Maglogiannis I, Zafiropoulos E, Kyranoudis C. Intelligent segmentation and classification of pigmented skin lesions in dermatological images. In: Proc. Adv. Artif. Intell., 4th Hellenic Conf. Heraklion, Crete; 2006. p. 214–23.
75. Zafar M, Sharif MI, Sharif MI, Kadry S, Bukhari SAC, Rauf HT. Skin lesion analysis and cancer detection based on machine/deep learning techniques: a comprehensive survey. Life. 2023;13(1):146.
76. Al-masni MA, Al-antari MA, Choi M-T, Han S-M, Kim T-S. Skin lesion segmentation in dermoscopy images via deep full resolution convolutional networks. Comput Methods Prog Biomed. 2018;162:221–31.
77. Mirikharaji Z, Abhishek K, Izadi S, Hamarneh G. "D-LEMA: Deep learning ensembles from multiple annotations-application to skin lesion segmentation", in Proc. IEEE/CVF Conf. Comput. Vis. Pattern Recognit. Workshops (CVPRW). 2021:1837–46.
78. Akyel C, Arıcı N. LinkNet-b7: noise removal and lesion segmentation in images of skin cancer. Mathematics. 2022;10(5):736.
79. Alahmadi MD. Multiscale attention U-Net for skin lesion segmentation. IEEE Access. 2022;10:59145–54.
80. Zhao C, Shuai R, Ma L, Liu W, Wu M. Segmentation of skin lesions image based on U-Net + +. Multimed Tools Appl. 2022;81(6):8691–717.
81. Mohammed MA, Bismark O, Alornyo S, Asante M, Essah BO. ResFCNET: a skin lesion segmentation method based on a Deep residual fully convolutional neural network. IETI Transactions on Data Analysis and Forecasting (iTDAF). 2023;1(1):4–19.
82. Kassem MA, Hosny KM, Damaševˇcius R, Eltoukhy MM. Machine learning and deep learning methods for skin lesion classification and diagnosis: a systematic review. Diagnostics. 2021;11:1390.
83. Farzad S, Rouhi A, Rastegari R. "The performance of deep and conventional machine learning techniques for skin lesion classification", In Proceedings of the 2021 IEEE 18th International Conference on Smart Communities: Improving Quality of Life Using ICT, IoT and AI (HONET), Karachi, Pakistan, 11–13 October 2021; New York: IEEE, 2021.

84. Hameed N, Shabut A, Hossain MA. "Computer-aided diagnosis system for classifying prominent skin lesions using machine learning", In Proceedings of the 2018 10th Computer Science and Electronic Engineering (CEEC), Colchester, UK, 19–21 September 2018; IEEE: New York, 2018; pp. 186–191.
85. Murugan A, Nair SAH, Sanal Kumar KP. Detection of skin cancer using SVM, random forest and kNN classifiers. J Med Syst. 2019;43:1–9.
86. Swamy KV, Divya B. Skin disease classification using machine learning algorithms. Proc. 2021 2nd Int. Conf. Commun. Comput. Ind. 4.0, C2I4 2021; 2021.
87. Nasiri S, Helsper J, Jung M, Fathi M. DePicT melanoma Deep-CLASS: a deep convolutional neural networks approach to classify skin lesion images. BMC Bioinform. 2020;21:1–13.
88. Ahmad B, Usama M, Ahmad T, Khatoon S, Alam CM. An ensemble model of convolution and recurrent neural network for skin disease classification. Int J Imaging Syst Technol. 2022;32:218–29.
89. Karthik R, Vaichole TS, Kulkarni SK, Yadav O, Khan F. Eff2Net: an efficient channel attention-based convolutional neural network for skin disease classification. Biomed Signal Process Control. 2022;73:103406.
90. Zia Ur Rehman M, Ahmed F, Alsuhibany SA, Jamal SS, Zulfiqar Ali M, Ahmad J. Classification of skin cancer lesions using explainable deep learning. Sensors (Basel). 2022;22:6915.
91. Ahmad B, Usama M, Huang CM, Hwang K, Hossain MS, Muhammad G. Discriminative feature learning for skin disease classification using deep convolutional neural network. IEEE Access. 2020;8:39025–33.
92. Wu ZHE, Zhao S, Peng Y, He X, Zhao X, Huang K, Wu X, Fan W, Li F, Chen M, et al. Studies on different CNN algorithms for face skin disease classification based on clinical images. IEEE Access. 2019;7:66505–11.
93. Hosny KM, Kassem MA. Refined residual deep convolutional network for skin lesion classification. J Digit Imaging. 2022;35:258–80.
94. Reis HC, Turk V, Khoshelham K, Kaya S. InSiNet: a deep convolutional approach to skin cancer detection and segmentation. Med Biol Eng Comput. 2022;60:643–62.
95. Cai G, Zhu Y, Wu Y, Jiang X, Ye J, Yang D. A multimodal transformer to fuse images and metadata for skin disease classification. Vis Comput. 2023;39:2781–93.
96. Liu J, Yan J, Chen J, Sun G, Luo W. Classification of vitiligo based on convolutional neural network. In: Proceedings of the International Conference on Artificial Intelligence and Security: 5th International Conference, New York, 26–28 July. Cham: Springer; 2019. p. 214–23.
97. Luo W, Liu J, Huang Y, Zhao N. An effective vitiligo intelligent classification system. J Ambient Intell Humaniz Comput. 2023;14:5479–88.
98. Sadik R, Majumder A, Biswas A, Ahammad B, Rahman M. An in-depth analysis of Convolutional Neural Network architectures with transfer learning for skin disease diagnosis. Healthc. Anal., vol. 3, p. 100143, Nov. 2023.
99. Magdy A, Hussein H, Abdel-Kader RF, El Salam KA. Performance enhancement of skin cancer classification using computer vision. IEEE Access. 2023;11:72120–33. https://doi.org/10.1109/ACCESS.2023.3294974.
100. Zhang J, Zhong F, He K, Ji M, Li S, Li C. Recent advancements and perspectives in the diagnosis of skin diseases using machine learning and deep learning: a review. Diagnostics. 2023;13(23)
101. Silberg J, Manyika J. Notes from the AI frontier: tackling bias in AI (and in humans). McKinsey Glob Inst. 2019:1.
102. Serte S, Serener A, Al-Turjman F. Deep learning in medical imaging: a brief review. Trans Emerg Telecommun Technol. 2022;33:33.

Pioneering AI in Dermatology Education: Recognizing the Initial Milestone

3

Emmanouil Karampinis, Christina Zoumpourli, and Zoe Apalla

3.1 Dermatology as a Field of Education: The Educational Needs

Dermatology is the specialty that includes a wide variety of diverse pathology entities that range from cancerous to inflammatory dermatoses. It also encompasses hair and nail disorders, as well as skin care approaches and aesthetic interventions. The dermatologists are asked to evaluate skin lesions thoroughly, recognize lesion patterns and distributions and give a precise description of what they see in the patients' skin. The precise observation is essential for diagnosis, since even small differences can lead to a different diagnosis. The ability to describe in detail does not limit to the macroscopic lesions (the skin diseases that the naked eye can catch) but also to dermoscopy or confocal microscopy, tools that dermatologists rely on, to recognize patterns that may facilitate accurate diagnosis. The different patterns of vessels or atypical features in dermoscopy can lead to the identification of a cancerous lesion. The dermatologist may also face challenging cases with diseases that present overlapping features, as in the scenario of inflammatory dermatoses [1]. The detailed medical history (time of onset, triggering factors, family history or patients' comorbidities, and age) can also provide valuable diagnostic clues. Finally, the treatment approach in dermatology may differ from that in other specialties, too.

E. Karampinis (✉)
Second Dermatology Department, School of Health Sciences, Aristotle University of Thessaloniki, Thessaloniki, Greece

Department of Dermatology, Faculty of Medicine, School of Health Sciences, University General Hospital of Larissa, University of Thessaly, Larissa, Greece

C. Zoumpourli
1st Department of Dermatology-Venereology, University of Athens, Athens, Greece

Z. Apalla
Second Dermatology Department, School of Health Sciences, Aristotle University of Thessaloniki, Thessaloniki, Greece

E. Karampinis et al. (eds.), *Artificial Intelligence Applications in Dermatology*,
https://doi.org/10.1007/978-3-032-15614-3_3

Those differences are mainly based on the different topical treatments and skin formulations that are used in dermatology, apart from the oral or injectable treatments. Also, the applications of lasers, as well as the skin surgery interventions, are included as a part of the dermatologists' expertise [2].

Concerning the aforementioned characteristics, dermatology is a specialty mainly based on image interpretation, let it be macroscopic or dermoscopic, as well as certain procedural skills, exceeding traditional internal medicine and overlapping with surgical practice. In the era of AI, there are essential raising questions, such as what are the educational needs that emerge to a doctor who desires to enter into the field of dermatology? And how, artificial intelligence (AI) can serve as a supplement to those needs?

3.2 Dermatology from Classrooms to Distance Learning: Is AI-Aided Education the Next Step?

Dermatology belongs to the curriculum of every medical school and represents a topic frequently tested in international exams such as USMLE. Usually, the student is presented with an image presenting a patient with a lesion pattern, known for a specific disease and is asked about diagnosis, next steps or treatment [3]. In case the diagnosis can be easily made solely by the macroscopic image, clues can also be found in the short medical history that accompanies the question [4]. Multiple choice questions and true or false sentences are usually utilized as evaluation forms, usually testing skin diseases that are commonly met in daily dermatology practice, such as psoriasis and atopic dermatitis, as well as skin infections, such as viral or fungal infections, that can be relevant in other specialties [5].

To be prepared, students usually read from their academic books, tutors' slides and their paperwork made during lectures. Tutors make presentations in front of classrooms full of students with slides highlighting the key features that students need to focus on. This interaction is essential as the students can make direct questions to the lecturer and discuss further the concerns regarding a specific topic, fueling spontaneous discussion in real time and reasoning with real world cases. Peers could also participate making a dynamic learning experience and discuss further uncertainties [6]. Apart from classrooms, discussions are also made during rounds in the clinic. The students have the opportunity to discuss with patients and see how the theoretical knowledge apply to the real-life cases. Also, the students can observe various procedures such as skin biopsies, cryotherapy, intralesional injections, excisions of benign and malignant lesions, laser treatments, and dermoscopic examinations [6, 7].

The COVID-19 pandemic significantly impacted students, particularly through the shift to remote learning. Medical students had to rely on screen-based images to learn how skin conditions appear, as access to hospitals was often restricted to minimize the spread of the virus. As a result, the students may miss valuable opportunities to observe skin lesions firsthand, examine them in detail, and follow their clinical evolution over time. Remote learning had many advantages. In many cases, teaching and learning did not require real-time interaction [8]. Asynchronous methods allowed educators more flexibility in creating content and gave students the ability to balance their academic responsibilities with home life. They could download the video with the video they wanted to watch it in their laptop any time. Advanced tools such as high-resolution images, dermoscopy videos, and 3D models provide an interactive and attractive method of learning dermatology as well, however, the danger of decreased social learning and the inability of certain students to have access to certain technology required to access remote learning should not be underestimated [9]. As the COVID-19 pandemic has been surpassed, the distance learning methods remained due to their convenient nature.

Gamifying learning is also a type of remote or direct learning, developed in the last decade, especially in dermatology. Using different apps, the contestants—users were asked a particular question, usually diagnosis of a pop-up dermatology image to their screens. For example, a pigmented lesion might appear with a question like, "Is this melanoma or a nevus?" and the student who answers it correctly and fastest win the competition [10]. Games and simulations in dermatology have been shown to effectively boost learner motivation, enjoyment, and performance [10, 11]. Early studies on gamified methods in dermatology education have shown improvements in diagnostic accuracy and increased interest in the specialty. Similarly, pilot studies using game-based interventions for melanoma detection have demonstrated positive effects on knowledge and efficacy. However, the small number of participants and significant variability in outcome measures suggest that the generalizability of these findings regarding the impact of gamification may be limited. Some of the apps used for gamifying education in dermatology are Kahoot!, Skinquizition and i-DERMIFY [12].

While gamified learning is engaging, it remains unclear how these methods truly enhance medical knowledge. Remote learning, while convenient, has not improved practical skills significantly, as hands-on experience remains limited. Moreover, turning medical knowledge into a game may downplay the seriousness of diseases and patients' health, potentially making them seem less critical than they are. While AI appears to be the next step in educational evolution, the integration of AI tools into traditional learning processes raises questions about how they can be incorporated and what the future implications of this integration might be.

AI-powered education in dermatology is more likely contain the features of:

(a) Personalized AI-assisted education: Students may be tested in topics of dermatologist and the AI program may detect their strengths and weaknesses and make recommendations to the students which additional sources and materials to read so they can improve their performance in the upcoming assessment [13, 14]. For instance, if the focus is on skin cancer, topics such as melanoma, basal cell carcinoma (BCC), squamous cell carcinoma (SCC), and rarer skin cancers like Merkel cell carcinoma are emphasized. The AI program analyzes the student responses to diagnostic questions, including the recognition of specific lesion characteristics, patterns, and distributions. For example, the AI might evaluate a student's ability to differentiate between a malignant melanoma and a benign nevus based on clinical presentation. If the student struggles with identifying features such as asymmetry, irregular borders, or the ABCDE criteria (asymmetry, border, color, diameter, and evolving), the AI presents more images of melanomas and blue nevus presenting with circles and arrows their structural differences. Also, the AI model may present images and texts regarding the Tyndall effect and the depth of melanin that reflects why this type of nevus presents with blue color. Following, it can present detailed case studies, high-resolution images, dermoscopic videos, and relevant research papers as well as relevant past examination questions [15].

(b) AI-driven chatbots can serve as virtual tutors, answering students' questions about dermatology topics. Virtual patients, another impressive example of AI technology, can simulate real patient interactions. Students can ask these AI patients about symptoms, disease onset, and other relevant details, with the AI providing responses. Additionally, students can compare the lesions they observe with those from previous AI patients through side-by-side image comparisons. For instance, if the topic is inflammatory dermatoses, students might examine a patient with psoriasis and, if uncertain about distinguishing it from other scale-like skin conditions such as tinea corporis, they can recall previous cases and directly compare the images made or found by AI algorithms. In this AI-driven, interactive environment, students also have the opportunity to make treatment decisions for the AI patients, gaining experience in a risk-free setting [13].

3.3 How AI Educates Medical Student in Dermatology?

AI models and particularly chatbots and large language models have invaded our lives significantly. Students tend to enter different chatbots such as ChatGPT and Gemini, asking about dermatology topics, as well as write essays and projects on dermatology topics.

3.3.1 Writing Projects on Dermatology in Cooperation with Large Language Models

A major concern within the research community is the potential for students to misrepresent LLM-generated content as their own or to rely on these tools in order to perform incomplete literature reviews with oversimplistic or inaccurate unreliable research outcomes. Importantly, LLMs cannot be listed as co-authors on academic papers or chapters, as authorship is in line with responsibility and accountability, which AI tools cannot assume [16]. Students who make use of LLMs should be transparent about this by including it in the methods or acknowledgements sections of their papers. However, this usage is often concealed, as disclosing it can diminish the perceived value of their work and has, in some cases, resulted in lower grades. While LLM-generated text can often be identified upon close examination, it tends to exhibit recognizable patterns, such as bland or overly generic language, as well as occasional basic errors, due to the statistical nature of how these models generate text based on their training data and prompts [17].

The overreliance on the AI chatbots to write projects on dermatology may limit critical thinking and creativity. As a result, the purpose of writing is not achieved and is replaced by copying and pasting the AI-generated text. This phenomenon and the long-term effects of AI on learning outcomes deserve more attention and may result in the creation of noncritical doctors. Medical students are particularly at risk of being tempted to cheat on assignments with AI tools, as they know this is the only "easy way". Also, the risk of plagiarism cannot be underestimated, as students who have not searched enough for the subject run the danger of replicating ideas or phrases from existing sources, leading to unintentional plagiarism and copyright concerns. Since AI lacks an understanding of citations or source material in the way a human writer does, additional mistakes may also appear. Therefore, clear guidelines for AI usage in academia are necessary [18].

On the other hand, large language models can serve as a source of inspiration, offering guidance on how a student might approach their work, which papers to consult, and how to structure their writing. When asked about the development of an idea, a chatbot typically provides a well-organized response that outlines the concept clearly [16, 17]. For instance, if a student asks a chatbot for help with writing a paper on cutaneous drug eruptions, the LLM can offer a structured overview of the topic, suggesting key subtopics to cover, including classifications of drug eruptions, underlying mechanisms, diagnostic approaches, treatment, prognosis, follow-up strategies, as well as key structure points (abstract, introduction, methods, conclusion) of the paper. AI may also recommend relevant literature or landmark studies, helping the student frame their argument and organize the paper in a more comprehensible way, not just listing information randomly, but building a structured and purposeful discussion throughout. This kind of support can be useful in the early stages of research, offering direction and clarity when tackling a complex medical subject, as the cutaneous drug reactions.

3.3.2 Simplifying Hard Topics in Dermatology and Summarize Large Texts

The success of prompt-based models like ChatGPT has raised new possibilities for summarizing medical evidence, including large texts in dermatology. Medical students can paste large texts or chapters or whole manuscripts to chatbots and ask for highlight points or brief summary. Medical evidence summarization involves extracting and synthesizing essential information from a large number of medical research studies and clinical trials into clear and concise summaries [19]. In a recent study, the authors reported the automatic (with machine translation evaluation techniques) and human evaluations of the summary quality of a text provided by GPT-3.5 (text-davinci-003) and ChatGPT. Regarding human evaluations, participants were shown the full abstract of a systematic review and four summaries: (1) the Authors' conclusion, (2) ChatGPT—Main Result, (3) ChatGPT—Abstract, and (4) GPT3.5—MainResult. The order was randomized to avoid bias. They evaluated each summary using a 5-point Likert scale, and if a summary received a low score, participants explained why in a text box. Participants also indicated their most and least preferred summaries, with reasons for their choices, providing insights into the potential of model-generated summaries for systematic reviews. ChatGPT-MainResult were reported to have significantly more summaries labelled with the Strongly Agree choice [20].

The ability of the chatbots to simplify hard topics has been extensively used by students. The input "Explain" or "Simplify" in front of the text in question orders the chatbot to break the text into smaller parts and analyze each term. For example, in case the student asked a chatbot to explain the following sentence "Cutaneous small-vessel vasculitis typically presents with palpable purpura, especially on the lower extremities", it would separate the key aspects of the condition (terminology of purpura and palpable purpura and lower extremities predisposition explanation as well as inflammation of small vessels pathophysiology). Students are encouraged to revisit this information by consulting additional sources. AI-generated content differs from online text in that the former is produced by algorithms, while the latter is authored by a person with identifiable credentials and contact information, giving it accountability for errors and making it more trustworthy. In contrast, AI-generated content, despite its factual basis, lacks accountability due to the "black box" nature of its algorithms, which raises concerns about its accuracy [21].

The AI-generated texts have also been assessed with different scores of readabilities. There are many studies that compare human and chatbot made texts regarding the simple measure of Gobbledygook (SMOG) index and automated readability index (ARI) scores. The SMOG grade is a readability metric that estimates the level of education required to comprehend a text. SMOG is calculated using samples of ten sentences from the text. In these sentences, the number of polysyllabic words (those with three or more syllables) is counted. The Flesch–Kincaid readability tests are designed to evaluate the difficulty level of a passage in English. There are two tests: the Flesch reading-ease and the Flesch–Kincaid grade level. While both tests rely on similar core factors (word length and sentence length), they apply different weighting methods. The results of these two tests are typically inversely related: a text with a higher score on the reading ease test generally corresponds to a lower score on the grade-level test [22]. Those scores were assessed in different purposes for example consent forms for aesthetic procedures and educational material. Generally, AI texts tend to be more quickly red and easy to digest to read compared to the human-made ones, however those observations depend on the kind of input and the level and expertise of the human-author [23].

Therefore, the collaboration between students and AI, and not the overreliance on the AI-generated knowledge, should be encouraged. Students may find various creative ways to exploit AI capabilities. For example, the students can ask the chatbot to create acronyms to remember hard topics (Fig. 3.1) or ask the AI to create visual aids, like diagrams or flowcharts, to clarify complex processes or

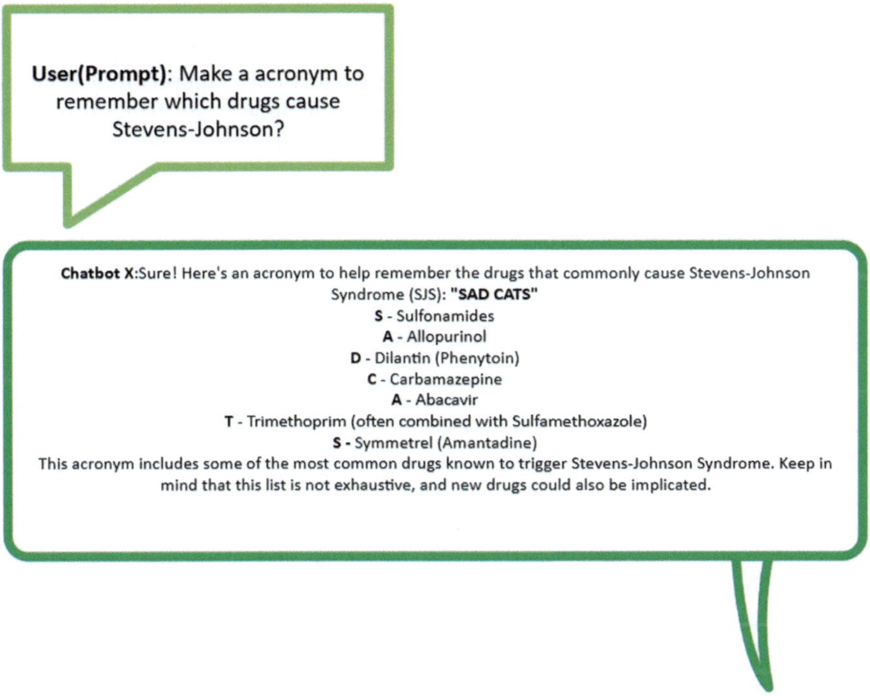

Fig. 3.1 A screenshot of chatbot X asking for an acronym to aid in understanding and remembering the challenging topic of cutaneous drug eruptions, specifically Stevens–Johnson syndrome. The proposed algorithm "SAD CATS" is indeed catchy and easy to remember. Chatbot x represents an AI chatbot available on the Internet, without any reference to a specific platform's interface and name to maintain neutrality

relationships between concepts. For instance, when studying dermatology, AI could generate a visual comparison of different skin conditions, aiding in quicker differentiation.

3.3.3 Tracking Performance in Dermatology

Skills like lesion identification have long been fundamental to a successful career in dermatology, but the swift pace of digital advancement over the past year, along with an increased focus on continuous learning and staying up to date with developments in the field, has made the development of effective teaching tools more crucial than ever for current learners. AI sets to play a major role in how dermatology is being taught and learnt. In many ways, AI can help streamline learning by tracking individual progress, highlighting areas where a student might need support, and identifying where tutor instruction is most essential. For educators, this AI progress detection offers tools to tailor teaching strategies based on each student's background and learning style. It can also handle time-consuming tasks like creating quizzes, grading, and providing feedback [13]. Beyond content recommendations, AI can shape how dermatology students learn, by pinpointing gaps in understanding, suggesting more effective teaching methods, and helping to keep learners engaged. In this evolving landscape, educators maintain their role using AI not to replace their expertise but to enhance it, and they can use AI insights and suggestions to better support and guide their students on the path to becoming skilled dermatology professionals [14].

3.3.4 Creating Dermatology Questions with AI Chatbots

Case-based scenarios, including multiple-choice questions, true or false assessments, and correlation exercises, are prevalent evaluation methods for medical students. Generally, students value exposure to a wide variety of lesions, conditions, presentations, and diagnostic, management, and referral issues as these reflect real-world clinical practice. Engaging and memorable cases are preferred, particularly for complex or less engaging topics, as they capture students' attention more effectively and enhance the learning experience [5]. Studies explored the effectiveness of chatbots in generating engaging educational materials in dermatology. AI-generated quizzes can quickly adapt to various learning styles and cover a wider array of scenarios, potentially matching or exceeding the effectiveness of human-created quizzes in promoting a deeper understanding of dermatological conditions. Given the high performance of chatbots in different exams, such as USMLE [4]. It is logical to assess how chatbots can create assessment materials, saving time for the tutors and professors who are responsible for creating tests for medical students. Also, chatbots have been assessed in other aspects of dermatology, such as dermatoscopy and dermatopathology, with encouraging results for the use of AI chatbots for educational purposes.

Table 3.1 presents AI-generated questions from two chatbots (ChatGPT-4 (OpenAI) and Perplexity (AI)). Comparing AI and non-AI questions, AI-generated cases typically present an analytical case description that includes a detailed analysis of medical history, clinical examination findings, and triggering factors. They often are modified according to the scenario depending on the specific question and may pose follow-up questions, occasionally providing answers to previous ones. Additionally, AI-generated cases tend to be difficult to distinguish from non-AI cases. On the other hand, non-AI cases have distinct features: they can combine multiple correct answer options, presenting D option as A and B, this approach is not made by AI-chatbots unless it is included in the input. Also, non-AI questions are generally more concise. These cases may also suggest alternative diagnoses using similar vocabulary for example, confusing students with terms that resemble each other such as psoriasis and parapsoriasis. Additionally, they feature direct and focused questions and present clinical practice dilemmas. Furthermore, they often include additional information within each question that alters the sequence of the medical history presented.

Table 3.1 Examples of AI-generated and non-AI examples of case-based multiple-choice questions regarding the topic of alopecia areata

ChatGPT-generated case	Question 1	Question 2	Question 3
A 32-year-old woman presents with sudden, patchy hair loss over the past month. She reports noticing smooth, round bald spots on her scalp that have progressively enlarged, causing her distress. She denies any recent illness, trauma, or changes in hair care practices. On examination, there are well-demarcated, round patches of hair loss with smooth skin and no signs of inflammation or scarring. Exclamation hairs are visible at the edges of the bald patches. She has no other significant medical history but mentions a family history of thyroid disease and rheumatoid arthritis. She asks about the diagnosis and possible treatment options	What is the most likely diagnosis for this patient? (A) Androgenic alopecia (B) Tinea capitis (C) Alopecia areata (D) Telogen effluvium. Answer: (C) alopecia areata	Which of the following is most strongly associated with alopecia areata? (A) Frequent hair dye use (B) Autoimmune conditions (C) Poor nutrition (D) Excessive sun exposure Answer: (B) autoimmune conditions	Which of the following is most strongly associated with alopecia areata? (A) Frequent hair dye use (B) Autoimmune conditions (C) Poor nutrition (D) Excessive sun exposure Answer: (B) autoimmune conditions
Human-generated	Question 1	Question 2	Question 3
A 58-year-old man with a history of medication-controlled hypertension, asthma, and chronic pruritis developed sudden appearance of four coin-sized lesions of the beard, loss of hair in the vertex, occiput and retro-auricular regions. Overall, 60% of scalp hair was lost. The sudden hair loss occurred over one week, with a second week of hair loss upon mild pulling	What is the most possible diagnosis? (A) Tinea capitis (B) Alopecia areata (C) Androgenic alopecia (D) Trichitilomania Answer is (B) alopecia areata	What is characteristic of alopecia areata? (A) Broken hair (B) Scale (C) Exclamation hair (D) Velous hair Answer is (C) exclamation hair	What is the pathophysiology of the hair disease presented in the case? (A) It is immune-mediated autoimmune disorder that affects hair follicles (B) It is a hormonal disruption disorder that affects the hair circle (C) It is a fungi-based hair disorder (D) None of the above Answer is (A) it is immune-mediated autoimmune disorder that affects hair follicles

(continued)

Table 3.1 (continued)

ChatGPT-generated case	Question 1	Question 2	Question 3
Perplexity—Generated	Question 1	Question 2	Question 3
A 27-year-old male patient presents with a 3-month history of asymptomatic hair loss on the scalp, which began as a small patch and gradually expanded into a larger, well-defined area of non-scarring alopecia at the occipital region. The patient has no significant family history of hair loss or systemic illness, and a KOH examination ruled out fungal infections. Histopathological analysis confirmed a diagnosis of alopecia areata (AA), characterized by broken hairs at the periphery, known as exclamation mark hairs. He was treated with intralesional injections of triamcinolone acetonide (5 mg/ml) every 4 weeks, leading to significant improvement after 3 months	What are the typical clinical features of alopecia areata? (A) Scarring hair loss (B) Well-defined patches of non-scarring hair loss (C) Diffuse thinning of hair across the scalp (D) Hair loss associated with itching and redness Answer: (B) well-defined patches of non-scarring hair loss	Which histopathological finding is most characteristic of alopecia areata? (A) Follicular hyperkeratosis. (B) Lymphocytic infiltrate around hair follicles (C) Sebaceous gland hyperplasia (D) Acanthosis Answer: (B) lymphocytic infiltrate around hair follicle	What is a common treatment option for alopecia areata? (A) Topical antifungals (B) Systemic antibiotics (C) Intralesional corticosteroids (D) Oral retinoids Answer: (C) Intralesional corticosteroids

Presenting the cases shown in Table 3.1 to students, we asked them to evaluate them in a Likert scale in terms of educational and motivational. The human-generated case has received the best scores (3.58 ± 1 vs 3.6 ± 0.49 vs 3.33 ± 0.58, $p < 0.05$), although without statistical significance. The sudden, coin-sized hair loss in multiple regions, including the beard and scalp, encourages differential diagnosis skills by requiring consideration of conditions like alopecia areata, tinea capitis, and telogen effluvium [24, 25]. Its complexity, involving comorbidities such as asthma, hypertension, and chronic pruritis, adds depth and mirrors the multifaceted nature of real clinical encounters. The psychosocial impact of sudden disfiguring hair loss highlights the importance of holistic, compassionate care, inspiring students to think beyond diagnosis and consider the patient's emotional well-being. The questions were about the most likely diagnosis, diagnostic clues, and pathophysiology correlations. In the AI-generated texts, the patient is portrayed in an idealized manner, presenting with a textbook example of alopecia areata, presenting with a single, well-defined, non-scarring patch of hair loss, no associated symptoms, no significant family or systemic history, and a clean diagnostic path with a negative KOH test and confirmatory histopathology. This observation also indicates that the narrative nature is important when tested by individuals as storytelling or contextual depth and logical sequence of events (as in case studies), participants appear to favor human-generated examples over AI-generated ones with the ideal presentation of events.

Worth noticing is the high performance for the motivational category of the human-made text (4.8 ± 0.4), compared to AI performances (3.2 ± 0.4 and 3.4 ± 0.71). AI-generated texts tend to be less motivational as they often lack the personal touch and emotional depth that make learning engaging. While AI can provide clear, accurate information, it does not capture the human aspects of medicine, like the real-world challenges, ethical dilemmas, or the personal stories that inspire students. Educators and clinicians bring their experiences, empathy, and passion into the material they create, which helps students connect on a deeper level and stay motivated.

It is also important to highlight the significance of the instructions provided to the chatbot. For example, consider the two instructions: "create a motivational case study report on BCC for medical students as a multiple-choice question" and "create a challenging case report on BCC for medical students as a multiple-choice question." The chatbot can generate different cases and questions, while the same is observed when the target audience is altered, such as changing from medical students to residents, indicating the AI flexibility (Figs. 3.2 and 3.3) This suggests that if students become accustomed to these types of questions, they may eventually lose their sense of challenge or educational value. Additionally, the influence of instructions can be seen in other instances [26]. For example, if a tutor asks the chatbot to create a case of lichen pigmentosus [27] in a light-skinned patient, the chatbot may generate a case, even though this condition is rare in such patients, potentially providing a misleading impression, as the result of the hallucination effect of AI.

In our survey, we also asked the students if they were able to recognize which case was made with chatbots and which by a clinician. For example, regarding the

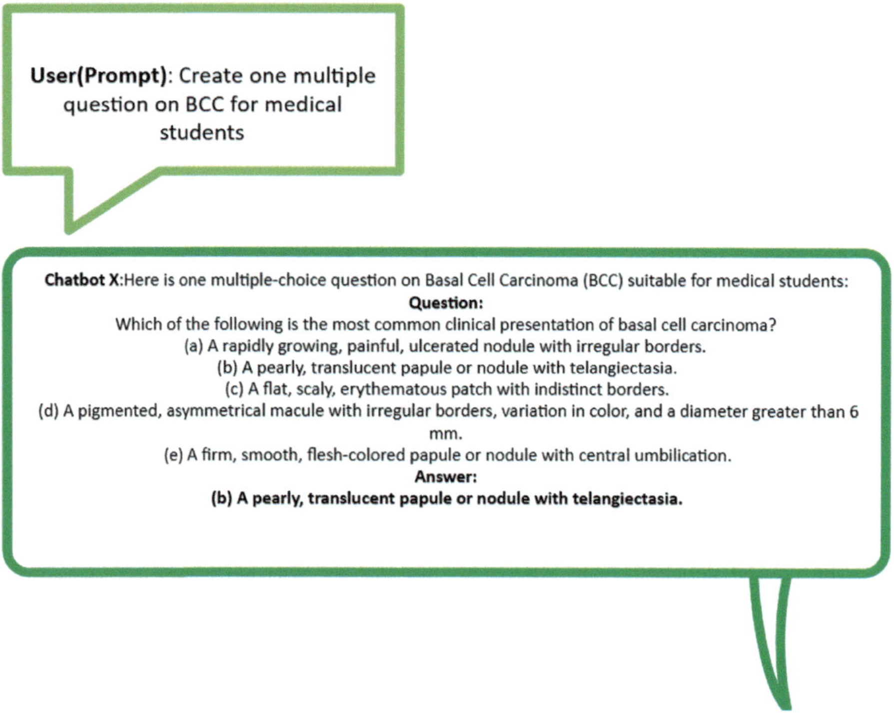

Fig. 3.2 The output text-question generated by the chatbot X, based on an inquiry about BCC for medical students, featuring a characteristic description of BCC in option B. The other options provided descriptions of conditions such as molluscum contagiosum, actinic keratosis, or squamous cell carcinoma

first case with alopecia areata presented in Table 3.1, 15 out of 45 answered that they were not sure while 17 did not manage to find each true origin, reporting that is human-made. Consequently, medical students struggled to reliably identify the origin of cases (AI vs. non-AI) across most scenarios. This phenomenon was also observed in other studies. The study revealed that previously suggested criteria, such as originality and comprehension, were ineffective in distinguishing between human-written and LLM-generated texts. These findings suggest that both humans and AI-detection software currently struggle to accurately identify the use of LLMs in academic literature. Additionally, the extent of undisclosed AI usage in academic publications is anticipated to be extensive [28].

Based on the points mentioned above, tutors are encouraged to create their own questions that reflect real-life clinical scenarios and actively challenge students, rather than relying solely on chatbots for the rapid generation of exercises. Questions crafted by clinicians can inspire students to engage more deeply with the material—potentially fostering empathy—and ultimately contribute to their development into more competent and compassionate healthcare

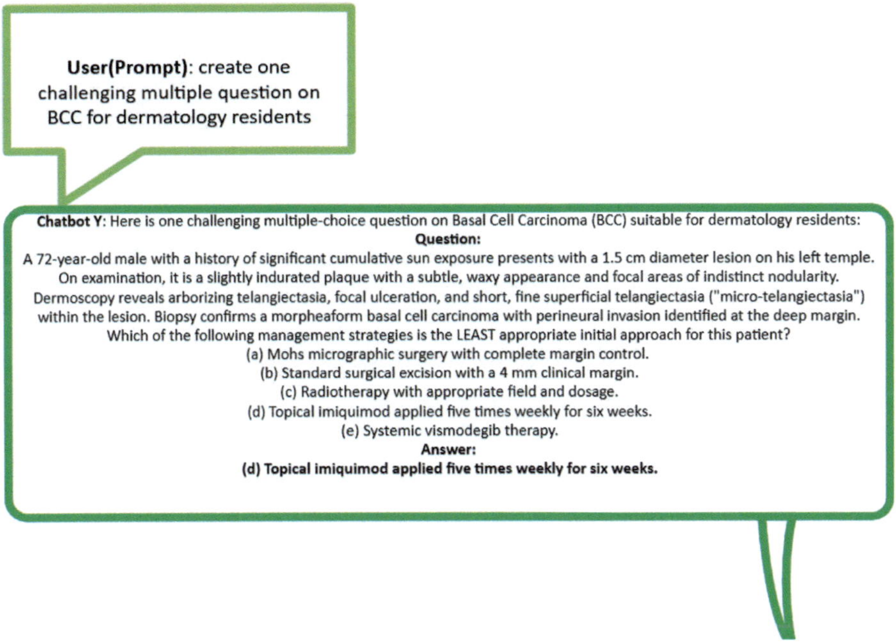

Fig. 3.3 The output text-question generated by the chatbot Y, based on an inquiry about a BCC challenging question for medical residents, presenting a case adding dermoscopy description and an aggressive subtype of BCC. The responder should know the treatment guidelines of the BCC to perform well in this test. Also, the question is focusing on the lease appropriate, possible confusing many residents

professionals. It's also worth noting the use of other AI-based tools by students, such as the AI Jungle website (https://jungleai.com/use-cases/ai-quiz-maker, n.d.) [29], where users can upload text for the system to generate multiple-choice questions. This platform serves as a valuable and engaging resource for both students and educators (Fig. 3.4).

3.3.5 Content-Based Image Retrieval Techniques for Educational Purposes in Dermatology

Content-based image retrieval (CBIR) is a valuable tool in medical practice that helps identify cases similar to the one being examined, effectively functioning like an automated literature search. General practitioners can use a CBIR system as a diagnostic aid by retrieving images from a database that closely resemble the clinical case in both appearance and confirmed pathological diagnosis. The image databases can be macroscopic or dermoscopic. Clinicians may also wish to compare more than one type of image, along with incorporating relevant

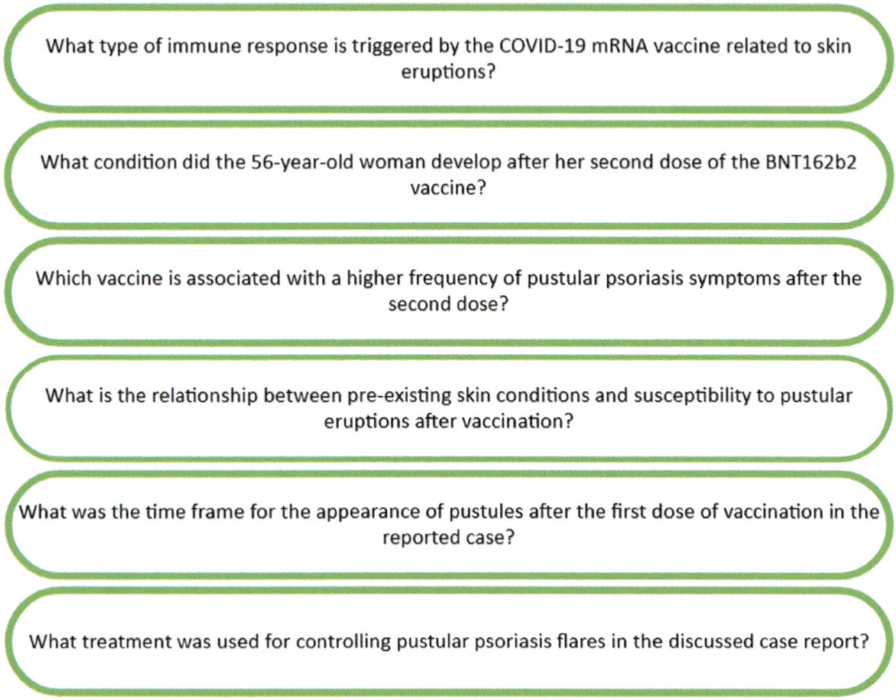

Fig. 3.4 AI-generated questions by using the AI automated creator website after uploading a case-based review of our clinic [32] regarding postvaccination psoriasis flares. Interesting questions occurred relevant to the topic and asking for the main features of the text. This type of AI model promises quick and efficient generation of educational content, allowing for the creation of relevant, targeted questions that align with specific topics. However, the ownership of the content uploaded to AI apps should always be considered

nonimage data to support their decision-making. Dermatology is particularly well-suited for this approach due to the traditionally large availability of image datasets [30]. Sadeghi M et al. found that CBIR was generally seen as user-friendly and engaging; however, it has yet to earn the level of trust required for regular clinical use. In another study assessing the effectiveness of CBIR as a decision-support tool, it was noted that users often gravitate toward other AI methods. The potential drawback of current CBIR systems is their limited interpretability, which may hinder user confidence. CBIR can also be used in the education of dermatology. Researchers developed an interactive user interface for a CBIR system designed to support decision-making using dermoscopic images and examined how 14 participants interacted with it and made decisions. The results showed that using the CBIR interface led to a noticeable improvement in both the accuracy of image classification and the users' confidence in their decisions compared to a version of the system without CBIR support. However, it also required more time to complete the tasks. Participants described the interface as highly educational, engaging, and easy to navigate [31].

3.4 Potential Risks Embedded in AI-Powered Dermatology Education

As AI models become more popular, they penetrate further in medical education of all specialties, including dermatology. This technology revolution has brought many opportunities to students to better understand hard topics and complicated cases without the presence of a tutor or mentor. While AI models are offering many advantages in the learning process, they also introduce several risks that learners must be aware when using them.

(a) Data Accuracy and Transparency: AI models are trained on specific datasets, and the information they provide is limited to what exists within those training sets. Due to the "black box" nature of most AI systems accessible to students, the training processes are not clearly explained. As a result, the origin of the information remains hidden, which is especially problematic for students who lack the expertise to critically assess the data. These learners may accept the output as fact without question, increasing the risk of misinformation. The lack of explainability significantly weakens the learning process, as students are given conclusions without understanding the reasoning behind them. This undermines the development of critical thinking—one of the main goals of education [33].

(b) Privacy Concerns: In dermatology, privacy risks are particularly concerning. Students and trainees may upload images of patients with visible skin lesions into AI applications or content-based image retrieval (CBIR) systems without obtaining proper consent. These images may include sensitive areas or facial features, raising ethical concerns, especially since it is unclear where these images are stored or how they are used. Without clear regulations in place, misunderstandings and potential privacy violations are very likely. Therefore, users must be cautious and should avoid uploading identifiable or intimate patient images [34].

(c) Hallucinations and Misinformation: AI-generated responses can sometimes include hallucinations—answers that appear factual but are entirely fabricated [35, 36]. A common example is the generation of false references, where AI tools may mix authors, titles, journals, dates, or DOIs. For instance, as shown in Fig. 3.5, one chatbot suggested a reference that not only cited the wrong journal but also included an incorrect order of authors and even listed names that were not part of the original study. In other cases, AI responses may not match the input request—for example, providing information about sun protection when the question asked for dermoscopic features. Incorrect DOIs, mislabeled skin conditions, inaccurate case descriptions, and flawed treatment suggestions are also common. Fig. 3.6 highlights how even small details in a prompt—such as stating that a patient with a rare skin condition common in darker skin types is Irish (and therefore likely fair-skinned)—can lead to misleading and unhelpful results. This shows how easily AI can generate unrealistic and educationally poor examples based on conflicting input details [27].

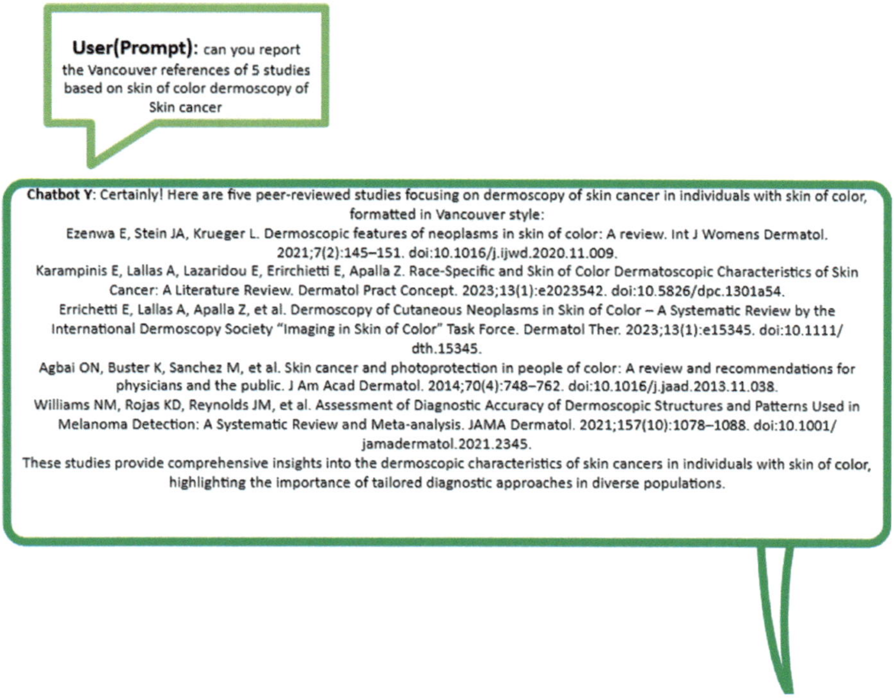

Fig. 3.5 Examples of flawed and inaccurate references generated by a chatbot Y. These errors may include incorrect author names, journal titles, author order, and DOIs. Students and researchers should remain cautious and recognize the potential for such AI-generated hallucinations

(d) Social and Interpersonal Impacts: The social and interpersonal effects of AI integration in education should not be underestimated. AI-driven tools may reduce opportunities for direct interaction between students and experienced dermatologists, which are essential for developing soft skills, clinical judgment, and nuanced understanding. Medicine, including dermatology, requires empathy, communication with the patient and contextual decision-making—elements that AI tools cannot fully replicate [37]. Without the guidance of tutors and mentors, students risk losing the human element of medical training, which is crucial for holistic patient care.

As a result of the threats and dangers explained, students may develop trust issues regarding AI answers and their incorporation into their learning material [38]. Forty-five students of our department were asked to consider a situation where they had to choose between multiple learning resources, including AI-based tools and traditional sources. The case examined how students make decisions when confronted with conflicting information from different sources. The results showed that 6.7% of students would trust the AI-generated answer, 68.9% would rely on information from the Internet, and 24.4% would seek further discussion with a tutor.

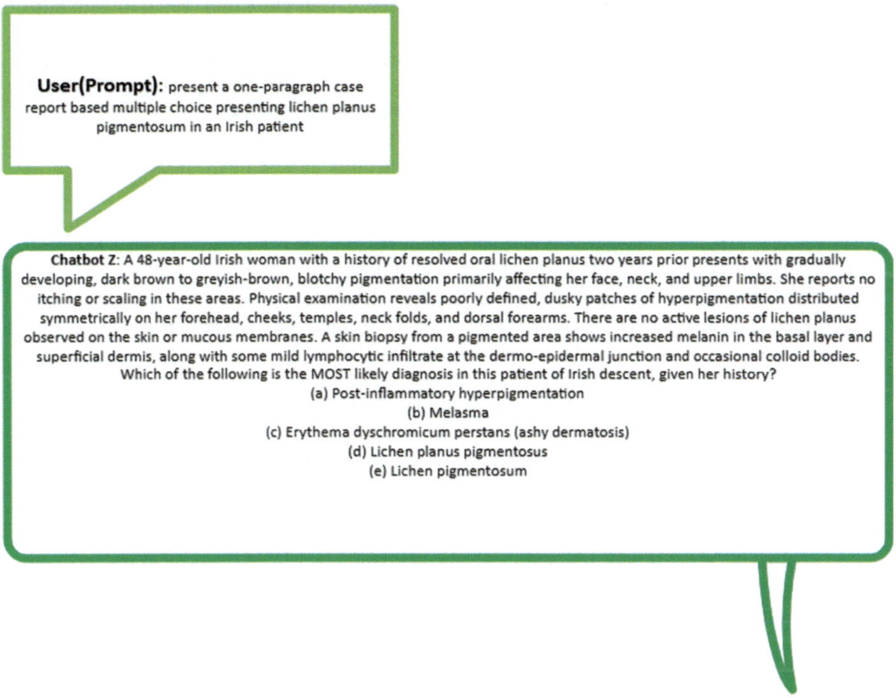

Fig. 3.6 A user request for a multiple-choice question involving a patient with a rare skin condition typically seen in individuals with darker skin tones, while also specifying that the patient is of Irish descent—implying a likely fair skin type. Also, lichen pigmentosum and lichen planus pigmentosum, also refer to the same clinical entity

These findings suggest that medical students do not yet fully trust AI-generated responses and tend to prefer Internet sources. However, it is important to note that some AI systems gather information from the Internet, combining and synthesizing this data to generate their answers.

References

1. Blattner CM, Sabic D, Murase JE. Understanding the importance of dermatology training in undergraduate medical education. Dermatol Pract Concept. 2015;5:95–6. https://doi.org/10.5826/dpc.0502a18.
2. Farajtabar Nashli N, Hatami P, Aryanian Z, Rahimi Foroushani A, Robati R, Goodarzi A, et al. Dermatologists communication skills and performance from point of view of patients. Dermatol Pract Concept. 2023:e2023120. https://doi.org/10.5826/dpc.1302a120.
3. Zuberi H, Ahmad N, Shalabi M, Hussain A. Comprehensive review of resources and strategy for dermatology board certification exams in the United States. Arch Dermatol Res. 2024;316:681. https://doi.org/10.1007/s00403-024-03421-2.
4. Passby L, Jenko N, Wernham A. Performance of ChatGPT on specialty certificate examination in dermatology multiple-choice questions. Clin Exp Dermatol. 2024;49:722–7. https://doi.org/10.1093/ced/llad197.

5. Comaish JS. Multiple choice questions in dermatology. Arch Dis Child. 1994;70:256. https://doi.org/10.1136/adc.70.3.256-a.
6. Ricco C, Rao BK, Pappert AS, Coppola KM. Brief teaching intervention improves medical students' dermatology diagnostic Skills and comfort in performing dermatology exams. Healthcare. 2024;12:1453. https://doi.org/10.3390/healthcare12141453.
7. Ting JSK, Tan YL, Veasuvalingam B, Yap AYM, Ghui SM, Yong JL, et al. Scaffolding dermatological learning with near-peer teaching for preclinical-year medical students. Clin Exp Dermatol. 2023;48:998–1006. https://doi.org/10.1093/ced/llad149.
8. Verheijden MJH, Martens H, Heeneman S. A dermatology E-learning programme is perceived as a valuable learning tool in postgraduate general practice training. Int J Med Educ. 2021;12:169–78. https://doi.org/10.5116/ijme.612f.3d6c.
9. Sil A, Das A, Patra A, Kumar R, Pandhi D, De D, et al. Impact of COVID-19 pandemic on dermatology teaching program in India: a survey on the faculty and residents' perspective. Indian Dermatol Online J. 2023;14:643. https://doi.org/10.4103/idoj.idoj_85_23.
10. Donoso F, Peirano D, Longo C, Apalla Z, Lallas A, Jaimes N, et al. Gamified learning in dermatology and dermoscopy education: a paradigm shift. Clin Exp Dermatol. 2023;48:962–7. https://doi.org/10.1093/ced/llad177.
11. Aponso S, Tan YTN, Jain S, Oh CC. Gamification of dermatoscopy education using a smartphone mobile platform: a pilot study. JAAD Int. 2024;16:91–6. https://doi.org/10.1016/j.jdin.2024.03.008.
12. Szeto MD, Strock D, Anderson J, Sivesind TE, Vorwald VM, Rietcheck HR, et al. Gamification and game-based strategies for dermatology education: narrative review. JMIR Dermatol. 2021;4:e30325. https://doi.org/10.2196/30325.
13. du Plooy E, Casteleijn D, Franzsen D. Personalized adaptive learning in higher education: a scoping review of key characteristics and impact on academic performance and engagement. Heliyon. 2024;10:e39630. https://doi.org/10.1016/j.heliyon.2024.e39630.
14. Lin H, Chen Q. Artificial intelligence (AI) -integrated educational applications and college students' creativity and academic emotions: students and teachers' perceptions and attitudes. BMC Psychol. 2024;12:487. https://doi.org/10.1186/s40359-024-01979-0.
15. Costa S, Byrne M, Pissaloux D, Haddad V, Paindavoine S, Thomas L, et al. Melanomas associated with blue nevi or mimicking cellular blue nevi. Am J Surg Pathol. 2016;40:368–77. https://doi.org/10.1097/PAS.0000000000000568.
16. Zhang Z, Zhang J, Duan L, Tan C. ChatGPT in dermatology: exploring the limited utility amidst the tech hype. Front Med (Lausanne). 2024;10 https://doi.org/10.3389/fmed.2023.1308229.
17. Goktas P, Grzybowski A. Assessing the impact of ChatGPT in dermatology: a comprehensive rapid review. J Clin Med. 2024;13:5909. https://doi.org/10.3390/jcm13195909.
18. Potestio L, Feo F, Martora F, Megna M, Napolitano M, D'Agostino M. The use of ChatGPT in the dermatological field: a narrative review. Clin Exp Dermatol. 2024; https://doi.org/10.1093/ced/llae546.
19. Nielsen JPS, Grønhøj C, Skov L, Gyldenløve M. Usefulness of the large language model ChatGPT (GPT-4) as a diagnostic tool and information source in dermatology. JEADV Clin Pract. 2024;3:1570–5. https://doi.org/10.1002/jvc2.459.
20. Tang L, Sun Z, Idnay B, Nestor JG, Soroush A, Elias PA, et al. Evaluating large language models on medical evidence summarization. NPJ Digit Med. 2023;6:158. https://doi.org/10.1038/s41746-023-00896-7.
21. Schwartz IS, Link KE, Daneshjou R, Cortés-Penfield N. Black box warning: large language models and the future of infectious diseases consultation. Clin Infect Dis. 2024;78:860–6. https://doi.org/10.1093/cid/ciad633.
22. Mac O, Ayre J, Bell K, McCaffery K, Muscat DM. Comparison of readability scores for written health information across formulas using automated vs manual measures. JAMA Netw Open. 2022;5:e2246051. https://doi.org/10.1001/jamanetworkopen.2022.46051.
23. Kirchner GJ, Kim RY, Weddle JB, Bible JE. Can artificial intelligence improve the readability of patient education materials? Clin Orthop Relat Res. 2023;481:2260–7. https://doi.org/10.1097/CORR.0000000000002668.

24. Xu L, Liu KX, Senna MM. A practical approach to the diagnosis and management of hair loss in children and adolescents. Front Med (Lausanne). 2017;4 https://doi.org/10.3389/fmed.2017.00112.
25. Sibbald C. Alopecia Areata: an updated review for 2023. J Cutan Med Surg. 2023;27:241–59. https://doi.org/10.1177/12034754231168839.
26. Karampinis E, Toli O, Georgopoulou K-E, Kampra E, Spyridonidou C, Roussaki Schulze A-V, et al. Can artificial intelligence "hold" a Dermoscope?—the evaluation of an artificial intelligence Chatbot to translate the Dermoscopic language. Diagnostics. 2024;14:1165. https://doi.org/10.3390/diagnostics14111165.
27. Ghosh A, Coondoo A. Lichen planus pigmentosus: the controversial consensus. Indian J Dermatol. 2016;61:482. https://doi.org/10.4103/0019-5154.190108.
28. Hakam HT, Prill R, Korte L, Lovreković B, Ostojić M, Ramadanov N, et al. Human-written vs AI-generated texts in orthopedic academic literature: comparative qualitative analysis. JMIR Form Res. 2024;8:e52164. https://doi.org/10.2196/52164.
29. https://jungleai.com/use-cases/ai-quiz-maker. n.d.; Last accessed on 13 Apr 2025.
30. Tschandl P, Argenziano G, Razmara M, Yap J. Diagnostic accuracy of content-based dermatoscopic image retrieval with deep classification features. Br J Dermatol. 2019;181:155–65. https://doi.org/10.1111/bjd.17189.
31. Sadeghi M, Chilana P, Yap J, Tschandl P, Atkins MS. Using content-based image retrieval of dermoscopic images for interpretation and education: a pilot study. Skin Res Technol. 2020;26:503–12. https://doi.org/10.1111/srt.12822.
32. Karampinis E, Gravani A, Gidarokosta P, Bogdanos DP, Roussaki-Schulze A-V, Zafiriou E. Pustular eruption following COVID-19 vaccination: a narrative case-based review. Vaccines (Basel). 2023;11:1298. https://doi.org/10.3390/vaccines11081298.
33. Sengupta D. Artificial intelligence in diagnostic dermatology: challenges and the way forward. Indian Dermatol Online J. 2023;14:782–7. https://doi.org/10.4103/idoj.idoj_462_23.
34. Yadav N, Pandey S, Gupta A, Dudani P, Gupta S, Rangarajan K. Data privacy in healthcare: in the era of artificial intelligence. Indian Dermatol Online J. 2023;14:788–92. https://doi.org/10.4103/idoj.idoj_543_23.
35. İnce Guliyev E, Üçok A. On the 'hallucinations' of artificial intelligence and the hallucination experience in human. Turk J Psychiatry. 2024; https://doi.org/10.5080/u27608.
36. Athaluri SA, Manthena SV, Kesapragada VSRKM, Yarlagadda V, Dave T, Duddumpudi RTS. Exploring the boundaries of reality: investigating the phenomenon of Artificial Intelligence hallucination in scientific writing through ChatGPT references. Cureus. 2023; https://doi.org/10.7759/cureus.37432.
37. Akgun S, Greenhow C. Artificial intelligence in education: addressing ethical challenges in K-12 settings. AI Ethics. 2022;2:431–40. https://doi.org/10.1007/s43681-021-00096-7.
38. Kauttonen J, Rousi R, Alamäki A. Trust and acceptance challenges in the adoption of AI applications in health care: quantitative survey analysis. J Med Internet Res. 2025;27:e65567. https://doi.org/10.2196/65567.

Medicolegal Issues Arising from the Use of AI in Dermatology

4

Vasiliki P. Karzi, Aikaterini Karampini, and Lillian Mitrou

4.1 Introduction

In dermatology, machine learning and deep learning are the most predominant types of AI employed. ML is a type of AI that allows computers to learn from human input data, which it analyses independently thanks to the generation of algorithms for decision-making. In latent terms, ML follows an algorithm based on input data with past observations, and by imitating the human cognitive process, it constructs a model for predicting and classifying new observations, unknown to the algorithm [2]. It is a prediction tool that can be applied dynamically to clinical decision-making that individualizes patient care rather than following a static algorithm [1].

Deep learning (DL) is the advancement of ML and comprises algorithms that create an artificial neural network simulating the human brain in terms of independent learning and decision-making, which is not dependent on human input since it can be trained to classify data on its own [3]. Dermatology, which emphasizes visual analysis, is well positioned to leverage DL to improve patient care. Chat boxes or large language models (LLMs), which are trained on text across the Internet, are DL AI. Popular DL AI such as OpenAI's ChatGPT or Google's Med-PaLM, or even AI Symptom Checker Apps such as Babylon or Ada, allow a patient to interact directly with an AI physician, sometimes outperforming human physicians [4, 5]. Even though most of these AI applications include a disclaimer that a human physician

V. P. Karzi
National and Kapodistrian University of Athens (Faculty of Law); Universiteit Leiden (Public International Law), Leiden, Netherlands

A. Karampini
National and Kapodistrian University of Athens (Labour Law), Athens, Greece

L. Mitrou (✉)
University of the Aegean - Department of Information and Communication Systems Engineeringn and, Samos, Greece
e-mail: l.mitrou@aegean.gr

E. Karampinis et al. (eds.), *Artificial Intelligence Applications in Dermatology*,
https://doi.org/10.1007/978-3-032-15614-3_4

should ultimately be consulted, it is becoming more and more likely that in the future, AI will play a major role in the diagnosis process and could ultimately improve access to high-quality medical care [5, 6]. AI technology in the medical field is progressing rapidly and aims to ultimately abolish medical error and prevent harm to patients. However, given that no AI system has a 100% success rate, and taking into consideration algorithmic bias, patient harm cannot be fully eradicated, and therefore, the new dynamics in medical practice give rise to questions on the current legal frameworks' ability to address such harm when AI technology is involved in a patient's care [7].

The present chapter aims to address the medicolegal issues arising from the use of AI in the field of dermatology, focusing specifically on the regulation of relevant AI technology and the attribution of liability for patient harm (physical or/and mental). It is structured into three primary sections. The first section examines existing legislation and its applicability to AI technology in healthcare, including in both European and US regulatory frameworks. The second section elucidates the types of AI tools employed in dermatology, methods of training AI models, and certification processes such as FDA and CE approvals. The third section addresses various liability schemes, including physician, manufacturer, vicarious, strict and common enterprise liability, and analyses case-studies to demonstrate these concepts.

The analysis shows that, in essence, existing regulations aim to ensure the safety, transparency, and reliability of the use of AI in dermatology with frameworks in place for data protection, cybersecurity, and ethics. Key legislations include the EU's Medical Devices Regulation (hereafter MDR), In Vitro Diagnostic Medical Devices Regulation (hereafter IVDR), and the Artificial Intelligence Act (hereafter AI act), along with the FDA's risk-based approach in the United States. On the other hand, current tort law primarily addresses patient harm through traditional medical professional liability, vicarious liability, and product liability. Questions arise, though, in relation to the applicability of these frameworks in light of AI's increasing autonomy. AI tools, such as image-based algorithms and chatbots, are widely applied in dermatology for diagnosing and treating skin conditions, with certification by the FDA and CE marks provided, adding proof of safety and effectiveness of these devices. By applying theories for liability, personal or harm-based, to certain case-studies, especially in the field of dermatology, the illustration of these concepts emphasizes the need for clear legal frameworks to address AI-related harm.

The methodology employed involves a comprehensive review of existing regulations, legal theories, and case law from various jurisdictions, supplemented by an analysis of the current state of AI technology in dermatology. This approach attempts to achieve a thorough evaluation of both the regulatory environment and the potential legal issues arising from the application of AI in this field.

4.2 Defining Legal Boundaries for AI in Dermatology

For the present analysis, it is important to examine whether the existing legal framework of the various national jurisdictions is already equipped to prevent or address physical or mental harm caused to patients from the application of AI technology.

4.2.1 Existing Legislation Pertinent to the Regulation of AI Use in Healthcare and Dermatology

Regulation is key to ensuring the safety, transparency, and reliability of AI. Comparative research shows that many jurisdictions have a legal framework in place for data protection, cybersecurity, and ethics that aims to address the challenges in the application of AI in healthcare [8]. This section aims to summarize the regulatory framework related to the manufacturing and development of AI-based medical technology as well as any relevant obligations of end-users, i.e., physicians.

In Europe, the relevant regulatory framework consists of the 2017/745 Medical Devices Regulation (MDR), which applies to AI devices used for medical purposes, including diagnosis, and the 2017/746 in vitro diagnostic medical devices regulation (IVDR), which applies specifically to devices used in genetic testing or in-vitro diagnosis [7, 8]. Together, these regulations provide a strict regulatory framework to ensure medical devices meet safety and performance standards. Under the MDR, AI-based medical devices must undergo certification by a designated body, which is also tasked with monitoring their performance prior to and after their market release. This regulatory framework is affected by the European Artificial Intelligence Act (EU AI Act), which entered into force in August 2024 (i.e., Regulation 2024/1689). The EU AI Act will be fully applicable in 3 years from its adoption, with some exceptions: prohibitions will take effect after 6 months, the governance rules and the obligations for general-purpose AI models will become applicable after 12 months, and the rules for AI systems—embedded into regulated products—will apply after 36 months. The Act aims to foster responsible artificial intelligence development and deployment in the EU.

Even though most obligations of the EU AI Act appear to coincide with those of the MDR, manufacturers of medical devices must also ensure protection from cyberattacks for AI-based systems and that in case of any system errors, these will be detected immediately, by humans, and traceable within the system. Manufacturers of high-risk AI systems must also undergo additional conformity assessment procedures. The EU AI Act includes legal obligations such as human intervention and surveillance, and consists of 113 Articles and 13 Annexes. It categorizes AI applications into various risk levels (prohibited, high-risk, limited risk, minimal risk). Under Article 6 and Recital 46 of the AI Act, high-risk AI systems are AI systems that pose a high risk to the health, safety or fundamental rights of EU citizens, but whose major socio-economic benefits outweigh these risks (which is why they are not banned). According to the European Commission, the AI Act considers the use of AI systems in medical diagnosis or health management as high-risk, and therefore, AI-based software intended for medical purposes must comply with several requirements, including risk-mitigation systems, high-quality data sets, clear user information and human oversight [9].

The EU AI Act does include a derogation in Article 6 para. 3, which states that if AI Systems do not pose a significant risk to the health, safety, or fundamental rights of natural persons are not considered high-risk. This derogation applies to AI systems that intended to perform a narrow procedural task; to improve the result of a previously completed human activity; to detect decision-making patterns or deviations from prior decision-making patterns and is not meant to replace or influence the previously completed human assessment, without proper human review; or to perform a preparatory task to an assessment relevant for the purposes of the use cases listed in Annex III of the Act.

Furthermore, subject to the provisions of EU AI Act are providers, deployers, importers, distributors, and manufacturers of AI products, which are based both within the EU and in third countries (in the latter case only where the output produced by the AI system is used in the Union). The Act defines "deployer" as a natural or legal person, public authority, agency, or other body using an AI system under its authority except where the AI system is used in the course of a personal nonprofessional activity (Article 3). It is crucial to highlight that under this broad definition, healthcare professionals and healthcare institutions using AI will fall within this definition when using AI, and therefore under Article 26 of the EU AI Act they must, inter alia, adhere to the systems' instructions for use and implement both technical and organizational measures to that effect; ensure human oversight; guarantee that the data used is relevant and representative; and ensure ongoing post-market monitoring, reporting any risks to providers and keeping detailed logs of AI system usage. Additionally, private entities must also conduct a thorough fundamental rights' impact assessment.

On the other hand, in the United States primary oversight is conducted by the Food and Drug Administration (FDA), which employs a risk-based approach to assess AI-based devices, with a focus on total product lifecycle surveillance to ensure patient safety [8]. There are approval pathways such as 510(k), pre-market approval (PMA) and de novo (another premarket petition) and in practice, most FDA-approved AI medical devices go through the faster approval pathway for low-risk devices, the 510(k). In India, the national regulatory body, the Central Drugs Standard Control Organization (CDSCO), regulates AI devices through local medical device regulations. Overall, each country has a different approach; however, the main focus is patient safety and effectiveness of AI-based medical devices [8].

4.2.2 Existing Liability Schemes for Harm Caused by AI-Based Diagnosis

In general, the current legal framework includes provisions to deal with cases where- due to AI-related medical errors - harm to a patient's health or death occurs. In this case, civil law will apply and provide the harmed patient or his/her relatives with the necessary means for achieving reparations. Liability for errors linked to AI-based diagnostics is still a matter of debate [10]. In most jurisdictions, patient harm is mainly addressed through traditional tort law and the medical professional's duty for upholding a standard of care [11, 12]. Depending on the specific national jurisdiction and whether they follow common law jurisdiction (such as most English speaking countries including the United Kingdom, United States, and Canada) or civil law jurisdiction (such as Continental European countries, East and Central Asia, Central and South America), the medical professional will either be judged according to what is done in practice, or according to what is required by normative imperatives [11] in order for the court to proceed to liability.

Liability under current liability rules must be attributable to a natural or legal person. This could be the medical professional, the clinic or hospital as an employer (due to vicarious liability) or even the manufacturer of the medical product used by the medical professional (based on product liability or consumer protection law). Introducing AI to the above equation already raises questions on the applicability of traditional tort law:

- What if the physician delivered a diagnosis based on a faulty AI?
- Is AI software a product that will lead to product liability?
- How can the manufacturer or developer be liable for a faulty AI if its algorithm has evolved?
- What if the AI applied a faulty diagnosis under the supervision of a human physician?
- What if the AI applied a faulty diagnosis while being used by a human physician not specialized in the relevant field (e.g., a primary-care provider)?
- What if the physician failed to apply the correct diagnosis of AI?
- What if the AI is fully autonomous and no human physician intervenes?

The above questions give rise to serious legal complications when applying a doctrine that was originally developed to apply exclusively to human conduct [12]. Tort liability schemes, which are the only available legal schemes at present, will need to undergo legislative amendment or extensive judicial interpretation in order to cover AI liability.

The courts in some jurisdictions have already produced case-law. In Canada, civil law is deemed sufficient and considered to foresee shared liability between the doctor using the AI and the developer of the technology, because developers are responsible for ensuring the safety and compliance of their AI devices with applicable regulations, while doctors must ensure that the devices are used safely and will not cause their patients any harm [8]. This is supported by Bourassa Forcier and others, who, by examining a hypothetical case, found that the current legal framework in Canada allows for a clear identification of the liability risks surrounding the use of AI as a medical decision-making tool; however, as they note, this still remains to be confirmed by case law [13].

A 2024 study, which examined 51 cases of injury caused by AI or software systems in the United States revealed that liability claims generally relate to harm caused by defects in software used to manage care or resources, physicians' use of software in making care decisions or the malfunctioning of software embedded in medical devices [14]. The study specifically cites the case of Lowe v. Cerner, where the court upheld the plaintiffs' claim that a drug-management software product had a defective user interface, which led physicians to mistakenly believe they had scheduled medication when in fact they had not; the case Sampson v. Heart Wise Health Systems Corporation where software wrongly classified a young adult with a family history of congenital heart defects as "normal" and where the court dismissed the ordinary negligence claim for his death because the developer's licensing agreement gave physicians final decision-making responsibility and the developer was not considered a "healthcare provider" under state law; and the Seargeant v. Orthopedic Associates Medical Clinic, where physicians, a technician, and a clinic were sued after a human error during a reprogramming of an infusion pump led to a lethal morphine dosing.

The authors of the above study found three emerging trends: (a) Plaintiffs struggle to sustain claims when they cannot identify specific design defects in software. Not only must plaintiffs show that the software produced an error, but they must also show how and why the error occurred (in other words, plaintiffs are unjustly burdened with proving a harmful error that requires an advanced understanding not only of how AI models operate but also of how potential errors may occur). (b) AI algorithms perform differently for different groups of patients, making it challenging to prove a physician should have known that the output was not reliable for a particular patient; and (c) Courts appear not to distinguish AI from traditional software. This raises the risk that cases about one kind of software will have impacts on other kinds, even if they are distinct and should be treated as such.

In the EU, there is limited information on case law and liability in the event of harm against a patient related to the use of AI as a decision-making tool. However, the EU has introduced a strict liability (no-fault) regime through the Product Liability Directive (hereafter PLD) 85/374/EC, which is repealed by the new PLD 2024/2853, which came into force in December 2024. Strict liability is a liability that does not depend on actual negligence or intent to harm.

It is important to highlight that so far, courts have refrained from applying the previous PLD because they do not consider software that is not embedded in hardware a "product". This was exactly what the European Court of Justice determined in the case of VI v KRONE—Verlag Gesellschaft mbH & Co KG (C-65/20, Judgement of 10 June 2021) by stating that the PLD only refers to tangible products. As such, there is uncertainty as to whether intangible code underpinning an AI process would be a "product", leaving a gap in the law.

The EU decided to address this gap by revising the PLD. Indeed, the most important innovation of the new PLD is its broader scope, which specifically includes software and AI, irrespective of the mode of supply, usage, whether embedded in hardware or distributed independently. This broader remit is significant as it means AI system providers, third-party software developers and other players in the supply chain can be held liable where a defective AI system causes harm (including damage to mental health or destruction or irreversible damage to data for the first time) [15]. This is even if the defect was not their fault. To this end, the EU AI Act will play an integral part, especially if a breach of safety standards identified during the monitoring procedure will also be considered a defect under the PLD.

As opposed to EU regulations, which have direct effect, the directive will first need to be transposed into the law of EU Member-States by December 2026. This means that during this transitional period, both the old as well as the new PLD will apply. Till then, a gap in the legal framework remains, and the national judges will decide on the liability formula applicable under national law and best suited for each case before them. Ultimately, this will lead to an inconsistency regarding the rules applicable in EU Member States. From their respective sides, attorneys will need to argue whether the current legal framework is equipped or not to cover harm caused to patients due to the application of AI technology.

4.3 AI Tools and Certification Procedures

Since the late 1990s, image-based AI tools have been developed and applied in dermatology for the diagnosis and treatment of skin-related conditions [16]. Today, there are several algorithms that incorporate AI and have been developed to help interpret both clinical and dermoscopic images for a variety of skin conditions, with multiple studies on the effect of AI-based support on dermoscopic images. Not only could AI assist primary care physicians (PCPs) and nurse practitioners (NPs) diagnose skin conditions from clinical images (i.e., taken without specialized equipment) [17], but also through the development of applications, every person can receive skincare and haircare assistance from the comfort of their homes [2].

4.3.1 The Application of AI in Dermatology

In dermatology, AI (both ML and DL) can be trained through three modes: supervised, unsupervised and by reinforcement [2]. Usually, in dermatological applications a supervised model is applied whereby the AI algorithm is trained with a set of examples labeled by an expert in which the output results are known [2]. Images labeled with the diagnosis or selected training parameter are "fed" to the AI, which is trained to recognize features and specific patterns and regions of interest, validated by a dermapathologist as a benign or malignant lesion. At a second phase, and thanks to DL algorithms, the AI can independently recognize patterns and regions of interest in lesions not previously analyzed and diagnose a lesion as a benign or malignant lesion based on these algorithms [2].

There are very few applications of unsupervised models in the field of dermatology, which is based on unlabeled data in which the output structure and results are not known beforehand [2]. An example of unsupervised learning would be the generation of classifiers for "melanoma versus nonmelanoma" by training a model that groups/classifies images through patterns detected by the algorithm itself.

In the last decade, the application of AI to classify skin lesions, particularly melanoma, has advanced rapidly [16]. More than 20 years ago, the use of two-dimensional (2D) total body photography (TBP) promoted the standardization of imaging, with some variability in its clinical application. The more recent introduction of three-dimensional TBP systems presents both challenges and opportunities to standardize both the image acquisition and labeling of clinical metadata for ML [16]. Existing systems, such as the VECTRA WB360 (Canfield Scientific), and emerging systems, such as the iToBoS (intelligent Total Body Scanner) funded by a European 2020 Horizons grant (grant identification 965221) aim to incorporate computer-aided diagnostic tools into user interface software [16]. Current VECTRA DermaGraphix software allows comparison between sequential images and is linked dermoscopy images. Likewise, the FotoFinder (FotoFinder Systems GmbH) 2D TBP system includes AI tools for new/changing lesions detected from TBP and a Moleanalyzer AI assistant, capable of lesion risk evaluation on linked dermoscopy images [16]. The fotofinder moleanalyzer tool is notably registered and licensed as a class II medical device in the European Union and has been shown to improve dermatologists' accuracy in classifying benign/malignant lesions in research studies [16].

Chat boxes, like ChatGPT, which is a large learning model (LLM), have also garnered attention concerning its application to dermatology. A study published in 2024 examined the diagnostic capabilities of ChatGPT using real-world anonymized medical dermatology cases [18]. Clinical information from 90 consecutive patients referred to a single dermatology emergency clinic between June and December 2022 were examined, and the suggested diagnosis made by ChatGPT was then compared with the diagnosis made by dermatologists. The study concluded that while ChatGPT has a diagnostic capability, in its current form, it did not significantly improve the diagnostic yield in primary or secondary care.

Another study published in 2020 examined the relevance of smartphone program applications (Apps) for dermatology [19]. The study found that smartphone Apps can be implemented responsibly when the image quality is good, the patient's history can be entered easily, transmission of the image, and results are assured and medicolegal aspects, as well as remuneration are clarified. Apps can be used for disease-specific information material and can optimize patient care by using teledermatology. Given the shortage of available dermatologists, teledermatology has been put forward as a means to ensure equitable and accessible healthcare [17, 20].

In the field of cosmetology, many companies have created intelligent questionnaires about skin and hair care that include questions about patient demographics, skin and hair characteristics, and desired aesthetic outcomes to generate personalized recommendations [2]. Companies such as L'oreal and Vichy offer web-based applications of augmented reality and age-prediction features, which is based on skin concerns, and also recommend products to users. Neutrogena developed a smartphone App where users upload images from their phone camera and receive skincare routine suggestions with monitoring features that check to see if the skin gradually improves. Dermatologists in 2020 developed the first independent application in the cosmetic industry, with the support of the European Commission within the Skiana Health and AI project (European Grants SME I 2020, Grant no. 885806) [2]. This virtual personal assistant is the first in its generation free of conflict of interest of any pharmaceutical or cosmetic company, which based on a questionnaire and information obtained from a facial analysis generated using AI algorithms, aims to improve wellbeing through healthy skin [2].

The above demonstrates that there is no shortage of the application of AI in dermatology. It can be applied to inflammatory diseases (psoriasis, atopic dermatitis, rosacea, acne, etc.), skin cancer, histologic diagnosis, such as mitosis count and assessment of positivity in immunohistochemical tests in skin radiology and ultrasound [2]. Broader application by physicians will depend on their approval by regulatory bodies, as discussed below.

4.3.2 Certification as a Basis of Legality—FDA and CE Approval

As noted above, the existing regulatory framework applicable to AI also includes certification or approval procedures. In the US certification is provided by the FDA through 510(k) pathway, PMA and de novo. The FDA evaluates the patient safety and effectiveness of Class III medical devices (Code of Federal Regulations, Title 21 Part 820 "Quality System Regulation") and companies wishing to sell medical devices in the United States that are or contain software may consult the several discussion and guidance documents published by the FDA on software validation, the use of Off-the-Shelf Software (OTSS), cybersecurity, etc. [21, 25].

In Europe, under the MDR, approval is carried out by notified bodies that evaluate medical devices. Manufacturers can place a Conformité Européenne (CE) mark on a medical device once it has passed a conformity assessment. The conformity assessment usually involves an audit of the manufacturer's quality system and, depending on the type of device, a review of technical documentation from the manufacturer on the safety and performance of the device [22, 28]. In the context of medical devices that use machine learning procedures, manufacturers should also pay particular attention to relevant International Organization for Standardization (ISO) and International Electrotechnical Commission (IEC) conformity standards.

Aside from what has been mentioned, the EU AI Act applies to most medical and in vitro diagnostic (IVD) medical devices that utilize artificial intelligence, especially machine learning. When these devices do not fall into the lowest risk class, their conformity assessment involves a notified body, and they are classified as "high-risk" devices under the AI Act.

It should be noted that there is no available database that lists all AI medical products with a CE mark relevant to dermatology, even though AI systems such as Skinive [23] or Derma AI [24] have received CE marks. The European database on medical devices provides a searchable database for issued certificates based on values such as certificate core data (notified body, certificate type, certificate number, etc.) or device data on the certificate, which is not particularly easy to use. Radiologists, on the other hand, can find any AI system with a CE mark through the AI for Radiology database, which makes the verification of MDR compliance much easier and user-friendly.

The FDA also has an online database for AI and ML enabled medical devices, which lists all medical devices that have met the FDA's applicable premarket requirements. This database is also more user-friendly. The first dermatology AI device to gain FDA authorization was MelaFind (multispectral spectroscopy) approved in 2017 via the PMA pathway, followed by the AI device, Nevisense (electrical impedance spectroscopy), also authorized under the PMA pathway in 2017 for use by dermatologists alone for melanoma detection; DermaSensor (elastic scattering spectroscopy), reviewed under FDA's de novo pathway remains on the market as of March 2025 [25, 26].

Conformity approvals, such as the ones mentioned above that guarantee patient safety, and the effectiveness of AI medical devices will not affect physician liability directly; however, indirectly they may provide potential benchmarks for courts in AI-related patient harm cases [27]. In other words, the fact that an AI product has received certification will not alter the physician's liability because, at present, liability does not include the physician's obligation to verify that certification shall guarantee patient safety and the effectiveness of the AI product, he/she chooses to use. It should be noted on the other hand, that stricter regulatory frameworks may minimize developer/manufacturer liability. In the event of a future autonomous AI system applicable to healthcare, without the intervention of human physicians, it will be interesting to see how liability for harm to patients will be addressed.

Finally, conformity approvals do not indemnify the physician of all obligations related to the deployment of AI. Apart from codes of ethics or relevant data protection rules, there are also obligations related to high-risk use of AI. As analyzed in the previous section, physicians—including dermatologists—under the EU AI Act must adhere to a comprehensive set of obligations when the AI system's output is employed within the EU (Article 26 of the EU AI Act). Considering the above applications of AI in dermatology, the following figure (Fig. 4.1) demonstrates which AI-related activities, depending on input or output data, in light of Article 6 para. 3 of the EU AI Act, could be potentially considered high or low risk.

As the above figure demonstrates, the AI system used by a dermatologist will be considered low risk because one of the following criteria are met: the AI system is intended to perform a narrow procedural task; the AI system is intended to improve the result of a previously completed human activity; the AI system is intended to

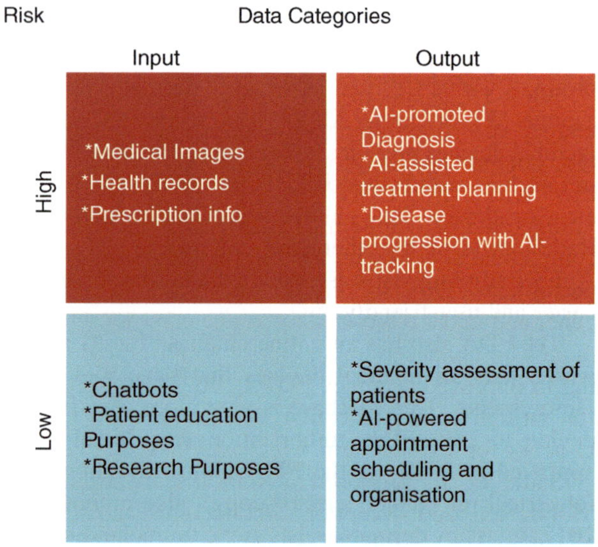

Fig. 4.1 Risk level depending on input and output data in dermatology

detect decision-making patterns or deviations from prior decision-making patterns and is not meant to replace or influence the previously completed human assessment, without proper human review; or the AI system is intended to perform a preparatory task to an assessment relevant for the purpose of the use cases. On the other hand, input or output data categorized as high-risk, do not meet any of the above criteria and could pose a significant risk to the health, safety or fundamental rights of the patient. In this case, the dermatologist must also ensure the safe and compliant use of the AI system, take appropriate measures to ensure compliance with provider instructions, ensure human oversight, monitor the system, report incidents, etc., as per the requirements of Article 23 of the EU AI Act.

4.4 Liability Schemes in Practice: Protecting the Patient from Harm

As noted above, there are many theories put forward for liability in the application of AI systems. In 2023, Cestonaro et al. [10] performed a review of the literature using the public electronic database PubMed and by searching with the terms "medical liability diagnostic algorithm". After sifting through a total of 97 articles to examine the most relevant articles available in English the authors were left with a total of 23 articles. This literature highlighted that the issue of liability in case of AI-related error has received growing attention in recent years. Nevertheless, liability is mainly discussed in position papers and non-systematic review whilst in-depth analysis is scarce. Morales Santos et al. [28] published in September 2024 a practical guide for radiologists with a more in-depth analysis on liability within the European legal regulatory framework for AI. It is a rare exception that could reflect the extended use of AI technology and liability concerns in the specific medical field of AI application (radiology).

4.4.1 Potential Liability Schemes for the Use of AI in Dermatology

As noted above, the existing liability framework which addresses harm caused to a patient from the application of AI, is national tort law. Given that the existing liability framework is still falling short in light of the challenges AI application creates in healthcare, legal practitioners will have to resort to theory-based argumentation and hope that the courts will start producing the necessary case law that will define liability in cases of AI-based harm. Unfortunately, this means that each national jurisdiction could adopt a different approach leading to the fragmentation of liability rules on an international level.

The literature converges on the same liability schemes: physician liability (fault-based liability), manufacturer liability (product liability), vicarious liability (hospital or clinic liability) and strict liability (harm-based liability). Note that in jurisdictions with public health systems, liability may be addressed by administrative courts. Criminal liability will not be covered by the present analysis however; it refers to cases where the physician commits a crime defined in criminal law (e.g., crimes of manslaughter or reckless injury).

Finally, it should be noted that some authors have also proposed no-fault insurance as an option for mitigating and overcoming liability issues. Such an insurance scheme requires the healthcare system or the medical insurance to indemnify the patients regardless of the establishment of liability [29]. An example of such a system includes the New Zealand Accident Corporation, which receives claims from individuals that have suffered injury from medical misadventures, and the Swedish Patient Injury Act which also provides compensation for medical injuries [29]. Mezrich [7] even proposes the imposition of a special tax on AI products which will be used for the creation of fund from which compensation could be administered, akin to that used for childhood vaccines in the US (i.e., the National Vaccine Injury Compensation Program-NVICP).

4.4.1.1 Physician Liability

Liability for medical errors falls under a negligence framework (malpractice); a fault-based liability which requires physicians to compensate patients for injuries for which the physician is responsible [12]. To establish a fault-based claim, the plaintiff must prove: that the defendant owed him/her the duty of care, was in breach of this duty and that it caused damages to the plaintiff [29]. Therefore, the first element is the duty of care which refers to the healthcare professional's commitment to delivering treatment to a patient that satisfies the medical community standards. The physician-patient relationship establishes this responsibility of care, a cornerstone of which is the patient's right to be informed [29]. The second element is a breach of duty, which happens when the healthcare provider fails to deliver treatment that complies with acceptable medical standards, i.e., the standard of care. As noted earlier, depending on the jurisdiction, the medical professional will either be judged according to what is done in practice, or according to what is required by normative imperatives [11] for the court to proceed to liability. The third element is causation, i.e., the causal link between the medical act or omission and the harm suffered by the patient [29]. Within the context of AI, it is important to distinguish the degree of control (autonomy) or the ultimate decision-maker. When the primary use of AI is simply a decision support tool for the physician, who thereafter makes the final determinations as to the diagnosis, the issue is simple. Medical malpractice or negligence law is well established and sufficient [7]. However, the more autonomous the AI, the more liability could possibly be shifted from the physician.

4.4.1.2 Manufacturer Liability

Another discussed model is the product liability model which requires the existence of a defect in the product and provides that the manufacturer of the defect product is presumed to be responsible [10]. The application of product liability is heavily dependent on whether AI software or algorithms are considered products (see above). Moreover, it should be highlighted that manufacturing companies should clearly provide the indications and possible adverse effects when using an AI algorithm and should be held liable for harms produced by a device that was used properly and on label [10]. If the autonomous AI is being used by a non-specialized primary care physician, he/she should not be held accountable for incorrect results. Instead, AI creators or the selling company should assume medical liability. Product liability is problematic in cases where the initial AI algorithm has evolved from the one created by the AI creator or developer and is no longer identical to that which ultimately causes harm. In this case, liability could be subject to the learned intermediary exception whereby the physician will be liable if he/she had the chance to review the findings and detect errors before they could cause a patient harm [7]. This theory, however, envisions a less autonomous AI system that will always need to be supervised or at least monitored by human physicians.

4.4.1.3 Vicarious Liability

The model of vicarious liability, whereby the negligence of an assistant or a subordinate is attributed to the supervisor, is proposed by multiple authors [10]. This theory treats the AI system as an employee in a clinical setting, of a hospital or a physician group. Malpractice of an employee using an AI program will similarly also be attributable to clinics, hospitals, and physician groups [10]. The rationale behind this liability scheme aims to distribute costs for any injury caused among hospitals or other relevant parties to fully compensate a patient [29]. The vicarious liability theory could prove useful for autonomous AI. As algorithms become more complex and independent, the vicarious theory may become the courts' preferred approach, reflecting the supervising physicians having essential fictitious control over the AI, setting the AI in motion and reaping the benefits of its use [7]. Such an approach would generate liability for human defendants that bear the risk, avoiding the murky scenarios of patients suing AI algorithms directly.

4.4.1.4 Strict Liability

In certain limited cases, national legal systems provide for strict or no-fault liability rules [30]. When strict liability rules are foreseen, the person who has suffered damage is not burdened with proving a fault (or defect) as in the case of physician liability above. The existence of the damage alone is sufficient. In strict liability situations, the person to whom strict liability rules attribute a risk will be liable for any damage caused. Conditions subject to strict liability refer to situations of a significant danger or increased public risk, or responsibility for the acts of minors, employees, or persons with limited capacities. The New Product Liability Directive of the EU foresees a strict liability regime whereby AI system providers, third-party software developers and other players in the supply chain can be held liable where a defective AI system causes harm (including damage to mental health or destruction or irreversible damage to data for the first time). This is even if the defect was not their fault [15].

4.4.1.5 Common Enterprise Liability

Common enterprise liability has also been put forward by some authors [10–12]. This theory proposes that the physician, manufacturers, and hospitals be treated as a common enterprise for the purpose of liability. This approach seeks to shift away from individualistic notions of responsibility embodied by negligence and products liability toward a more distributed conception. A common enterprise strict liability approach would also create strong incentives for the relevant actors to take care [10].

4.4.2 Case Studies

Following the above analysis, it is interesting to examine how various liability theories could apply in the case studies below (strict liability is excluded because the liable party will always be determined based on the relevant strict liability rule):

Case Study 1 A patient was diagnosed with an AI-misevaluated pigmented lesion that proved to be melanoma. Due to the delay of actual diagnosis and in receiving treatment, the patient files a claim for damages.

Physician Liability: If the physician was a specialized dermatologist and had the opportunity to review the AI-based diagnosis, the physician could be liable.

Manufacturer Liability: If it is an autonomous AI and the manufacturers' device was used properly, and on label, both the physician and the manufacturers could be liable. If the physician is a primary care physician who does not have specialized knowledge, then he/she should not be liable; only the AI creators and the selling company.

Vicarious Liability: If the misevaluation happened in a clinical setting, the hospital and physicians' group could also be jointly liable either for the AI-system employed or the physician using the AI-system.

Common Enterprise Liability: The physician, the manufacturer, and the hospital (if within such a setting) could also be jointly liable.

Case Study 2 Lip augmentation was performed on a patient who proposed a specific lip shape according to the Book Before You Look AI App. The patient is not satisfied with the end results, blaming both the App as well as the clinician.

The specific case is of a cosmetic nature, and the patient will have to establish that the result amounts to claimable injury or harm.

Physician Liability: If the physician failed to inform the patient of the possible end results, this is a violation of the patient's right to be informed and a possible breach of the duty of care [31]. If the physician was a specialist who could review the results of the AI App and propose an alternative and failed to do so, this could lead to liability.

Manufacturer Liability: If it is an autonomous AI and the manufacturers' device was used properly, and on label, both the physician and the manufacturer could be liable.

Vicarious Liability: If the AI-based harm occurred in a clinical setting, the hospital and physicians' group could also be held jointly liable either for the AI-App employed or the physician using the AI-system.

Common Enterprise Liability: The physician, the manufacturer, and the hospital (if within such a setting) could also be jointly liable.

Case Study 3 A patient with stage II melanoma diagnosed by an AI personalized program which also correlates patients with treatment options, follows the proposed treatment plan and fails to recover.

The present case depends on whether there was an error in the AI-based diagnosis or the proposed treatment plan. If the AI-based diagnosis and the proposed treatment plan were correct and ultimately followed by a specialized physician, it would be difficult to establish AI-related liability.

Physician Liability: If the physician was a specialized dermatologist and had the opportunity to review an incorrect AI-based diagnosis and proposed treatment plan, the physician could be liable.

Manufacturer Liability: If it is an autonomous AI and the manufacturers' device was used properly, and on label, both the physician and the manufacturers could be liable. If the physician is a primary care physician who does not have specialized knowledge, then he/she should not be liable, only the AI creators and the selling company.

Vicarious Liability: If the misevaluation happened in a clinical setting, the hospital and physicians' group could also be jointly liable either for the AI-system employed or the physician using the AI-system.

Common Enterprise Liability: The physician, the manufacturer, and the hospital (if within such a setting) could also be jointly liable.

Case Study 4 A patient follows an acne skincare plan from an AI App, which worsens his/her skin condition, causing pigmentation lesions, psychologically affecting the patient.

The present case depends on whether the AI App was supervised by a physician or within clinical settings, or a just a general user cosmetic App. In the latter case it falls outside the scope of the present analysis and will be regulated by consumer protection law and product liability rules. If the AI App is used within a healthcare provision setting, it is important to establish (a) whether there was an error in the AI diagnosis and skincare plan and (b) whether the mental harm suffered by the patient amounts to a claimable harm or injury in the given jurisdiction.

Physician Liability: If the AI App was being employed under the supervision of a physician within a healthcare setting which was a specialized dermatologist that had the opportunity to review the incorrect AI-based diagnosis and proposed treatment plan, the physician could be liable.

Manufacturer Liability: If it is an autonomous AI and the manufacturers' App was used properly and on label, the manufacturers (AI creators and selling companies) could be liable.

Vicarious Liability: If the misevaluation happened in a clinical setting, the hospital and physicians' group could also be jointly liable either for the AI-system employed or the physician using the AI-system.

Common Enterprise Liability: The physician, the manufacturer, and the hospital (if within such a setting) could also be jointly liable.

4.5 Conclusion—Addressing the Need for Further AI Regulation

This chapter showed that in recent years the application of AI in the medical field is spreading rapidly. The regulation of AI is currently under development at a global level. At EU level, the introduction of the EU AI Act, which promotes the importance of human–AI collaboration, will play an important role in future applications of AI in the field of dermatology. Even though AI holds vast capabilities, for now it only remains a supporting diagnostic and treatment tool for the modern medical practitioner. AI has the potential to significantly enhance the accuracy of disease diagnosis and identify the best available treatment, including in the field of dermatology. Yet AI technology has not advanced to the degree of eliminating harm to patients and, given that the ultimate decision-maker will be the medical professional, it is necessary to explore how medical liability is affected by the use of AI. Research demonstrates that there is no definitive legal solution to be applied to AI-based diagnosis that causes a patient harm. There is a lack of harmonization regarding liability related issues, which has led to the proposal of various theories. Ultimately, the realization of these legal theories will come down to two scenarios: a practice-based approach or a normative-based approach. In other words, it will either be left to the courts to formulate the necessary legal framework, which is time-consuming and may lead to legal uncertainty that will inadvertently interrupt innovation in AI development, or it will be left to legislators to introduce a comprehensive legal framework, which will be developed in tandem with relevant stakeholders specialized in the application of AI in healthcare, i.e., medical professionals, medical institutions, AI developers, and legal professionals.

At an EU level it is important to note that in September 2022 the European Commission released a proposal for an Artificial Intelligence Liability Act [32]; a new liability regime that aimed to ensure legal certainty, enhance consumer trust in AI, and assist consumers' liability claims for damage caused by AI-enabled products and services. The proposal recognized that without a harmonizing act in place, Member-States will proceed to adapt their existing national liability rules to the challenges of AI, leading to further legal uncertainty, fragmentation and increased costs for businesses across the EU. In February 2025 the European Commission withdrew the proposal while it was still being debated in the European Parliament and scheduled for voting in 2026 [32]. It remains to be seen if the European Commission will introduce a new proposal or choose an alternative approach. For the time being pertinent literature underscores the lack of clear and unified legislation concerning the liability of healthcare professionals employing AI and there are no universal rules for the distribution of medical liability in case of harm to patients [33]. AI technology continues to advance at a rapid pace, and it remains to see when the regulatory and legal frameworks will eventually catch up.

References

1. Kaul V, Enslin S, Gross SA. History of artificial intelligence in medicine. Gastrointest Endosc. 2020;92:807–12. https://doi.org/10.1016/j.gie.2020.06.040. PMID: 32565184
2. Martorell A, Martin-Gorgojob A, Ríos-Vinuela E, Rueda-Carnero JM, Alfageme F, Taberner R. [Translated article] Artificial intelligence in dermatology: a threat or an opportunity? Actas Dermo-Sifiliográficas. 2022;113:T30–46. https://doi.org/10.1016/j.ad.2021.07.014.
3. Li J, Jiang P, An Q, Wang G-G, Kong H-F. Medical image identification methods: a review. Comput Biol Med. 2024;169:107777., ISSN 0010-4825. https://doi.org/10.1016/j.compbiomed.2023.107777.
4. Reardon S. AI Chatbots can diagnose medical conditions at home. How good are they? Sci Am. 2024;
5. Zawati MH, Lang M. Does an app a day keep the doctor away? AI symptom checker applications, entrenched bias, and professional responsibility. J Med Internet Res. 2024;26:e50344. https://doi.org/10.2196/50344. PMID: 38838309, PMCID: 11187504
6. Li J. Security implications of AI Chatbots in health care. J Med Internet Res. 2023;25:e47551. https://doi.org/10.2196/47551. PMID: 38015597; PMCID: PMC10716748
7. Mezrich JL. Is artificial intelligence (AI) a pipe dream? Why legal issues present significant hurdles to AI autonomy. AJR Am J Roentgenol. 2022;219(1):152–6. https://doi.org/10.2214/AJR.21.27224.
8. Naili YT, Mangkunegara IS, Purwono, Baballe MA. Regulatory challenges in ai-based diagnostics: legal implications of AI use in medical diagnostics. BIO Web Conf. 2025;152:01034. https://doi.org/10.1051/bioconf/202515201034.
9. European Commission, official website on "Artificial Intelligence in healthcare". https://health.ec.europa.eu/ehealth-digital-health-and-care/artificial-intelligence-healthcare_en
10. Cestonaro C, Delicati A, Marcante B, Caenazzo L, Tozzo P. Defining medical liability when artificial intelligence is applied on diagnostic algorithms: a systematic review. Front Med (Lausanne). 2023;10:1305756. https://doi.org/10.3389/fmed.2023.1305756. PMID: 38089864; PMCID: PMC10711067
11. Rimkutė D. AI and liability in medicine: the case of assistive-diagnostic AI. Balt J Law Polit. 2024;16:64–81. https://doi.org/10.2478/bjlp-2023-0013.
12. Sullivan HR, Schweikart SJ. Are current tort liability doctrines adequate for addressing injury caused by AI? AMA J Ethics. 2019;21(2):E160–6. https://doi.org/10.1001/amajethics.2019.160. PMID: 30794126
13. Bourassa Forcier M, Khoury L, Vézina N. Liability issues for the use of artificial intelligence in health care in Canada: AI and medical decision-making. Dalhousie Med J. 2020;46 https://doi.org/10.15273/dmj.Vol46No2.10140.
14. Mello MM, Guha N. Understanding liability risk from healthcare AI, understanding liability risk from using health care artificial intelligence tools. N Engl J Med. 2024;390(3):271–8. https://doi.org/10.1056/NEJMhle2308901. PMID: 38231630
15. Howarth M, Chandler K, Behrendt P. AI liability—who is accountable when artificial intelligence malfunctions? Insights, TaylorWessing. 2025;07:01.
16. Clare A, Primiero, Rezze GG, Caffery LJ, Carrera C, Podlipnik S, Espinosa N, Puig S, Janda M, Soyer HP, Malvehy J. A narrative review: opportunities and challenges in artificial intelligence skin image analyses using total body photography. J Invest Dermatol. 2024;144:1200–7., ISSN 0022-202X. https://doi.org/10.1016/j.jid.2023.11.007.
17. Jain A, Way D, Gupta V, et al. Development and assessment of an Artificial Intelligence–based tool for skin condition diagnosis by primary care physicians and nurse practitioners in teledermatology practices. JAMA Netw Open. 2021;4(4):e217249. https://doi.org/10.1001/jamanetworkopen.2021.7249.
18. Stoneham S, Livesey A, Cooper H, Mitchell C. ChatGPT versus clinician: challenging the diagnostic capabilities of artificial intelligence in dermatology. Clin Exp Dermatol. 2024;49:707–10. https://doi.org/10.1093/ced/llad402. PMID: 37979201

19. Blum A, Bosch S, Haenssle HA, et al. Künstliche Intelligenz und Smartphone-Programm-Applikationen (Apps). Hautarzt. 2020;71:691–8. https://doi.org/10.1007/s00105-020-04658-4. PMID: 32720165
20. Young AT, Xiong M, Pfau J, Keiser MJ, Wei ML. Artificial intelligence in dermatology: a primer. J Invest Dermatol. 2020;140:1504–12., ISSN 0022-202X. https://doi.org/10.1016/j.jid.2020.02.026.
21. U.S. Food and Drug Administration—FDA, Regulatory Information and Medical Devices.
22. European Medicines Agency—EMA, Medical Devices, updated on 24.03.2025.
23. Skinive, Delivering quality: CE-mark and ISO 13485 certificate, 11.12.2020.
24. Medical Device Network, Advanced Human Imaging's Derma AI gains CE mark approval, 28.05.2021.
25. Venkatesh KP, Kadakia KT, Gilbert S. Learnings from the first AI-enabled skin cancer device for primary care authorized by FDA. npj Digit Med. 2024;7:156. https://doi.org/10.1038/s41746-024-01161-1.
26. U.S. Food and Drug Administration—FDA, Artificial Intelligence and Machine Learning (AI/ML)-Enabled Medical Devices.
27. Maliha G, Gerke S, Cohen IG, Parikh RB. Artificial Intelligence and liability in medicine: balancing safety and innovation. Milbank Q. 2021;99:629–47. https://doi.org/10.1111/1468-0009.12504.
28. Santos ÁM, Lendoiro SL, Cañellas MR, Solís PV. The legal regulation of artificial intelligence in the European Union: a practical guide for radiologists. Radiologia. 2024;66:431–46., (English edition) ISSN 2173-5107. https://doi.org/10.1016/j.rxeng.2023.11.011.
29. Eldakak A, Alremeithi A, Dahiyat E, et al. Civil liability for the actions of autonomous AI in healthcare: an invitation to further contemplation. Humanit Soc Sci Commun. 2024;11:305. https://doi.org/10.1057/s41599-024-02806-y.
30. Evas T., Civil liability regime for artificial intelligence, European Parliament Research Service, September 2020.
31. Pallocci M, Treglia M, Passalacqua P, Tittarelli R, Zanovello C, De Luca L, Caparrelli V, De Luna V, Cisterna AM, Quintavalle G, Marsella LT. Informed consent: legal obligation or cornerstone of the care relationship? Int J Environ Res Public Health. 2023;20(3):2118. https://doi.org/10.3390/ijerph20032118. PMID: 36767485; PMCID: PMC9915667
32. European Parliament, AI liability directive.
33. Sablone S, Bellino M, Cardinale AN, Esposito M, Sessa F, Salerno M. Artificial intelligence in healthcare: an Italian perspective on ethical and medico-legal implications. Front Med. 2024;11:1343456. https://doi.org/10.3389/fmed.2024.1343456.

Bioethics in the Use of AI in Dermatology 5

Anna Mavrophorou

5.1 AI Model Integration in Dermatology Practice

The technologically advanced world is rapidly changing our lives, bringing opportunities, challenges, threats, and risks. Dermatology, as a technologically dependent medical specialty heavily relying on visual diagnosis, could not remain unaffected by these developments. Artificial intelligence (AI) is a computational method that in some way mimics the human thought process. The integration of AI applications in dermatology, such as image analysis applications and teledermatology, especially for the diagnosis of conditions such as melanoma, other forms of skin cancer and chronic diseases, has already started to change the way dermatology is practiced, both in daily clinical practice and in research [1, 2].

Additionally, the development of telemedicine applications makes access to dermatological services easier for patients, particularly in areas where specialists are scarce. Through smart apps, patients can send photos of their lesions for initial assessment, suggesting further diagnostic or therapeutic approaches [3].

Big data analytics technologies enable both the automatic identification of skin lesions with an accuracy that often compares or exceeds the expertise of specialists and the study of billions of clinical and research data for a deeper understanding of the causes of skin conditions. The analysis of this data contributes to the discovery of new prognostic indicators or new therapeutic targets. Technological platforms offer access to students and dermatology residents to virtual patients, enhancing interactive learning.

The use of bioinformatics and AI algorithms helps to personalize treatments, considering the genetic profile, skin type, and individual needs of the patient. Data from clinical studies are used to predict response to specific drugs, such as biological agents for the treatment of psoriasis [3].

A. Mavrophorou (✉)
Deontology and Bioethics Laboratory, Faculty of Nursing, School of Health Sciences, University of Thessaly, Larissa, Greece

E. Karampinis et al. (eds.), *Artificial Intelligence Applications in Dermatology*,
https://doi.org/10.1007/978-3-032-15614-3_5

Through classic examples of the everyday use of AI applications in dermatology, we can explore how these facilitate the processes of diagnosis, monitoring, and treatment of patients in clinical practice, as well as address the legal and ethical issues raised for the users and recipients of these applications [4, 5]. AI has inevitably produced certainties and uncertainties in healthcare [6]. Are AI applications always reliable? What issues are raised when they address rare conditions or unusual clinical data? Are patients' personal data protected? Can AI replace the human dimension of medical science?

5.2 Bioethics Approach of AI Integration on Dermatology—Practical Examples

Example 1: *A dermatologist prescribes a patient with resistant psoriasis a new treatment regimen while encouraging him to download an AI app on his mobile phone to better monitor his disease*

Problems arise from this patient monitoring option, such as:

1. Patient's ability to handle the application of AI in a correct way.

   People with limited experience on smart devices or applications, etc. and with low digital literacy, may find it difficult to understand the process of their operation. But also, applications with complex interfaces or incomplete instructions for use may confuse patients. For example, if the app itself does not provide clear examples of how to enter data (e.g., through questions, pictures, and text), the patient may enter incomplete information. If the patient is not familiar with smartphone technology, adapting to a new potentially complex app with AI services may seem difficult. If the app does not provide immediate confirmation or correction, or instructions to the user, the patient may be unsure of the usefulness of the app [7, 8].
2. Uncertainty and anxiety arising from the fear of incorrect application of the AI.

   When the patient is not familiar with these technologies, they may feel uncertainty and anxiety about their usability. He or she may reasonably wonder whether he or she will be able to handle it and indeed whether he or she will be able to handle it in the right way. The fear of misuse of the application by him or her causes anxiety about whether this will have an impact on his or her correct diagnosis or treatment and, more generally, on the outcome of the disease and his or her health [6, 7].
3. Concern for preserving the privacy of the patients, as some users are reluctant to provide personal health data for fear of privacy violations. The use of AI applications often involves the collection and processing of sensitive personal data. Patients are concerned about the security of this information and possible misuse [6, 9].
4. Concern about alienation of the patient from the doctor.

   Medicine is a field that combines science with the art of understanding human beings, and a full understanding of a patient's health cannot be limited solely to measurable quantities and mechanically interpretable terms. Laboratory tests, imaging methods, and other technological approaches provide critical information about human physiology and pathology. Indicators such as blood pressure, blood glucose level, and enzyme values are objective data that are essential for the diagnosis and monitoring of the disease. However, these data, although useful, are not sufficient for a complete understanding of a person's health, which is multidimensional. Pain, fatigue, stress, and quality of life are experiences that are often not fully captured by measurements. A patient's mental and emotional state can affect their health, but cannot always be quantified or interpreted mechanically. The doctor–patient relationship is crucial. The patient's narratives about their illness experience, their history, and their social circumstances often provide information that is not captured in the tests. A doctor must understand the human dimension and consider factors such as the patient's environment, values, and fears. The human dimension and personal interaction remain irreplaceable. Personal contact and trust are crucial elements of the therapeutic process. The use of technology must not create the impression in the patient that the doctor is withdrawing from his or her care, leaving the fate of the patient's health to the applications of AI and technology in general.

How can the problems arising from the physician's recommendation to the patient to use AI applications be addressed? First, it is worth noting that the patients' concerns are reasonable, as health technology is constantly evolving, and it takes time to become fully accepted. Human guidance remains critical and can be provided in many ways, such as:

- With education and support from the physician. Requiring the physician to take the time to explain in a simple way how the app works and help with the app's installation, as well as with patient testing of the AI app in the presence of the physician. This process helps the patient to gain practical experience in using the app, which reduces the fear of making mistakes. In fact, the presence of the doctor gives the patient a sense of security and increases his/her confidence in the procedure. The doctor also adapts the app to the patient's needs, making it more efficient to use, and can identify any obstacles the patient faces and suggest alternatives. It requires the doctor to take the time to explain in a simple way how the app works and to offer help in setting it up as well as having the patient test the AI app in the presence of the doctor. This process helps the patient to gain practical experience in using the application which reduces the fear of making mistakes. In fact, the presence of the doctor gives the patient a sense of security and increases his/her confidence in the procedure. The doctor also adapts the app to the patient's needs, making it more efficient to use, and can identify any obstacles the patient faces and suggest alternatives.
- With reassurance from the doctor that their personal data will be safe. It is important to explain that the data stored in the AI application is secure and will be processed in a privacy-preserving manner. It should also be made clear that AI does not replace the doctor but helps him/her to be guided to the correct diagnosis and make the decisions needed to safeguard his/her health.

- With the understanding that the application of AI also ensures the patient's autonomy and communication with the doctor. If the patient does not understand how the AI model works, they may question whether the system can actually help their health. The patient may think, "can a machine understand my condition better than a human?". On the contrary, if the patient sees the application of AI as an opportunity to stimulate autonomy in managing their health, they may feel curious or even excited about the experience. Also, some apps allow for direct data sharing with the doctor, facilitating remote monitoring of their psoriasis control and treatment effectiveness without constant visits to the doctor [6–10]. Understanding the benefits of implementing AI includes: (i) Early detection of changes; (ii) Speed; (iii) Accuracy; and (iv) Prediction (sees trends that are difficult to observe without advanced tools). All those features assist in making optimal decisions.

Prerequisites for the proper use of AI applications include the following: (a) appropriate application: it is important that the application is scientifically validated and protects patient data; (b) cooperation with the doctor: the doctor must guide the patient on the correct use of the application; and (c) familiarity with the technology: the patient must be comfortable using his/her mobile device.

Examples of applications that can be used in the specific example are PsoHappy, MyPsoriasisTeam, or general skin condition monitoring systems with artificial intelligence, such as SkinVision can help patients with psoriasis.

Example 2: *In a patient with a suspicious pigmented lesion and a history of melanoma, the doctor uses an AI system for screening to diagnose if he/she has cancer (melanoma)*

The use of an AI system to screen a patient with a history of melanoma for a pigmented lesion raises important legal and ethical dilemmas.

(i) Legal Dilemmas

Liability for misdiagnosis is a major concern. If the diagnosis is wrong (false positive or false negative), who is liable? The doctor, the developer of the AI system, or the technology provider? In Greece, the doctor has the ultimate responsibility for medical decisions. However, the use of AI may create situations where the division of responsibility may be indistinguishable.

Compliance with data protection legislation also represents a major legal dilemma. Patient data, such as skin images, may be subject to General Data Protection Regulation (GDPR). It must be ensured that patient data is collected, stored, and used with their consent and in a strictly secure manner.

The lack of transparency (black box AI) aspect lies on the fact that the AI system operates as a black box, without a clear explanation of the decision. This can create problems in legal proceedings if the diagnosis is challenged.

Medical device regulation should also be considered by the user. The AI system must meet standards and be approved by competent authorities as a medical device. Essentially, the AI system must comply with specific legal, technical, and ethical requirements that ensure that it is safe, reliable, and suitable for use in medical applications [11–13].

These requirements vary depending on the country or region where it is used, but typically include the following:

A. Compliance with international standards (the AI system must follow internationally recognized standards such as those set by organizations such as ISO (International Organization for Standardization)).
B. Control by competent authorities (AI systems used as medical devices must be controlled and approved by organizations such as FDA, EMA, National Health Authority of the country where it is applied).
C. Safety and effectiveness assessment (the AI system must demonstrate through clinical studies or trials that it provides accurate and reliable results, that it does not pose any risks to users or patients, and that it works properly even under different conditions of use).
D. Transparency and documentation (the AI system must be transparent about how it works—e.g., how it makes decisions, especially if it is involved in clinical decisions—i.e., detailed documentation on its design, development, and testing is required).
E. Continuous monitoring and updates (even after approval, the AI system must be monitored for any problems, such as malfunctions or adverse effects).
F. Categorization as a medical device, i.e., depending on its use, the AI system is classified into different categories. There are high-risk or low-risk AI systems. The most critical systems, such as those involved in diagnosis or treatment, are subject to stricter requirements.
G. Approval by the competent authorities ensures that the AI protects the health and safety of patients and avoids false or inaccurate results that could lead to wrong medical decisions [6, 10, 14].

(ii) Ethical Dilemmas

The ethical dilemmas in the above-mentioned case include:

A. Patient Autonomy: The patient has the right to know that the AI application is being used for diagnosis and to decide whether to consent. Transparency is essential. The patient is adequately informed about the use and limits of the system.
B. Trust in Technology: The patient or even a doctor may rely too much on the system, underestimating the need for human judgment. Is there a risk of dehumanizing medical care?
C. Impartiality and Fairness: AI systems may have been trained on data that is not representative of all populations, which may lead to discrimination. There is a risk of misdiagnosis in patient groups not adequately covered by the AI system training data.
D. Substitution of the Role of the Physician: If the system takes the place of human judgment this may reduce the physician's responsibility and commitment to investigate the patient's case in depth.

E. Risk of Causing Distress and Social Stigma: A wrong diagnosis can cause extreme distress to the patient or affect their psychological and professional situation, and can also lead to social stigmatization.
F. Equity of Access: If such technologies are not affordable and geographically accessible to all, there is a risk of inequalities in healthcare.

To address the legal and ethical dilemmas, it is important to have: (a) A clear legislation in defining the liability of doctors and providers of AI applications. (b) Transparency and information to provide an adequate explanation of how the limitations of the AI system work to the patient. (c) Compliance with ethical principles to ensure that AI is used to improve patient health while respecting patient autonomy, and (d) Continuous education of physicians on the advantages and limitations of AI so that human judgment remains at the center. AI is not a panacea, and doctors need to be aware of its limitations. The results of AI systems are only as good as the data used to train them. If the data is incomplete or biased, incorrect recommendations can be produced [1, 5, 6, 9].

In conclusion, AI works with algorithms but lacks the ability to integrate the legal framework and lacks empathy to understand the ethical principles governing medicine in different socio-economic environments. AI cannot replace the emotional understanding and communication that a doctor provides to the patient. Therefore, it should be seen as a support tool that enhances his/her work, not a replacement for human judgment. Doctors are the only ones who can make holistic decisions, taking into account the personal and psychological aspects of the patient and interpreting the results of AI based on their medical background and experience. Their central role in patient care should therefore not be undermined.

Example 3: *A patient presents to a doctor with a lesion in the genital area, reporting a medical history of careless sexual intercourse. The doctor wishes to upload the image of the lesion to an AI program or chatbot and ask what can be done. A doctor's intention to upload an image of a sensitive area of a patient's body to an AI program or an online platform such as a chatbot to seek diagnostic advice raises serious ethical and legal dilemmas*

(i) Legal Dilemmas
   A. Personal Data Breach: According to the General Data Protection Regulation, medical data, such as images of bodily injuries, are considered sensitive data and require explicit patient consent for their collection, processing, and transmission. If the doctor uploads the image without the patient's consent, he or she may find himself or herself legally exposed.
   B. Ensuring Anonymity: Even if the image does not include obvious personal details such as name, body part, and history, it may reveal other visible details on the patient's body. e.g., a tattoo on the shin, can lead to identification. If the inability to identify him or her is not fully ensured, then there is a risk of a breach of privacy.

C. Liability in Case of Misdiagnosis: If the AI model provides incorrect and misleading advice, there is always the question of who is liable, the doctor or the system provider? The doctor must ensure that the advice received from the AI is reliable and confirm the diagnosis through traditional medical methods.

D. Setting Up the AI as a Medical Tool: The AI platform must be approved for medical use and comply with the standards applicable to medical devices. The AI law [EU Regulation 2024/1689] recently adopted by the European Commission sets out the conditions required to ensure that AI systems respect the fundamental rights of citizens and businesses and ensure the safety and ethical principles that arise from the use of very powerful and effective AI models [5, 6, 9].

(ii) Ethical Dilemmas

A. Patient Consent: The doctor must inform the patient and obtain the patient's consent before uploading the image. Lack of informed consent violates the bioethical principle of patient autonomy.

B. Privacy and Dignity: Posting an image of such a sensitive part of the patient's body can be considered an affront to the patient's dignity, especially if it is not clear how the image will be used and by whom.

C. Accuracy of Diagnosis: If the AI is not adequately trained for such lesions, it may give inaccurate results in violation of the principle of utility.

D. Substitution of the Doctor's Role: If the doctor relies too much on AI, neglecting his or her own clinical judgment, there is a risk of failure to provide quality care.

E. Justice in the use of technology? The use of AI technologies must be fair, transparent and without bias. The physician has a responsibility to choose systems that are ethically and technically appropriate [6, 15].

Suggestions for mitigating the dilemmas include patient's information and consent. The patient should be made aware of the purpose and potential risks of using AI and should give written consent and anonymization of data: Any element that could in any way identify the patient must be removed from the image. The use of approved AI systems is necessary. The AI platform must be certified for medical use with known levels of accuracy as defined by an AI law [EU Regulation 2024/1689] recently adopted by the European Commission. AI should function as a tool to support medical judgment and not as an exclusive diagnostic method replacing it. Additionally, the doctor must ensure that the data is not stored or used for purposes by the AI platform other than those for which the patient has given consent.

The use of AI in medicine has significant advantages, but it must be done with full respect for patients' personal data and rights and with the application of strict legal and ethical rules.

Example 4: *A minor patient with a facial lesion enters a dermatology clinic with his father. Can the doctor upload photographs of his face to a AI model available on the Internet asking for the child's medical problem?*

The use of facial photographs of a minor patient by a dermatologist for medical purposes (e.g., diagnosis, archiving, education, or publication) is subject to legal and ethical offences, given the sensitive nature of the data and the age of the patient.

(i) Legal Dilemmas
   A. Parental/guardian consent, as under the law, minors' data are particularly protected. The use of photographs of the person requires the explicit and written consent of the parent or legal guardian, as the minor cannot give valid legal consent.
   B. Consent of the Minor: Although parental consent is necessary, it is important to take into account the minor's point of view, especially if he or she is mature enough to understand the process.
   C. General Data Protection Regulation and Sensitive Data: Photographs showing the patient's face are considered sensitive personal data as they can lead to the identification of the individual. Therefore, the collection, storage, and use of these photographs must be in accordance with the principles of the GDPR, such as:
      (i) Purpose: The use of the photographs must be limited to the purpose for which they were collected (e.g., for diagnosis).
      (ii) Data Minimization: Data need to be stored only if necessary.
      (iii) Security: It must be ensured that photographs are protected from unauthorized access.
      (iv) Use in Research or Publications: If photographs are intended for education, publication, or conferences, specific consent is required, describing the purpose and how they will be used.
      (v) Third-Party Access: Photos must not be shared with third parties (e.g., technology platforms, other professionals) without parental consent [16].

(ii) Ethical Dilemmas
   A. Respect for Privacy: If the person is readily identifiable and the publication of images even without a name can damage the privacy and self-esteem of the minor.
   B. Patient Consent: The minor patient has the right to express his/her opinion if taking pictures without his/her consent violates the principle of autonomy.
   C. Stigmatization: The use of images of a person with obvious problems (e.g., severe skin conditions) may lead to social stigmatization if they are leaked or used incorrectly.
   D. Ethical Use of Data: There is a risk that photographs may be used for purposes other than those stated (e.g., commercial use and training without anonymization).
   E. Long-Term Consent: A minor may not fully understand the implications of using their images in the future. What happens when they become an adult and disagree with the use made? [16].

Suggestions for ensuring ethical and legal compliance:

A. Informed Consent: The parent/guardian and the minor must be informed of the purpose of taking and using the photograph, the retention period and how it will be stored, and their rights (withdrawal of consent and deletion).
B. Anonymization: If the photograph is used for research or education, avoid identification of the patient (e.g., processing to hide identifiable data).
C. Restriction of Use: Photographs should only be used for the purpose stated and deleted after the end of use.
D. Secure Storage: Photographs should be stored in secure databases with restricted access.
E. Respect for the Minor: Obtaining the minor's opinion, even if it is not legally binding, is useful to ensure respect for the minor's privacy.
F. The use of photographs of minors is an area that requires special attention both to protect privacy and to ensure that the doctor's actions are legally and ethically sound [16].

Example 5: *A young adult patient wishes to have her lips augmented with fillers and her physician shows her the final future image in a program. How will it look when she undergoes the requested "Book before you look" technique?*

Cosmetic dermatology is a distinct field that does not address an illness, either fatal or posing direct threat to a patient's physical health. Nevertheless, beauty related problems such as wrinkles, age spots, acne, freckles, and melasma may have important psychological implications to individuals resulting in diminished self-esteem and confidence with long-term mental effects.

The use of AI in the field of cosmetic dermatology may provide tools of three-dimensional facial reconstruction and models for predicting clinical outcomes. This in fact may assist dermatologists to close the gap between the patient and the unknown outcome of the treatment plans. AI and deep learning are integral parts of computer vision technology allowing computers to learn and improve the identification and classification of objects accurately within the provided images. This technology may be used to appropriately identify and classify facial rhytids before treatment with neuromodulators or soft tissue fillers [17–20].

While the use of this technology to show patients for instance the final image after a cosmetic intervention such as lip augmentation with fillers shows promising future in delivering a tailored patient experience it may raise significant legal and ethical dilemmas.

(i) Legal Dilemmas
   A. Liability for the Result: If the result differs from the simulation the patient can take legal action claiming that he/she was misled by the doctor or the program.
   B. Data and Personal Information Security: The use of programs that include photographs of the patient's face poses privacy risks if the data is stored or leaked.

   C. Informed Consent and Documentation: The doctor must clearly record that the simulation is an indication and not a guarantee of the outcome in order to be legally protected.
   D. Advertising and Misrepresentation: If the simulation is presented as an advertising or service promotion tool it may be considered misleading, especially if it is not an accurate representation of the outcome [17–20].

(ii) Ethical Dilemmas
   A. Patient Expectations: The program may create unrealistic expectations of the outcome. If the result is not the same as what was presented the patient may feel disappointed or experience depression even though the procedure was successful.
   B. Personal Perception of Beauty: The projection of an image may affect the patient's self-perception and create concerns about their appearance or create a need for more cosmetic procedures potentially stimulating psychological disorders such as dysmorphophobia.
   C. Informed Consent: The patient should be aware that the image is only a simulation and not a guarantee of the result. There is a risk that the image may be seen as a binding promise the ethics of intervention; in young adults, the question arises whether it is ethical for the doctor to proceed with aesthetic interventions, especially if the patient does not have a fully developed perception of his/her body image [17–20].

5.3 Conclusions and Recommendations

A. Focusing on Ethics

The doctor should bear in mind that if data sets used to train the model is not diverse and representative it might disproportionately favor specific traits or futures. This is why it is important to inform the patient of the limitations of simulation. Additionally, the use of the program should be accompanied by a written consent stating that the image is indicative. The decision to intervene should consider the psychological-emotional maturity and needs of the patient, avoiding the reinforcement of unrealistic expectations. Finally, it is important that privacy and protection of patient data is ensured.

Balancing ethical and legal obligations requires transparency, empathy, and professional responsibility. The phrase "Book before you look" in medicine can be applied in situations where patients are asked to make an appointment for a cosmetic intervention without having full information or access to details about the service, the doctor or the results. Scheduling cosmetic procedures in areas such as botox treatments, fillers, FG plastic surgery procedures, patients may be asked to make appointments for specialist medical tests and surgical procedures without first having thorough information about the doctor, the procedure and the possible outcome. In medicine, the patient must be fully informed about the procedure, risks, benefits, and alternatives. "Book before you look" undermines this principle, especially if adequate information is not provided in advance of what to expect, leading to a risk of disappointment and legal claims if the results do not meet expectations. Particularly in cosmetic procedures, patients may rely on advertising from photographs that do not reflect reality. This strategy may create pressure on the patient to commit before they have all the information. It is important for the patient to feel confident about the quality of care and lack of information before it can shake confidence [17–20].

B. How Will "Book Before You Look" Become Ethically Acceptable?

To make 'book before you look' ethically acceptable, it is necessary to ensure that patients receive adequate and transparent information, that their consent is genuinely informed, and that their trust is safeguarded.

Patients must receive detailed information about the nature of the procedure or test (what it involves, what the steps are, what the potential risks and benefits are), alternatives (i.e., to know if there are noninvasive or less costly options). The cost and cancellation policy (clear reference to prices, prepayments, and cancellation rights), effects, and limitations. Especially in the case of aesthetic interventions, it should be stressed that the results may differ from the images. The patient's consent prior to the intervention must be documented and adequately informed. The patient should sign a form explicitly stating that he/she has been informed of all risks and potential benefits. Allow time for the patient to express questions and concerns before making an appointment for the intervention. Especially for cosmetic procedures, doctors should show realistic examples of their work (e.g., before and after photos, having the approval of previous patients).

The patient should have the opportunity to meet the doctor before committing. There should be a flexible policy for changing or cancelling the appointment, especially if the patient changes their mind after further information. If images or personal data are used for simulation, privacy legislation must be respected.

Finally, it is important to have personalized counselling for patients provided free of charge or at a very low cost for their assessment. Doctors should take the patient's mental state into serious consideration to avoid interventions based on unrealistic or impulsive decisions [17–21].

5.4 Ethical and Privacy Considerations in Personalized Medicine

Secure processing of genetic data through advanced encryption and federated learning can be enhanced to ensure data privacy. At the same time, it may facilitate large-scale analysis, addressing concerns about the sensitive nature of genetic information.

Characteristic examples of this facility provided by AI are the following:

- Oncology: AI-driven tools like IBM Watson for Genomics analyze genetic mutations in cancer patients to recommend specific treatments.

- Rare Diseases: Platforms like DeepMind's AlphaFold help predict protein structures from genetic sequences, aiding in understanding genetic disorders.
- Pharmacogenomics: Companies like 23andMe and Foundation Medicine use AI to analyze DNA for personalized drug recommendations.

As AI is a very dynamic technology, major evolutions in the future are expected. Thus, several platforms may develop to enable real-time monitoring of genetic changes (e.g., in cancer progression), predictive models for disease outbreaks based on genetic epidemiology and fully personalized preventive medicine based on both genetics and lifestyle factors. Nevertheless, for the ethical deployment of AI, governance models and bias evaluation checklists remain an important challenge [22–27].

5.5 AI and Physician–Patient Relationship

In the modern era, we have witnessed a transition from paternalism to a more patient-centered relationship in which both physician and patient are considered as partners in the decision-making and execution of healthcare choices. The physician holds the role of the expert who has clinical knowledge, and the patient has the authority to express his values and preferences. While the integration of AI into healthcare provides important advantages, there are still issues of concern as it is the way that it affects the physician–patient relationship. Its integration into clinical practice can interfere with this relationship in several ways, both positively and negatively [5–8, 28–30].

On one hand, positive interference, enhancing the physician–patient relationship includes:

- Improved diagnostic accuracy and efficiency by analyzing vast datasets (e.g., imaging, lab results, and genetic information) quickly and accurately, assisting physicians in making precise diagnoses. This allows physicians to focus more on communication and patient care rather than data analysis, enhancing trust and satisfaction.
- Personalized care plans by enhancement of patient data analysis, enabling highly tailored treatments, fostering a sense of individualized care that strengthens the physician–patient bond.
- Better time management as AI-powered automation reduces administrative burdens (e.g., charting, scheduling, and billing), giving physicians more time to engage directly with patients.
- Enhanced patient education as tools, like chatbots or virtual assistants, can provide patients with easy-to-understand explanations about their conditions and treatments, promoting transparency and informed decision-making.
- Proactive and preventive care through the prediction of health risks and suggesting preventive measures, which enable physicians to build trust by focusing on long-term health outcomes for their patients.

On the other hand, there might be some negative interference with the physician–patient relationship, such as:

- Loss of human connection because of the overreliance on AI, which might reduce face-to-face interaction between physicians and patients, leading to a perceived lack of empathy and personal touch. In addition, patients may feel neglected if there is a lack of adequate direct communication.
- Erosion of trust, as patients may feel uncomfortable relying on machine-driven recommendations instead of their physician's judgment.
- Dehumanization of care is another negative interference of AI if patients perceive that this has replaced the emotional and relational aspects of care. While, for instance, AI-driven chatbots might answer patient queries, they lack the emotional intelligence to provide genuine reassurance.
- Bias and errors as all AI systems are inherent to because they are based on the data they are trained on, potentially leading to inequities in care. Thus, incorrect predictions or recommendations may undermine trust in the physician's expertise.
- Reduction in physician autonomy as AI-generated recommendations or protocols could limit their ability to exercise clinical judgment and adapt to the unique needs of their patients.
- Privacy concerns because AI requires significant patient data. This inevitably raises concerns about data security and privacy breaches. If patients feel their information is not secure, it can strain their relationship with their healthcare provider.
- Technology dependency for both physicians and patients might potentially lead to challenges if technology fails or produces ambiguous results.

To control the potential dangers from the use of AI in healthcare, it is of great importance to set certain strategies to preserve a healthy physician–patient relationship. Attention should be placed on maintaining human oversight by using AI as a supportive tool and not as a replacement for the physician's clinical judgment or personal connection with the patient. Also, transparent communication with patients remains crucial to explaining how AI is used and ensuring that patients understand how the decisions are made. Technology and empathy should be balanced in a way that physicians should use the time saved by AI to build trust and address patients' emotional and psychological needs. Additionally, the implementation of ethical guidelines to minimize bias, ensure transparency, and maintain patient privacy and data security all play an important role. Finally, physicians should be trained in AI tools to be aware of their limitations, interpret results effectively, and integrate them seamlessly into patient care.

The Council of Europe, and in particular the Steering Committee for Human Rights in the fields of Biomedicine and Health, has produced a report on the impact of AI on the doctor–patient relationship, underlining the importance of this issue in the disintegration of AI in modern healthcare [5–8].

To summarize, AI has undoubtedly the potential to enhance the physician–patient relationship by improving care quality and efficiency. However, its misuse or overuse could create barriers. To ensure that the use of AI tools will be for the benefit of the patients, they should be used in a complementary way and by no means replace the human involvement in healthcare decisions. A balance between technology and empathy is crucial to ensure that patient trust and satisfaction remain intact.

References

1. Omiye JA, Gui H, Daneshjou R, Cai ZR, Muralidharan V. Principles, applications and future of artificial intelligence in dermatology. Front Med. 2023;10:1278232.
2. Pai VV, Pai RB. Artificial intelligence in dermatology and healthcare: an overview. Indian J Dermatol Venereol Leprol. 2012;87:457–67.
3. Trettel A, Eissing L, Augustin M. Telemedicine in dermatology: findings and experiences worldwide – a systematic literature review. J Eur Acad Dermatol Venereol. 2017;32:215–24.
4. Hogarty DT, Su JC, Phan K, Attia M, Hossny M, Nahavandi S, et al. Artificial intelligence in dermatology-where we are and the way to the future: a review. Am J Clin Dermatol. 2019; https://doi.org/10.1007/s40257-019-00462-6.
5. Liopyris K, Gregoriou S, Dias J, Stratigos AJ. Artificial intelligence in dermatology: challenges and perspectives. Dermatol Ther (Heidelb). 2022;12:2637–51.
6. Tretter M, Ott T, Dabrock P. AI-produced certainties in healthcare: current and future challenges. AI Ethics. 2025;5:497–506.
7. Sohail N, Puyana C, Zimmerman L, Tsoukas M. Artificial intelligence in dermatology: bridging the gap in patient care and education. Clinica Dermatol. 2024;42:434–6.
8. Herrick G, Frasier K, Li V, Fritts H, Woolhiser E, Vinagolu-Baur J. Enhancing patient education and engagement through digital intelligence tools in dermatology. Int J Res Dermatol. 2024;10:391–400.
9. Yadav N, Pandey S, Gupta A, Dudani P, Gupta S, Rangarajan K. Data privacy in healthcare: in the era of artificial intelligence. Indian Dermatol Online J. 2023;14:788–92.
10. Nelson C, Perez-Chada LM, Creadore A, et al. Patient perspectives on the use of artificial intelligence for skin cancer screening. JAMA Dermatol. 2020;156:501–12.
11. Esteva A, Kuprel B, Novoa RA, Ko J, Swetter SM, Blau HM, et al. Dermatologists-level classification of skin cancer with deep neural networks. Nature. 2017;542:115–8.
12. Hekler A, Utikal JS, Enk AH, Berking C, Klode J, Schadendorf D, et al. Pathologist-level classification of histopathological melanoma images with deep neural networks. Eur J Cancer. 2019;115:79–83.
13. Chichi N, Takwoingi Y, Dinnes J, Matin RN, Bassett O, Moteau JF, et al. Smartphone applications for triaging adults with skin lesions that are suspicious for melanoma. Cochrane Database Syst Rev. 2018;12:CDO13192.
14. Fliorent R, Fardman B, Podwojniak A, Javaid K, Tan IJ, Ghani C. Artificial intelligence in dermatology: advancements and challenges in skin color. Inter J Dermatol. 2024;63:455–6.
15. Grzybowski A, Jin K, Wu H. Challenges of artificial intelligence in medicine and dermatology. Clinics Dermatol. 2024;42:210–5.
16. Fan BE, Chow M, Winkler S. Artificial intelligence-generated facial images for medical education. Med Sci Educ. 2024;34:5–7.
17. Elder A, O'Donnel Cappelli M, Ring C, Saedi N. Artificial intelligence in cosmetic dermatology: an update on current trends. Clin Dermatol. 2024;42:216–20.
18. Kania B, Montecinos K, Goldberg DJ. Artificial intelligence in cosmetic dermatology. J Cosmetic Dermatol. 2024;23:3305–11.
19. Vatiwutipong P, Vachmanus S, Noraset T, Tuarob S. Artificial intelligence in cosmetic dermatology: a systematic literature review. IEEE Access. 2023; https://doi.org/10.1109/ACCESS.2023.3295001.

20. Zhang AD, Shirazi R, Vashi NA. Cosmetic dermatology in the digital age. J Clin Med. 2024;13:6953.
21. Park HJ. Patient perspectives on informed consent for medical AI: Aweb-based experiment. Digit Health. 2024;10 https://doi.org/10.1177/20552076241247938.
22. Wildan Gifari M, Samodro P, Wahyu Kurniawan D. Artificial intelligence toward personalized medicine. 2012;8:65–72.
23. Schork NJ. Artificial intelligence and personalized medicine. Cancer Treat Res. 2019;178:265–83.
24. Taherdoost H, Ghofrani A. AI's role in revolutionizing personalized medicine by reshaping pharmacogenomics and drug therapy. Intell Pharm. 2024;2:643–50.
25. Gallo C. Artificial intelligence for personalized genetics and new drug development: benefits and cautions. Bioengeneering. 2023;10:613.
26. Parekh ADE, Shaikh OA, Simran MS, Hasibuzzaman MA. Artificial intelligence (AI) in personalized medicine: AI-generated personalized therapy regimens based on genetic and medical history: short communication. Ann Med Surg. 2023;85:5831–3.
27. Carini C, Seyhan A. Tribulations and future opportunities for artificial intelligence in precision medicine. J Transl Med. 2024;22:411.
28. Aminololama-Shakeri S, Lopez JE. The doctor-patient relationship with artificial intelligence. AJR. 2019;212:308–10.
29. Sauerbrei A, Kerasidou A, Lucivero F, Hallowell N. The impact of artificial intelligence on the person-centred, doctor-patient relationship: some problems and solutions. BMC Med Inform Decis Mak. 2023:1–14. https://doi.org/10.1186/s12911-023-02162-y.
30. Mittelstadt B. The impact of artificial intelligence on the doctor-patient relationship. Report commissioned by the Steering Committee for human rights in the fields of biomedicine and health. Council of Europe, December 2021, pp 1–67.

Part II

Artificial Intelligence in Skin Cancer Diagnosis and Management

6 Artificial Intelligence in Non-melanoma Skin Cancer

Dimitrios Sgouros, Melpomeni Theofilli, and Georgia Pappa

6.1 Introduction

Non-melanoma skin cancers (NMSC)—primarily basal cell carcinoma (BCC) and cutaneous squamous cell carcinoma (cSCC)—represent the most frequently diagnosed malignancies worldwide [1]. Together, they account for over five million new cases annually, with BCC alone comprising nearly 80% of all skin cancer diagnoses [2]. Despite their generally low metastatic potential and favorable long-term prognosis, NMSC contribute significantly to morbidity, recurrence rates, and rising healthcare costs, largely due to their high prevalence and potential for local tissue destruction when not promptly treated [2–4].

The incorporation of artificial intelligence (AI) into clinical diagnosis and subsequent work-up has brought about a substantial change in dermatological practice nowadays. Once considered a theoretical innovation, AI has become a practical and crucial tool in dermatology. Image-based diagnostics, histopathological analysis, clinical decision-making, surgical planning, and patient education are just a few of the areas of skin cancer care that AI technologies are starting to impact [5]. Although

D. Sgouros (✉)
2nd Department of Dermatology and Venereology, "Attikon" General University Hospital, Medical School, National and Kapodistrian University of Athens, Athens, Greece

M. Theofilli
1st Department of Dermatology-Venereology, "Andreas Syggros" Hospital for Cutaneous and Venereal Diseases, National and Kapodistrian University of Athens, Medical School, Athens, Greece

G. Pappa
2nd Department of Dermatology and Venereology, "Attikon" General University Hospital, Medical School, National and Kapodistrian University of Athens, Athens, Greece

1st Department of Dermatology-Venereology, "Andreas Syggros" Hospital for Cutaneous and Venereal Diseases, National and Kapodistrian University of Athens, Medical School, Athens, Greece

E. Karampinis et al. (eds.), *Artificial Intelligence Applications in Dermatology*,
https://doi.org/10.1007/978-3-032-15614-3_6

melanoma has been the primary focus of AI research in dermatology, mainly due to its high mortality rate and distinctive clinical presentation, NMSC present an equally important yet less explored area. NMSC have predictable biological behavior, high frequency, and well-defined clinical and histological features, and they are technologically feasible and accessible due to their high incidence [1, 2]. These characteristics make them ideal candidates for machine learning systems that rely on large datasets for accurate prediction.

AI systems are continuously improving at supporting clinicians with every aspect of care, from identifying suspicious lesions early on to assisting with individualized treatment choices. As AI continues to evolve, its role in the management of NMSC is becoming more prominent, offering the potential to improve diagnostic precision, reduce unnecessary biopsies and/or excisions, and ultimately enhance patient outcomes across various clinical settings.

In the following sections, we explore how AI has been integrated across various stages of NMSC management, including diagnostic support, therapeutic decision-making, prognostic assessment, and emerging clinical applications.

6.2 NMSC Diagnosis

One of the most well-developed uses of AI in NMSC is in image-based diagnosis. These AI tools are usually trained on large collections of preexisting images collected from real-world clinical settings. The quality of training data used for AI in NMSC varies widely. Some images are generated by patients using their smartphones, often accompanied only by a clinical diagnosis. Others are high-resolution clinical or dermoscopic photos that have been confirmed by histopathologic examination. While both types of images can be useful, dermoscopic images are especially important; they provide the level of detail that AI needs to accurately detect and differentiate subtle features in NMSC that basic smartphone photos might fail to capture.

At the core of many of these AI systems is machine learning, a field of AI where algorithms learn to recognize patterns and improve over time by analyzing data, rather than explicit programming. A more advanced branch of this is convolutional neural networks (CNNs), which play a key role in analyzing dermatologic images. These deep learning models are designed to process visual information and automatically identify important features. Thus, they are particularly useful in distinguishing between benign and malignant skin lesions. In a head-to-head comparison, a dual CNN model performed significantly better when analyzing dermoscopic images than smartphone-captured photos [6]. The AI system achieved an area under the curve (AUC) of 0.911 with dermoscopic images versus 0.821 for smartphone images, along with a much higher sensitivity (95.3% vs. 75.3%, $p < 0.001$) [6]. These findings demonstrate that although AI can be useful in telemedicine, the quality of the images it receives, greatly affects its performance.

In real-world settings, AI diagnostic technologies are increasingly being used to assist in clinical decision-making. These systems analyze skin lesions and generate risk scores, helping clinicians decide whether a biopsy is necessary or if the patient should be referred to a specialist. In more advanced healthcare settings, AI has been integrated into dermoscopy platforms to assist in identifying early signs of keratinocytic tumors, such as BCC and cSCC, even when their features are subtle and easy to miss [6]. Meanwhile, some smartphone applications are evolving to do more than flag high-risk lesions; they can also offer preliminary differential diagnoses, providing clinicians with an extra layer of insight. This can be particularly beneficial in primary care or remote settings where access to dermatologic expertise may be limited [7].

Despite the advantages of dermoscopic imaging, AI has demonstrated strong diagnostic capabilities even when evaluating smartphone-acquired images. In certain studies, these algorithms achieved AUC values exceeding 80% when distinguishing BCC from benign lesions, and sensitivity greater than 90% when classifying lesions as benign or non-benign [8]. However, the sensitivity for explicitly identifying malignant lesions has been lower, around 76%, highlighting the ongoing need for clinical monitoring, particularly in ambiguous lesions or high-risk patients [8].

Beyond conventional photography, AI is being increasingly paired with non-traditional imaging and diagnostic technologies to further improve the accuracy of skin cancer detection. Reflectance confocal microscopy (RCM) allows in vivo imaging of skin architecture at nearly histological resolution, reaching from the stratum corneum down to the upper dermis [9]. This modality enables clinicians to examine skin lesions at the cellular level without the need for a biopsy. In recent years [9], AI has been applied to RCM for a variety of purposes, including automated localization of skin layers, detection of the dermal–epidermal junction, and classification of atypical cellular or vascular features associated with NMSC [10]. These tools have shown potential to increase diagnostic consistency, reduce interobserver variability, and support faster image interpretation. However, challenges remain, particularly related to image quality degradation, the large file size of RCM datasets, and phenotypic variability of lesions, which may limit algorithm performance in more heterogeneous populations.

A recent multicenter study introduced laser-induced plasma spectroscopy (LIPS) as an AI-compatible diagnostic tool. By capturing elemental and molecular emissions from the skin surface and analyzing them through a deep neural network, LIPS enabled the real-time, noninvasive classification of skin tumors. In a cohort of over 600 histologically confirmed lesions—including BCC, cSCC, and melanoma—the system achieved 94.6% sensitivity and 88.9% specificity, with subtype sensitivities of 95.2% for BCC and 93.8% for cSCC [11]. Notably, the technique was safe, with no reported tissue damage, and revealed unique emission spectra (e.g., calcium, iron, copper, sodium, and CN bands) that may reflect underlying tumor biology [11]. These findings highlight AI-coupled LIPS, as a promising, objective tool with potential applications in clinical and remote settings.

One of the most promising techniques involves combining complementary imaging modalities using AI-driven analysis. For example, the integration of spectroscopy with RCM, analyzed through a unified deep learning framework, has resulted in significant diagnostic advances. In this setup, sensitivity remained 100%, while specificity increased from 84.2% (using spectroscopy alone) to 92.4% [12]. This demonstrates the synergistic potential of multimodal AI systems, which combine morphological, cellular, and biochemical data to provide a more thorough and reliable diagnosis.

Infrared thermal imaging is another developing area of study, as it detects temperature differences across the skin's surface, which are typically indicative of underlying vascular or metabolic abnormalities linked with cancer [13]. When combined with deep learning, IRT has shown area under the curve (AUC) values ranging from 0.901 to 0.950, with sensitivity reaching 95% and specificity 83%, providing a practical, noninvasive alternative for use in settings where traditional dermoscopic evaluation is limited or unavailable [13, 14].

Beyond surface-based and optical modalities, AI is also increasingly being used in histopathological analysis to assist pathologists in identifying key features such as tumor margins, perineural invasion, and mitotic activity, hence improving diagnostic precision. In recent years, several research teams have developed deep learning algorithms capable of classifying a wide range of dermatopathologic entities [15–19]. One such model, trained on over 300 histologic slides covering 40 distinct skin tumor types, was able to detect BCC with 99% sensitivity and 100% specificity [20, 21]. Another algorithm showed comparable results, achieving 97.2% sensitivity for BCC and 95.3% for atypical cSCC [20, 21]. What makes these developments especially exciting is that the role of AI goes beyond simply flagging a lesion as benign or malignant. Some models are now capable of assessing degrees of atypia [22], identifying nuclear chromatin differences between actinic keratoses and early cSCC [23], and even supporting pathologists in margin assessment during surgical excisions [24]. These are areas where clinical interpretation can often be subjective and influenced by experience or context. AI can act as a consistent second opinion, offering objective analysis to support the clinician's assessment. While it doesn't replace clinicians, it can definitely enhance confidence in decision-making, especially in cases where features are subtle or ambiguous.

6.3 Screening and Triage

The integration of AI into the screening and triage processes for NMSC has shown promising advancements in enhancing early lesion detection. One such device, DermaSensor, employs elastic scattering spectroscopy combined with AI to evaluate lesions non-invasively. In a multicenter clinical validation study, DermaSensor demonstrated a sensitivity of 97.0% for detecting skin cancer, including 97.0% for both BCC and cSCC, comparable to the performance of expert dermatologists [25]. However, its specificity for benign lesions was only 22%, suggesting a higher rate of false positives. In public healthcare setting, the DERM AI platform developed by skin analytics has been adopted across multiple sites within the UK's National Health Service [26]. This AI-driven triage tool assists clinicians by analyzing lesion images submitted via teledermatology and flagging suspicious lesions for priority review. Evaluations have shown that DERM achieves a sensitivity of 97% for malignant melanoma, while also effectively identifying high-risk NMSC, resulting in reduced referral times and improved diagnostic pathways [26]. Recent large-scale data, spanning from December 2023 to October 2024, showed that AI systems achieved a sensitivity of 98% for cSCC (N = 529) and 98% for BCC (N = 1075), underscoring their reliability in identifying keratinocyte carcinomas [26]. These sensitivity levels are comparable to specialist performance, indicating AI's potential to support general practitioners and nonspecialist settings where dermatologic expertise may be limited.

In addition, the negative predictive value across all skin cancers reached 99.93%, suggesting strong reliability in ruling out malignancies when lesions are classified as benign [26]. However, specificity varied considerably depending on the reference standard: It was 79% among clinically and histologically confirmed benign lesions but dropped to 24% when only biopsy-confirmed benign cases were considered [26]. This variation highlights the importance of context in evaluating AI outputs and suggests that while AI tools are highly sensitive for detecting NMSC, their relatively lower specificity may contribute to increased false-positive rates. Despite these results, the consistently high sensitivity and negative predictive value underscore the utility of AI in triage settings, where the primary objective is to avoid missed malignancies. Consequently, AI technologies are being progressively integrated into teledermatology and primary care screening protocols to support early identification of high-risk NMSC and to facilitate more efficient referral to specialist care.

Moreover, in a recent meta-analysis, researchers compared AI models with clinicians and reported that AI achieved an overall sensitivity of 87.0% and specificity of 77.1%, comparable to expert Dermatologists [27]. Notably, AI significantly outperformed general practitioners, who had a sensitivity of 64.6% and specificity of 72.8%, underscoring the value of AI-assisted tools in primary care and underserved areas [27].

While these findings highlight the promise of AI in enhancing NMSC detection and streamlining triage, especially in settings with limited access to dermatologic care, its integration into everyday practice requires careful, ongoing evaluation. Real-world implementation studies, continuous algorithm refinement, and collaboration between clinicians and developers will be essential to ensure these tools are both clinically meaningful and easily incorporated across diverse healthcare settings.

6.4 NMSC Treatment

Artificial intelligence is increasingly being recognized not only as a diagnostic aid but also as a valuable tool in the therapeutic management of NMSC. While the majority of current AI applications focus on lesion recognition, several systems are emerging that assist with treatment decision-making, surgical planning, intraoperative guidance, and follow-up care. These technologies are not intended to replace clinical expertise, but rather to support it—organizing workflows efficiently, enhancing precision, and allowing for more personalized treatment strategies.

In surgical dermatology, particularly during Mohs micrographic surgery, time and accuracy are of paramount importance. To this end, deep learning models—most commonly CNNs—have been trained to identify residual tumor tissue on digitized histological slides. These models can assist the Mohs surgeon by rapidly flagging areas suspicious for remaining cancer, supporting real-time margin assessment. Notably, a recent study demonstrated that an AI-driven BCC detection and tumor mapping algorithm achieved a 94% accuracy rate in identifying tumor presence and location, showing high concordance with surgeon-generated maps [28]. Although slightly below the gold-standard human accuracy, the system performed well enough to be integrated in a non-autonomous manner, meaning it assisted but did not replace the surgeon in decision-making [28].

The impact of this integration goes beyond accuracy. In a simulated 20-day implementation, the algorithm reduced slide waiting time by 35.6% and led to an 18% reduction in both staff and histotechnician waiting times [28]. These efficiencies were most pronounced on days involving complex reconstructions or multiple tumor removal stages. By shortening these critical waiting periods, the algorithm allowed nurses and histotechnicians to anticipate next steps earlier and enabled the surgeon to move between cases more efficiently. Furthermore, by enabling multiple workflow steps to occur in parallel rather than sequentially, this approach streamlines the surgical process, reduces overall procedure duration, and optimizes resource use.

Beyond the microscope, AI has also been used to predict the complexity of surgical procedures [29]. By analyzing variables such as lesion size, anatomical location, patient age, and whether the cancer is primary or recurrent, machine learning algorithms can estimate the likelihood of requiring multiple Mohs stages or advanced reconstruction techniques like flaps or grafts [29]. This helps surgeons better prepare for challenging cases, allows for more accurate scheduling, and improves patient counseling before surgery.

Another area where AI shows promise is in guiding treatment selection. Not all NMSC require the same approach; some lesions may be treated effectively with excision or cryotherapy, while others warrant referral for MMS or consideration of nonsurgical options. AI-based decision-support systems have been developed to recommend treatment strategies by synthesizing clinical, histologic, and demographic data. In one study focused on nasal BCCs—a particularly challenging site due to its functional and cosmetic importance—a supervised machine learning algorithm was able to predict multidisciplinary team recommendations with notable accuracy [30]. The model reliably triaged 37.5% of patients to Mohs micrographic surgery based on factors such as tumor location and patient age, and predicted the overall multidisciplinary team recommendations treatment decision in 45.1% of cases [30]. While these tools are still in early phases of adoption, they suggest a future in which AI may help standardize care and reduce treatment variability, especially in resource-limited settings.

For patients with locally advanced or inoperable tumors, AI has also been explored in the context of radiotherapy planning and response prediction. Neural networks trained on patient profiles, tumor characteristics, and treatment outcomes have been able to predict who is most likely to respond favorably to radiation therapy. For example, a study applying fourth-generation artificial neural networks to patients with cSCC of the scalp uncovered four distinct response profiles that were not identifiable using conventional statistical methods [31]. These profiles included: (a) patients aged 70–80 years with stage T2 tumors, (b) patients under 70 with frontal scalp lesions, (c) those with nonrecurrent, nodular, or nodulo-ulcerated stage T3 tumors of the vertex treated with doses above 60 Gy, and (d) patients with flat, occipital, stage T1 tumors treated with 50–59 Gy [31]. The predictive model achieved impressive performance metrics, with 85.7% sensitivity, 97.6% specificity, and 91.7% overall accuracy [31]. These findings suggest that machine learning may serve as a valuable tool in patient stratification, potentially guiding more personalized therapeutic decisions and helping clinicians better assess the risk–benefit balance of radiotherapy, particularly in complex or borderline cases.

6.5 NMSC Prognosis and Follow-Up

As mentioned earlier, the role of AI has expanded to histopathology, where it is beginning to redefine how we assess tumor behavior and thus, guide patient management. In cSCC, where accurate risk stratification is essential yet often complex, AI-driven analysis of routine slides offers a novel approach. A notable advancement in this area is the development of the Cellular Morphometric Risk Score (CMRS), an AI-derived tool that quantifies morphologic features at the cellular level to classify cSCC into prognostically relevant subgroups [32]. When integrated with the established Brigham and Women's Hospital (BWH) staging system, prognostic accuracy improves substantially [32]. The combined model achieves concordance indices of 0.92 for predicting local recurrence and 0.91 for nodal metastasis—metrics that highlight its clinical value [32]. Additionally, it improves key performance indicators: negative predictive value increases from 94.4% to 96.0%, positive predictive value from 36.4% to 41.7%, and overall accuracy from 86.8% to 89.2% [32].

AI is also playing an increasingly meaningful role in the post-treatment surveillance of patients with NMSC [33]. Given the probable relapsing nature of these malignancies, especially in patients with a history of multiple lesions, field cancerization, or genetic syndromes such as Gorlin-Goltz, ongoing follow-up can be both labor-intensive and time-consuming. AI-powered algorithms are being developed to analyze sequential clinical and dermoscopic images over time, aiming to identify subtle morphologic changes that may indicate early recurrence or the development of new lesions [33]. This approach is particularly promising in teledermatology, where remote monitoring can be combined with AI triage systems to prioritize follow-up for lesions that demonstrate worrisome patterns over time.

6.6 Patient Education

Large language models (LLMs) like ChatGPT are starting to transform how both clinicians and patients interact with medical information, even in fields where they weren't originally designed to operate, such as dermatology. While these models weren't built with skin cancer in mind, they've already shown surprising utility in several dermatologic contexts. For instance, they can help rephrase complex pathology reports into language that patients can actually understand, or guide someone searching online about a new diagnosis of cutaneous cancer with relatively clear and informative responses [34]. Some studies have even explored using LLMs to draft treatment summaries or support clinicians in building patient education materials [35].

These models can sometimes generate information that sounds convincing but is factually arbitrary or inaccurate, a phenomenon known as "hallucination" or "confabulation" [36]. Moreover, these models, while impressive, lack the depth of clinical reasoning inherent to medical professionals, and as a result, they might miss important details [37]. Their responses can vary depending on how a question is phrased or what version of the model is being used, which may create confusion or even misinformation if used without supervision [38]. That said, we are rapidly moving into a space where more specialized models, such as Med-PaLM, or fine-tuned versions of ChatGPT trained specifically on dermatology or oncology data, may begin to bridge these gaps [39–41]. These tailored systems could eventually become useful companions in clinical settings: helping with documentation, automating routine patient communications, or supporting decision-making through evidence-informed suggestions.

6.7 Pitfalls

While AI has shown impressive performance in identifying NMSC, it still faces important limitations, especially in anatomically complex sites, rare histologic variants, and clinically ambiguous presentations. One of the fundamental weaknesses of current AI models is their dependence on training datasets, which are often skewed toward common tumor types and lack adequate representation of adnexal neoplasms, traumatized lesions, and tumors located on special anatomic sites. As a result, the generalizability of these models is inherently restricted across diverse clinical scenarios that may fall outside their "learned" spectrum.

Trained on more than 66,000 annotated dermoscopic images, DEXI (Dermoscopy EXplainable Intelligence) is an AI-powered diagnostic engine developed by Canfield that assists clinicians by scoring lesions, generating explainable image-based assessments. In our clinical practice, we utilize the Canfield platform, incorporating DEXI, which has shown high diagnostic sensitivity and specificity for keratinocytic malignancies, particularly basal cell carcinoma (BCC), even under routine, real-world conditions. The algorithm reliably detects lesions with classic dermoscopic features such as arborizing vessels, blue-gray ovoid nests, and

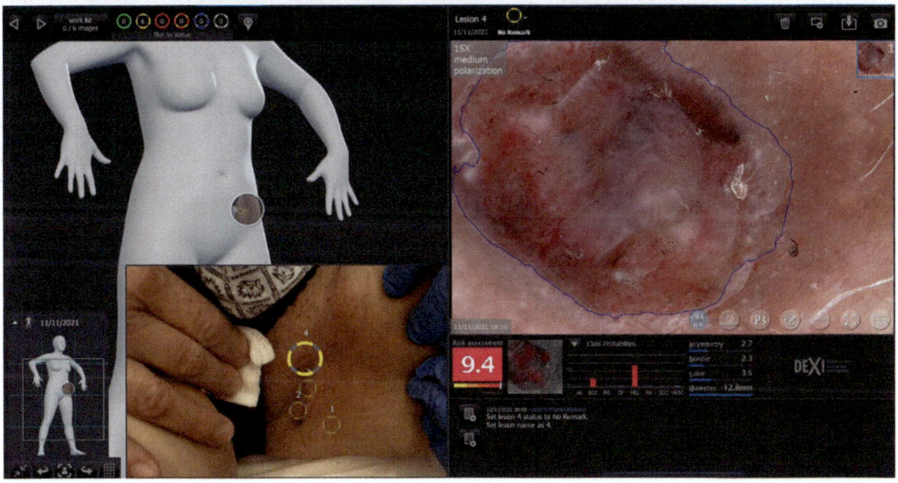

Fig. 6.1 AI misclassification of pigmented basal cell carcinomas on the vulvar region as melanomas in a 56-year-old female patient

ulceration. However, we have observed limitations in specific contexts, especially in intertriginous regions or mucosal areas (e.g., genitalia and lips), where lesion morphology may differ from that typically seen in training datasets.

In one such case (Fig. 6.1), involving a 56-year-old female with three pigmented BCCs on the outer labia, the system correctly identified the lesions as malignant but erroneously classified all three as melanomas, a diagnosis that would be considered highly improbable by an experienced dermatologist. Nonetheless, trauma-induced changes remain a confounding factor for the algorithm. In one such case (Fig. 6.2), a keratoacanthoma, dermoscopically characterized by the typical white circles, was misclassified, likely due to surface crusting and hemorrhagic features that disrupted pattern recognition. Technical factors can also impact diagnostic accuracy. In one example, when the imaging probe was not firmly or evenly attached to the lesion surface, the system produced an initial result suggestive of BCC (Fig. 6.3a). However, once the probe was repositioned with proper contact and lighting, the same lesion was confidently classified as BCC (Fig. 6.3b). This case underscores the importance of consistent probe application, lighting conditions, and pressure—all of which can influence image quality and, in turn, algorithmic interpretation.

Equally noteworthy is a case (Fig. 6.4) in which a patient correctly suspected the development of a new BCC at the site of a previously excised lentigo maligna on the upper back. Clinically and dermoscopically, the lesion had several features that could have easily raised suspicion for melanoma recurrence, particularly given the location on a scar and the presence of pigmentation. Nonetheless, the AI system correctly classified the lesion as a BCC, an outcome that aligned with histopathologic confirmation.

While these examples are isolated and derived from a single system in a specific clinical setting, they underscore a broader issue: the evolving yet imperfect nature

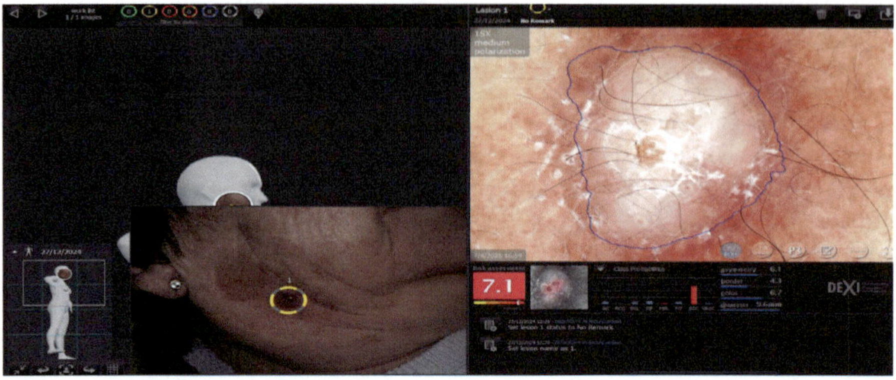

Fig. 6.2 A keratoacanthoma on the right cheek of an 81-year-old female, showing surface crusting and hemorrhagic changes due to repeated manipulation of the lesion. Trauma-related changes prevented AI's ability to provide accurate lesion identification

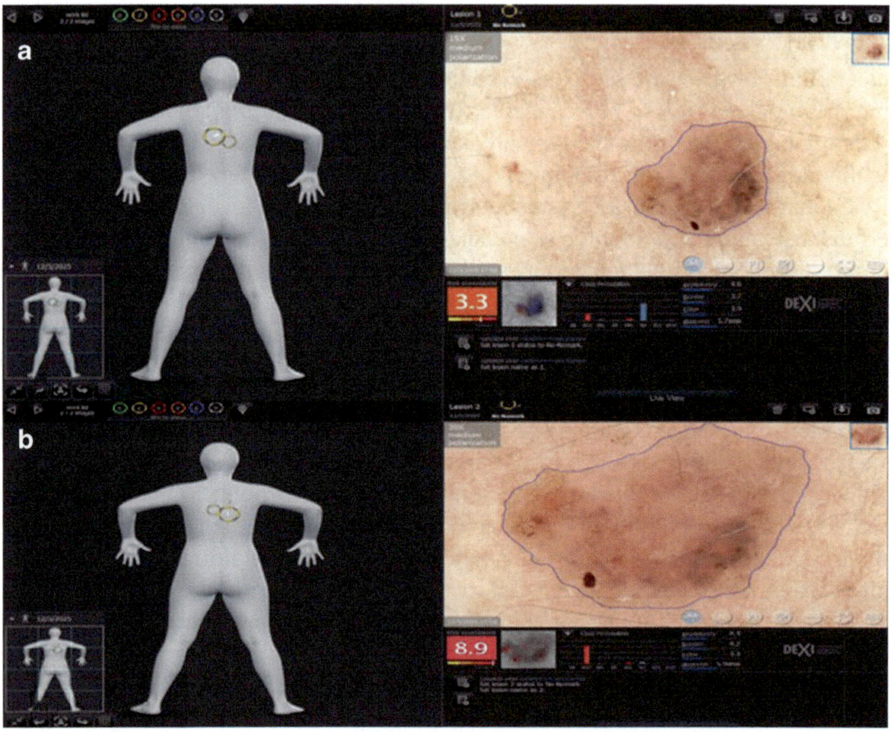

Fig. 6.3 (**a**) Initial scan of a lesion with poor probe contact, resulting in an uncertain suggestion of basal cell carcinoma. (**b**) Better contact and lighting enabled accurate classification of the same lesion as basal cell carcinoma with a higher AI-derived risk score of 8.9 vs 3.3 on the initial scan

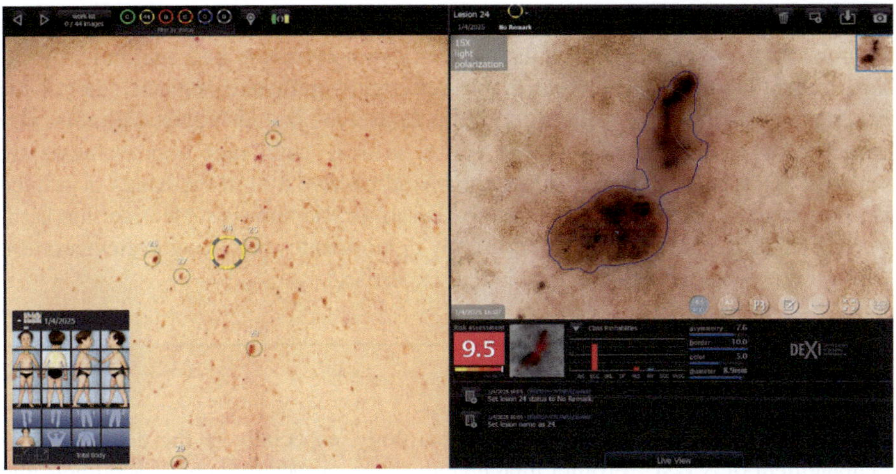

Fig. 6.4 Pigmented lesion on a scar from prior lentigo maligna excision. Despite clinical and dermoscopic features suggestive of melanoma recurrence, AI accurately identified the lesion as basal cell carcinoma

of current AI systems in cutaneous oncology. Indeed, although AI can augment visual inspection and dermoscopic interpretation, it remains insufficient as a standalone diagnostic tool, particularly in diagnostically ambiguous or rare presentations.

AI systems may misdiagnose BCC by confusing it with other lesions that exhibit similar dermoscopic features. For example, adnexal tumors (e.g., desmoplastic trichoepithelioma or trichoblastoma) may display arborizing vessels or shiny white structures, which can closely resemble the dermoscopic appearance of BCC. Likewise, microcystic adnexal carcinoma may present with nonspecific vascular patterns or white areas, leading to misclassification. In heavily pigmented dermatofibromas, the blue-gray areas or homogeneous dark pigmentation can mimic the blue-gray globules or ovoid nests of pigmented BCC, especially in anatomical areas where image quality and pattern clarity may be suboptimal.

Similarly, cSCC may be incorrectly identified as actinic keratosis or seborrheic keratosis, particularly when dominated by scaling, crusting, or surface keratin, which can obscure malignant clues. AI may also confuse cSCC with keratoacanthoma, as both may show central keratin, white circles, and vascular structures such as hairpin or dotted vessels. Inflammatory dermatoses, such as psoriasis or eczema, may further complicate classification due to overlapping features such as erythema, scale, or erosion, which are common in both malignant and benign lesions under dermoscopy. Additionally, certain poorly differentiated BCCs, especially in the spectrum of basosquamous carcinoma, may exhibit dermoscopic features such as central ulceration, crust, or nonspecific vascular patterns, making them difficult to distinguish from cSCC. These overlapping features can lead to significant misclassification when context is not accounted for.

Moving forward, future AI systems must be designed with greater contextual awareness. Incorporating metadata such as lesion evolution and anatomical location, patient history, and previous diagnoses could significantly enhance diagnostic accuracy. Furthermore, expanding training datasets to include adnexal tumors, rare variants, and diverse skin types will also be critical. Until such improvements are realized, AI should be viewed as a valuable adjunctive tool in the hands of trained Dermatologists, particularly for common keratinocytic tumors such as actinic keratosis, BCC, and cSCC, where dermoscopy demonstrates high diagnostic accuracy. However, it is not a substitute for clinical expertise.

6.8 Conclusion

AI is becoming a valuable asset in dermatology, especially in the diagnosis and management of NMSC. Prompt image analysis, improved diagnostic accuracy, and expanded support for clinicians in both specialized and resource-limited settings are just a few of its useful benefits. AI is best suited to support human judgment rather than replace it, helping to expedite processes and offering assistance in complicated or unclear cases. The limitations of the training data are frequently reflected in current systems, which can negatively affect performance when dealing with diverse patient populations and unusual presentations. These systems also lack the clinical context that dermatologists routinely use, such as lesion history, patient risk factors, and subtle visual cues—factors that are difficult to quantify but often crucial to the correct diagnosis. Developing more representative and clinically integrated models is the way forward. As these technologies advance, their function will likely develop into an incorporated tool of everyday clinical practice in the overall NMSC management.

References

1. Bashline B. Skin cancer: squamous and basal cell carcinomas. FP Essent. 2019;481:17–22.
2. Chen JT, Kempton SJ, Rao VK. The economics of skin cancer: an analysis of Medicare payment data. Plast Reconstr Surg Glob Open. 2016;4(9):e868. https://doi.org/10.1097/GOX.0000000000000826.
3. Barton V, Armeson K, Hampras S, Ferris LK, Visvanathan K, Rollison D, et al. Nonmelanoma skin cancer and risk of all-cause and cancer-related mortality: a systematic review. Arch Dermatol Res. 2017;309(4):243–51. https://doi.org/10.1007/s00403-017-1724-5.
4. Lazareth V. Management of non-melanoma skin cancer. Semin Oncol Nurs. 2013;29(3):182–94. https://doi.org/10.1016/j.soncn.2013.06.004.
5. Puri P, Comfere N, Drage LA, Shamim H, Bezalel SA, Pittelkow MR, et al. Deep learning for dermatologists: part II. Current applications. J Am Acad Dermatol. 2022;87(6):1352–60. https://doi.org/10.1016/j.jaad.2020.05.053.
6. Dascalu A, Walker BN, Oron Y, David EO. Non-melanoma skin cancer diagnosis: a comparison between dermoscopic and smartphone images by unified visual and sonification deep learning algorithms. J Cancer Res Clin Oncol. 2022;148(9):2497–505. https://doi.org/10.1007/s00432-021-03809-x.

7. Kränke T, Tripolt-Droschl K, Röd L, Hofmann-Wellenhof R, Koppitz M, Tripolt M. New AI-algorithms on smartphones to detect skin cancer in a clinical setting—a validation study. PLoS One. 2023;18(2):e0280670. https://doi.org/10.1371/journal.pone.0280670.
8. Kalwa U, Legner C, Kong T, Pandey S. Skin cancer diagnostics with an all-inclusive smartphone application. Symmetry. 2019;11(6):790. https://doi.org/10.3390/sym11060790.
9. Takiddin A, Schneider J, Yang Y, Abd-Alrazaq A, Househ M. Artificial intelligence for skin cancer detection: scoping review. J Med Internet Res. 2021;23(11):e22934. https://doi.org/10.2196/22934.
10. Patel RH, Foltz EA, Witkowski A, Ludzik J. Analysis of artificial intelligence-based approaches applied to non-invasive imaging for early detection of melanoma: a systematic review. Cancers (Basel). 2023;15(19) https://doi.org/10.3390/cancers15194694.
11. Pyun SH, Min W, Goo B, Seit S, Azzi A, Yu-Shun Wong D, et al. Real-time, in vivo skin cancer triage by laser-induced plasma spectroscopy combined with a deep learning-based diagnostic algorithm. J Am Acad Dermatol. 2023;89(1):99–105. https://doi.org/10.1016/j.jaad.2022.06.1166.
12. Chen M, Feng X, Fox MC, Reichenberg JS, Lopes F, Sebastian KR, et al. Deep learning on reflectance confocal microscopy improves Raman spectral diagnosis of basal cell carcinoma. J Biomed Opt. 2022;27(6) https://doi.org/10.1117/1.JBO.27.6.065004.
13. Godoy SE, Ramirez DA, Myers SA, von Winckel G, Krishna S, Berwick M, et al. Dynamic infrared imaging for skin cancer screening. Infrared Phys Technol. 2015;70:147–52.
14. Magalhaes C, Tavares JMRS, Mendes J, Vardasca R. Comparison of machine learning strategies for infrared thermography of skin cancer. Biomed Signal Process Control. 2021;69:102872.
15. Thomas SM, Lefevre JG, Baxter G, Hamilton NA. Non-melanoma skin cancer segmentation for histopathology dataset. Data Brief. 2021;39:107587. https://doi.org/10.1016/j.dib.2021.107587.
16. Kriegsmann K, Lobers F, Zgorzelski C, Kriegsmann J, Janssen C, Meliss RR, et al. Deep learning for the detection of anatomical tissue structures and neoplasms of the skin on scanned histopathological tissue sections. Front Oncol. 2022;12:1022967. https://doi.org/10.3389/fonc.2022.1022967. Erratum in: Front Oncol. 2023 May 18;13:1201237. https://doi.org/10.3389/fonc.2023.1201237.
17. Zhou Y, Koyuncu C, Lu C, Grobholz R, Katz I, Madabhushi A, et al. Multi-site cross-organ calibrated deep learning (MuSClD): automated diagnosis of non-melanoma skin cancer. Med Image Anal. 2023;84:102702. https://doi.org/10.1016/j.media.2022.102702.
18. Duschner N, Baguer DO, Schmidt M, Griewank KG, Hadaschik E, Hetzer S, et al. Applying an artificial intelligence deep learning approach to routine dermatopathological diagnosis of basal cell carcinoma. J Dtsch Dermatol Ges. 2023;21(11):1329–37. https://doi.org/10.1111/ddg.15180.
19. Le'Clerc Arrastia J, Heilenkotter N, Otero Baguer D, Hauberg-Lotte L, Boskamp T, Hetzer S, et al. Deeply supervised UNet for semantic segmentation to assist dermatopathological assessment of basal cell carcinoma. J Imaging. 2021;7(4) https://doi.org/10.3390/jimaging7040071.
20. Requa J, Godard T, Mandal R, Balzer B, Whittemore D, George E, et al. High-fidelity detection, subtyping, and localization of five skin neoplasms using supervised and semi-supervised learning. J Pathol Inform. 2023;14:100159. https://doi.org/10.1016/j.jpi.2022.100159.
21. Brodsky V, Levine L, Solans EP, Dola S, Chervony L, Polak S. Performance of automated classification of diagnostic entities in dermatopathology validated on multisite data representing the real-world variability of pathology workload. Arch Pathol Lab Med. 2023;147(9):1093–8. https://doi.org/10.5858/arpa.2021-0550-OA.
22. Fischman S, Perez-Anker J, Tognetti L, Di Naro A, Suppa M, Cinotti E, et al. Non-invasive scoring of cellular atypia in keratinocyte cancers in 3D LC-OCT images using deep learning. Sci Rep. 2022;12(1):481. https://doi.org/10.1038/s41598-021-04395-1.
23. Krouse RS, Alberts DS, Prasad AR, Yozwiak M, Bartels HG, Liu Y, et al. Progression of skin lesions from normal skin to squamous cell carcinoma. Anal Quant Cytol Histol. 2009;31(1):17–25.

24. Wako BD, Dese K, Ulfata RE, Nigatu TA, Turunbedu SK, Kwa T. Squamous cell carcinoma of skin cancer margin classification from digital histopathology images using deep learning. Cancer Control. 2022;29:10732748221132528. https://doi.org/10.1177/10732748221132528.
25. Manolakos D, Patrick G, Geisse JK, Rabinovitz H, Buchanan K, Hoang P, et al. Use of an elastic-scattering spectroscopy and artificial intelligence device in the assessment of lesions suggestive of skin cancer: a comparative effectiveness study. JAAD Int. 2024;14:52–8. https://doi.org/10.1016/j.jdin.2023.08.019.
26. Skin Analytics. DERM AI performance in the NHS pathway. 2023. Available from: https://skin-analytics.com/ai-pathways/derm-performance/. Last accessed on 18 May 2025.
27. Salinas MP, Sepúlveda J, Hidalgo L, Peirano D, Morel M, Uribe P, et al. A systematic review and meta-analysis of artificial intelligence versus clinicians for skin cancer diagnosis. NPJ Digit Med. 2024;7(1):125. https://doi.org/10.1038/s41746-024-01103-x. Erratum in: NPJ Digit Med. 2024 May 24;7(1):141. https://doi.org/10.1038/s41746-024-01138-0.
28. Chacko R, Davis MJ, Levy J, LeBoeuf M. Integration of a deep learning basal cell carcinoma detection and tumor mapping algorithm into the Mohs micrographic surgery workflow and effects on clinical staffing: a simulated, retrospective study. JAAD Int. 2024;15:185–91. https://doi.org/10.1016/j.jdin.2024.02.014.
29. Shoham G, Berl A, Shir-Az O, Shabo S, Shalom A. Predicting Mohs surgery complexity by applying machine learning to patient demographics and tumor characteristics. Exp Dermatol. 2022;31(7):1029–35. https://doi.org/10.1111/exd.14550.
30. Andrew TW, Hamnett N, Roy I, Garioch J, Nobes J, Moncrieff MD. Machine-learning algorithm to predict multidisciplinary team treatment recommendations in the management of basal cell carcinoma. Br J Cancer. 2022;126(4):562–8. https://doi.org/10.1038/s41416-021-01506-7.
31. Damiani G, Grossi E, Berti E, Conic RRZ, Radhakrishna U, Pacifico A, et al. Artificial neural networks allow response prediction in squamous cell carcinoma of the scalp treated with radiotherapy. J Eur Acad Dermatol Venereol. 2020;34(6):1369–73. https://doi.org/10.1111/jdv.16210.
32. Perez-Baena MJ, Mao JH, Perez-Losada J, Santos-Briz A, Chang H, Canueto J. Artificial intelligence-empowered cellular morphometric risk score improves prognostic stratification of cutaneous squamous cell carcinoma. Clin Exp Dermatol. 2024;49(7):692–8. https://doi.org/10.1093/ced/llad264.
33. Sharma AN, Shwe S, Mesinkovska NA. Current state of machine learning for non-melanoma skin cancer. Arch Dermatol Res. 2022;314(4):325–7. https://doi.org/10.1007/s00403-021-02236-9.
34. Aydin S, Karabacak M, Vlachos V, Margetis K. Large language models in patient education: a scoping review of applications in medicine. Front Med (Lausanne). 2024;11:1477898. https://doi.org/10.3389/fmed.2024.1477898.
35. Mondal H, Panigrahi M, Mishra B, Behera JK, Mondal S. A pilot study on the capability of artificial intelligence in preparation of patients' educational materials for Indian public health issues. J Family Med Prim Care. 2023;12(8):1659–62. https://doi.org/10.4103/jfmpc.jfmpc_262_23.
36. Farquhar S, Kossen J, Kuhn L, Gal Y. Detecting hallucinations in large language models using semantic entropy. Nature. 2024;630(8017):625–30. https://doi.org/10.1038/s41586-024-07421-0.
37. Lievin V, Hother CE, Motzfeldt AG, Winther O. Can large language models reason about medical questions? Patterns (NY). 2024;5(3):100943. https://doi.org/10.1016/j.patter.2024.100943.
38. Shiferaw MW, Zheng T, Winter A, Mike LA, Chan LN. Assessing the accuracy and quality of artificial intelligence (AI) chatbot-generated responses in making patient-specific drug-therapy and healthcare-related decisions. BMC Med Inform Decis Mak. 2024;24(1):404. https://doi.org/10.1186/s12911-024-02824-5.
39. Anisuzzaman DM, Malins JG, Friedman PA, Attia ZI. Fine-tuning large language models for specialized use cases. Mayo Clin Proc Digit Health. 2025;3(1):100184. https://doi.org/10.1016/j.mcpdig.2024.11.005.

40. Singhal K, Tu T, Gottweis J, Sayres R, Wulczyn E, Amin M, et al. Toward expert-level medical question answering with large language models. Nat Med. 2025;31(3):943–50. https://doi.org/10.1038/s41591-024-03423-7.
41. Singhal K, Azizi S, Tu T, Mahdavi SS, Wei J, Chung HW, et al. Large language models encode clinical knowledge. Nature. 2023;620(7972):172–80. https://doi.org/10.1038/s41586-023-06455-0.

Melanoma and Artificial Intelligence

7

Olga Toli, Cristian Navarrete-Dechent,
Emmanouil Karampinis, and Alexander Stratigos

7.1 AI in Melanoma Diagnosis

The diagnosis of melanoma is based on clinical and histopathologic examination. Conventional methods such as visual inspection and dermoscopy have improved diagnostic precision, but these approaches are still limited by the variability in physician expertise and subjective interpretation of dermoscopic and histopathologic features. Additionally, many areas of the world are underserved, making dermatological evaluations unavailable. The integration of artificial intelligence (AI) and particularly deep learning and convolutional neural networks (CNNs), into clinical settings is transforming skin cancer diagnostics. Unlike traditional computer-aided diagnostic (CAD) systems, which rely on handcrafted features, CNNs autonomously learn and refine patterns through exposure to large image datasets, which lead to high diagnostic accuracy.

O. Toli
Dermatology Department, Oncoderm Center One Day Clinic, Ioannina, Greece

C. Navarrete-Dechent
Department of Dermatology, Escuela de Medicina, Pontificia Universidad Católica de Chile, Santiago, Chile

Melanoma and Skin Cancer Unit, Escuela de Medicina, Pontificia Universidad Católica de Chile, Santiago, Chile

E. Karampinis (✉)
Second Dermatology Department, School of Health Sciences, Aristotle University of Thessaloniki, Thessaloniki, Greece

Department of Dermatology, Faculty of Medicine, School of Health Sciences, University General Hospital of Larissa, University of Thessaly, Larissa, Greece

A. Stratigos
First Department of Dermatology-Venereology, Medical School, National and Kapodistrian University of Athens, 'A. Sygros' Hospital for Skin and Venereal Diseases, Athens, Greece

E. Karampinis et al. (eds.), *Artificial Intelligence Applications in Dermatology*,
https://doi.org/10.1007/978-3-032-15614-3_7

7.2 AI in Melanoma Diagnosis: Image-Based Detection and Dermoscopic Analysis

Over the last decades, the melanoma incidence rates have risen sharply, leading to a high focus on early detection and prevention. It is proven by several studies that dermoscopy significantly improves the diagnostic accuracy compared to the naked eye examination. Pocket dermoscopy enables the bedside evaluation of suspicious lesions. Additionally, for patients with multiple nevi, digital dermoscopy has improved the evaluation of the so-called atypical mole syndrome. A two-step method was initially introduced to assist in identifying new or changing melanocytic lesions through comparison of baseline images with subsequent images over time via the combination of total body photography (TBP) and sequential digital dermoscopy (SDD) [1, 2]. This method proved to be very specific and sensitive, was able to decrease significantly the number of excisions, especially in high-risk melanoma patients and improved the detection of thin melanomas [3, 4]. However, two of the major limitations of the TBP–SDD are that it is very time-consuming and that it is dependent on the level of dermatologists' and medical practitioners' expertise and the image quality. Consequently, this has highlighted the need for standardization and objective evaluation of melanocytic lesions. Nowadays, these limitations have been addressed, and recent technological advancements have been introduced in clinical practice. High-resolution polarized 2D TBP systems, automated lesion identification, risk scoring, and the advent of 3D full-body scanners offer innovative approaches for patient imaging, producing avatar-like reconstructions that enable rapid lesion analysis and monitoring (Figs. 7.1 and 7.2) [5, 6].

The classification of single lesions, particularly melanocytic neoplasms, using image-based inputs is one of the most well-studied applications of AI in dermatology. Clinical and dermoscopic images are used to train these models to distinguish between benign and malignant lesions. Within this framework, AI applications are able to classify the lesion, taking into account mainly the dermoscopic and clinical macroscopic image analysis but also in some cases by integrating metadata such as age, lesion site, or risk factors. Landmark studies by *Esteva* et al *(2017), Tchandl* et al *(2019),* and *Haenssle* et al. *(2018)* have shown that deep learning models—when applied to single-lesion classification tasks—can achieve diagnostic performance same as board-certified dermatologists or even outperform expert dermatologists [7–9]. However, these AI applications reflect a controlled diagnostic setting far from the routine clinical complexity, because they have been primarily validated in controlled clinical scenarios and retrospective clinical studies, involving biopsy-proven lesions and fixed image inputs.

In contrast, when dealing with patients with high nevus counts, atypical mole syndrome, or a personal/family history of melanoma, a different and arguably more holistic clinical approach is needed, such as longitudinal monitoring. This can be achieved by applying AI-enhanced TBP systems that are designed to process wide-field, full-body images and track changes over time rather than assessing and classifying each lesion solely. Lesion segmentation and localization, change detection across sequential images, skin phenotype quantification, and

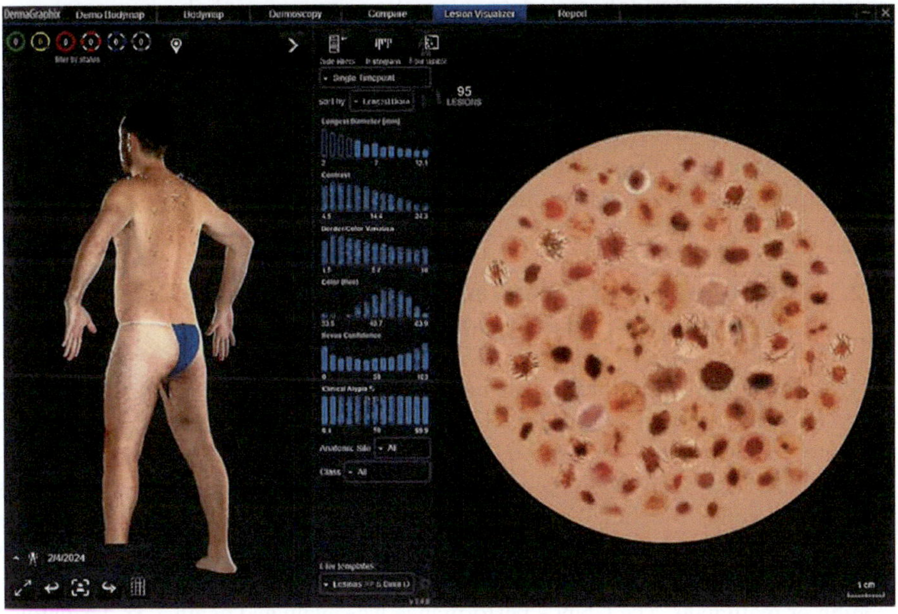

Fig. 7.1 Canfield's lesion visualizer identifies and measures lesions greater than 2.0 mm in 3D and 2D TBP [94]. The comprehensive display helps clinicians identify outlying lesions that merit further investigation. Integrated AI and ML models provide valuable metrics on nevus confidence and clinical atypia [95, 96]. Large, worldwide challenges have been built atop of Canfield's WB360 lesion visualizer lesion images and measurements for further development of AI models to identify melanoma [97]. (Image reproduced with permission from Canfield© All rights retained)

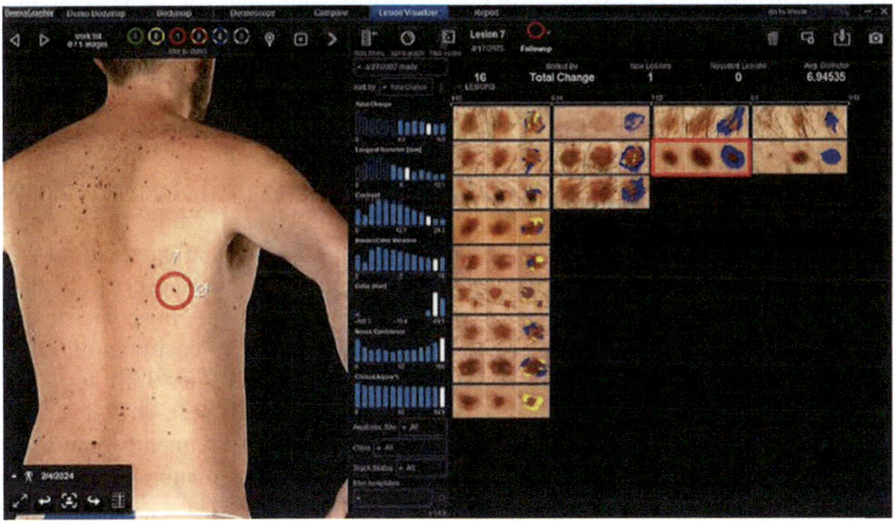

Fig. 7.2 Canfield's lesion visualizer change module uses markerless tracking to register 3D or 2D total body images, allowing the measurement of lesion change and identification of new or evolving lesions. Promising results have been obtained by combining this lesion change algorithm with Canfield's dermoscopic AI, DEXI [98]. (Image reproduced with permission from Canfield © All rights retained)

risk stratification through metadata integration are some of the key categories within AI-TBP applications, that enable these systems to detect automatically new lesions, flag the changes, and recognize pattern outliers ("ugly duckling" lesions) within a patient's overall nevus phenotype. Notably, while AI has already proven to be highly effective at analyzing individual skin lesions, its expansion into TBP represents a significant step toward personalized and proactive monitoring for people at risk of melanoma [10].

7.2.1 Performance of CNNs Versus Clinicians and the Role of Augmented Intelligence

Over the past years, multiple studies have demonstrated the impressive capabilities of AI and particularly CNNs in classifying skin lesions. Their performance levels are often comparable to or exceed even those of experienced dermatologists. As already mentioned, among the pioneering studies exploring AI in dermatology was the "Man Against Machine" study by *Haenssle* et al. in 2018 [9]. In this study a deep learning CNN based on GoogleNet Inception v4 architecture was trained on over 100,000 dermoscopic images to classify exclusively melanocytic lesions as benign or malignant. The CNN's performance was evaluated against 58 dermatologists from 17 countries, 30 of which were experts. Both groups were assessed under two conditions: only dermoscopic images were provided in level I, while dermoscopic images along with clinical information such as patient history and lesion localization were included in level II. The performance of CNN showed sensitivity comparable to dermatologists and significantly higher specificity. The area under the curve (AUC) was higher for the CNN compared to the mean dermatologist. Notably, dermatologist performance improved with additional clinical context, particularly specificity, while there was variability based on experience, with some experts matching or exceeding CNN performance. However, this study failed to match a real-life clinical situation. This gap was identified, and an attempt to measure the performance of CNNs in a more realistic clinical setting was made a few years later by another landmark study, the "Man against machine reloaded" study in 2020 [11]. This study included a dataset of 100 cases comprised of pigmented/non-pigmented and melanocytic/non-melanocytic skin lesions, while the market-approved CNN's performance was evaluated against 96 dermatologists of various experience levels in two levels. The first level included only dermoscopic images, whereas the second level included clinical close-up photos, dermoscopic images and was accompanied by textual details. The CNN achieved a sensitivity of 95.0% and a specificity of 76.7%, while dermatologists improved from 89.0% to 94.1% sensitivity when given full clinical context, with specificity stable at 80.4%. This study also proved that more experienced dermatologists frequently surpassed CNN's performance and supported the role of AI as a decision-support tool rather than a replacement for human judgment.

Recent systematic reviews and metanalyses show that when compared to clinicians overall (sensitivity 79.8%, specificity 73.6%), AI algorithms were able to achieve higher sensitivity and specificity in the range of 87.0% and 77.1% in skin cancer classification. Notably, the difference was particularly evident against generalist clinicians, while AI and expert dermatologists showed comparable performance (AI sensitivity 86.3% vs experts 84.2%) [12]. However, this performance is often observed under ideal, highly curated experimental conditions, and this observation becomes more evident when CNNs are tested in real-world studies. In uncontrolled environments, when AI models trained on pristine datasets are tested on patient-submitted images, their diagnostic accuracy declines substantially due to their inability to generalize to the variability of clinical practice [13]. Additionally, the usefulness of AI among experienced dermatologists is less transformative compared to nonspecialists, that tend to rely on it in order to enhance their diagnostic abilities. Evidence supports that, AI tools appear to be more valuable in settings where diagnostic expertise is limited, proving that at least for the time being its primary role may be in leveling access to care rather than replacing specialist judgment [14].

The concept of augmented intelligence (AuI) emphasizes on the collaboration between AI systems and clinicians in the decision-making process and is emerging as the optimal model for AI integration [15–18]. Studies have shown that in high-risk populations, diagnostic performance is improved by the use of 2D and 3D TBP combined with CNNs. Remarkably, in the study by Goessinger et al. it was demonstrated that patients preferred AuI-assisted screening, compared to AI or dermatologists alone, reporting the highest subjective safety scores when dermatologist evaluations were supported by CNN analysis [16]. Nowadays, it is obvious that we are moving away from the concept of "Man against the machine" and we are entering the era of "Man with machine" [15]. Taking into consideration the limitations of CNNs, such as lower specificity, challenges in automated nevus counting, etc., we understand that AI tools are not yet capable of replacing clinical judgement, but they can serve as a valuable adjunct. Overall, the integration of AuI into melanoma screening enhances early detection while at the same time maintaining patient trust, underscoring its potential to transform dermatological practice (Table 7.1).

7.2.2 AI Models Across Different Melanoma Subtypes, Localizations, Sex, and Skin Tones

Dermatology has been revolutionized through the incorporation of AI, particularly deep learning and CNNs, which enable the automated classification of skin lesions without prior human-designed rules. Accurate classifications are led by abstract features such as color, texture, and shape from images that are learned autonomously by CNNs. These advances have been supported by efforts such as the international skin imaging collaboration (ISIC) that provide large datasets and host competitions that push the limits of automated skin lesion analysis and also by landmark studies showing AI matching or outperforming dermatologist performance [8, 86–89]. Although algorithm accuracy and performance have shown promising results, they often fail to mirror real-world clinical settings, where diagnosis relies on more than

Table 7.1 This is an overview of advanced AI models commonly utilized in melanoma diagnosis

Algorithm/AI model	Year	Applications
SVM (support vector machine) [19, 20]	1990	Efficiency in high-dimensional feature spaces. Popular in early medical image analysis.
Random forest [20, 21]	1990	Aggregates multiple decision trees for classification tasks.
AlexNet [20, 22–25]	2012	One of the earliest CNNs for image recognition. Assisted in bringing deep learning into the spotlight.
Inception/GoogLeNet [20, 26]	2014	Combines multiple convolution filter sizes at each layer to capture different spatial features. Improves pattern detection across scales.
VGG (visual geometry group) [20, 27–32]	2014	Straightforward, deep-layered structure using small convolution filters. Effective in feature extraction.
GAN (generative adversarial network) [20, 33–37]	2014	Generates realistic synthetic images to expand training datasets. Especially useful when real data is limited.
ResNet (residual network) [20, 38–51]	2015	Assists in the development of deep networks by allowing certain layers to skip others during training. Identifies complex patterns in dermoscopic images.
U-net [20, 52–56]	2015	Precise image segmentation.
YOLO (you only look once) [20, 57–62]	2016	Fast object detection model. Ability to locate and classify objects in real-time from a single pass over the image.
Xception [20, 37, 63–67]	2016	Uses depthwise separable convolutions for efficient image analysis. Needs fewer parameters than standard CNNs.
NASNet (neural architecture search network) [20, 68, 69]	2017	Applies neural architecture search to improve its design, boosting both speed and precision in classifying images.
DenseNet [20, 28, 70–73]	2017	Densely connected convolutional networks. Improve information transfer, helping preserve important features throughout the network.
MobileNet [20, 74, 75]	2017	Lightweight models. Made for mobile and embedded devices. Balancing performance with efficiency.
ResNeXt [20, 76]	2017	Based on ResNet. Uses grouped convolutions. More powerful feature extraction with less complexity.
Mask R-CNN [20, 77–81]	2017	Adds pixel-level segmentation on top of object detection. Enables precise region extraction in images.
EfficientNet [20, 82–85]	2019	Scales the model width, depth, and resolution.

This table summarizes key machine learning and deep learning algorithms, outlining their year of introduction and primary applications in medical image analysis. From efficient feature extraction and deep network training (e.g., ResNet and DenseNet) to real-time object detection (e.g., YOLO) and precise lesion segmentation (e.g., U-net and mask R-CNN), each model offers distinct advantages. Understanding the strengths and design principles of these models is essential for selecting appropriate architectures for skin cancer detection tasks, optimizing diagnostic accuracy, speed, and computational efficiency

Table 7.2 Summary of major publicly available datasets for melanoma

Dataset name		Number of images	Number of melanomas
PH2 dataset		200	200
ISIC (international skin imaging collaboration)			
	ISIC 2016	900	273
	ISIC 2017	2000	374
	ISIC 2018-HAM10000	10,015	1113
	ISIC 2019	25,333	4522
	ISIC 2020	33,126	584
	ISIC 2024 (SLICE-3D)	401,059	>10,000
DERMNET		22,500	635
MED-NODE		170	100
DERMQUEST		126	66
DERMIS		397	146

This table highlights key datasets commonly used to develop, train, and validate AI algorithms for skin lesion classification. The generalizability and diagnostic performance of AI models can be impacted by the variability in dataset composition, labeling standards, skin tones, and representation of rare melanoma subtypes. When interpreting algorithm outcomes and designing robust, clinically applicable AI systems, it is crucial that the characteristics of these datasets to be considered

just the visual analysis of a single lesion image, and involves evaluating additional factors like patient age, medical and family history, UV exposure, nevi patterns across the body, and genetic data [90, 91] (Table 7.2).

As discussed before, for patients with multiple nevi and atypical mole syndrome, TBP has been used for new or changing lesions. Traditional 2D TBP assisted in the standardization of dermatology imaging, and now the evolution to 3D TBP systems offers new opportunities and challenges for integrating detailed clinical metadata into AI workflows. Modern systems are equipped with AI tools for lesion analysis and risk evaluation and have shown the ability to enhance diagnostic accuracy, sometimes even outperforming standalone dermatologists (Figs. 7.1, 7.2, 7.3, 7.4, 7.5, 7.6 and 7.7). Current imaging systems like VECTRA WB360 (Canfield Scientific, Parsippany, NJ, USA) and the upcoming iToBoS (intelligent total body scanner, City, Country), are designed to integrate advanced computer-aided diagnostic tools directly into their user interface software. Capabilities like automatic detection and quantification of nevi larger than 2 mm, tracking changes across sequential images, and linking dermoscopic data for a more comprehensive lesion assessment are already offered by the VECTRA DermaGraphix system (Figs. 7.1 and 7.2). Canfield's DEXI (dermoscopy explained intelligence) is an AI-based dermoscopic research tool, consisting of an overall risk assessment score on a scale of 0–10, as well as several explainable components including a spatial heatmap indicating where DEXI is focusing on, and a probability graph showing individual probabilities for the five benign classes (nevi,

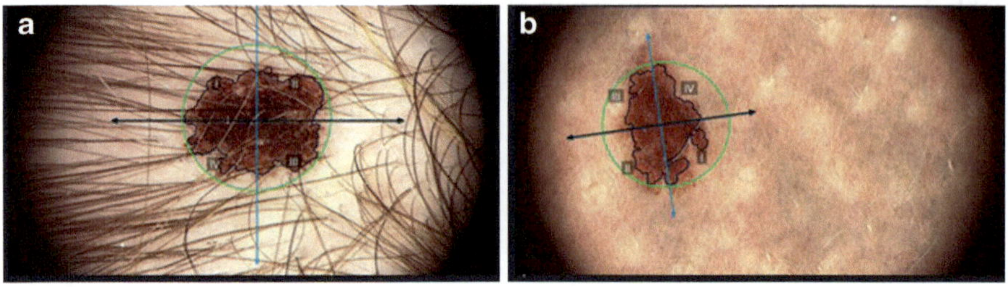

Fig. 7.3 Screenshots of dermoscopic images, captured by a lesion classification system. (**a**) Dermoscopic image of a melanocytic nevus located on the scalp of a 6-year-old girl, captured using the lesion classification system. The AI analysis assigned a low malignancy risk score of 0.1. Despite the challenging location within hair-bearing skin, the AI algorithm successfully identified and delineated the lesion borders with high accuracy. This case highlights the capability of advanced AI systems to maintain performance in complex anatomical sites where image artifacts, such as hair occlusion, could otherwise interfere with lesion assessment. Accurate border detection is critical for reliable feature extraction and risk stratification in pediatric dermatology. (**b**) Dermoscopic image of a melanocytic nevus on the back of a 45-year-old male with Fitzpatrick skin type III, captured using the lesion classification system. The lesion was situated on an area of old and faded tattoo pigment. The AI system assigned a low malignancy risk score of 0.1 and accurately delineated the lesion borders despite the presence of underlying tattoo ink and background skin tone variation. This case underscores the robustness of modern AI algorithms in complex scenarios, where pigmentary artifacts and darker skin tones can challenge traditional image analysis and potentially confound feature detection

vascular lesions, benign keratosis-like lesions, dermatofibromas, and actinic keratosis, though it is clinically recognized as a precursor to SCC) and three malignant classes (melanoma, BCC, and SCC) (Fig. 7.6). Similarly, the FotoFinder 2D TBP system (FotoFinder Systems GmbH, Bad Birnbach, Germany) incorporates AI-driven features that can identify new or evolving lesions from TBP. Its Moleanalyzer AI Assistant also evaluates lesion risk using linked dermoscopic images, is accredited as a class II medical device in the European Union and has demonstrated its ability to enhance dermatologists' diagnostic accuracy in differentiating between benign and malignant lesions in multiple studies [10, 15, 92]. MoleAnalyzer Pro AI assistant provides a risk analysis on subsequent dermoscopy images, evaluating changes and irregularities in the lesion area, perimeter, and diameter. The numerical measurements of these parameters and calculated differences between images are presented, and then an AI risk score ranging from 0 to 1 is provided, with any score > 0.5 considered high risk (Figs. 7.3 and 7.7).

A significant variation in diagnostic performance of AI tools across melanoma subtypes, anatomical localizations, patient sex, and skin tones has been documented and highlights both the potential and the limitations of our current technology. To improve the generalizability, reliability, and clinical utility of AI tools, it is important to understand these dimensions.

In more common melanoma types such as superficial spreading melanoma (SSM), nodular melanoma (NM), and lentigo maligna melanoma (LMM), CNNs exhibit high diagnostic accuracy, achieving sensitivities above 93%, specificities

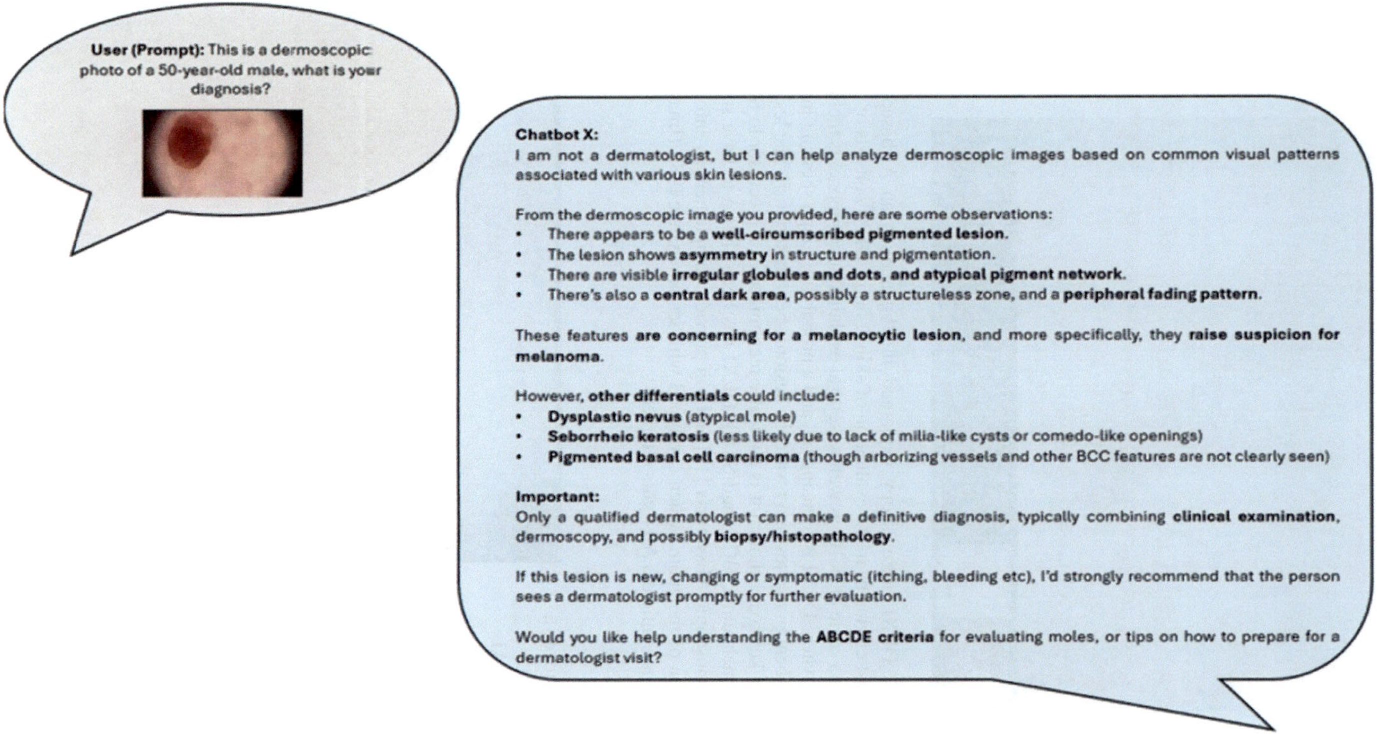

Fig. 7.4 Evaluation using a chatbot-X integrated AI tool suggests the possibility of melanoma, highlighting a significant discrepancy in AI diagnostic outputs. A screenshot of the same dermoscopic photo using a lesion classification system indicated a low malignancy risk with a score of 0.1, suggesting a benign lesion. This emphasizes the variability in risk stratification depending on the algorithm used and underlines the critical need for clinical validation and cautious interpretation of AI-based skin lesion assessments

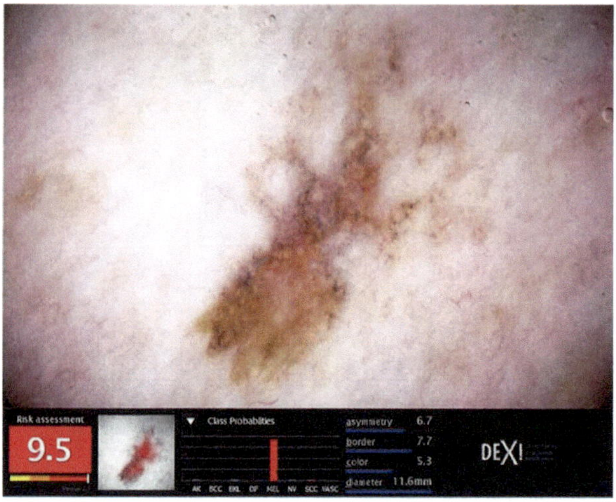

Fig. 7.5 Canfield's DEXI (dermoscopy explained intelligence) is an AI-based dermoscopic research tool to assist clinicians in the evaluation of skin lesions. DEXI consists of an overall risk assessment score on a scale of 0–10, as well as several explainable components including a spatial heatmap indicating where DEXI is focusing on, and a probability graph showing individual probabilities for the five benign classes (nevi, vascular lesions, benign keratosis-like lesions, dermatofibromas and actinic keratosis, though it is clinically recognized as a precursor to SCC) and three malignant classes (melanoma, BCC, and SCC). DEXI has been shown to have superior performance vs other dermoscopic AI systems [17] and can provide complementary information to aid in the early detection of melanoma when combined with lesion change [98]. (Image reproduced with permission from Canfield© All rights retained)

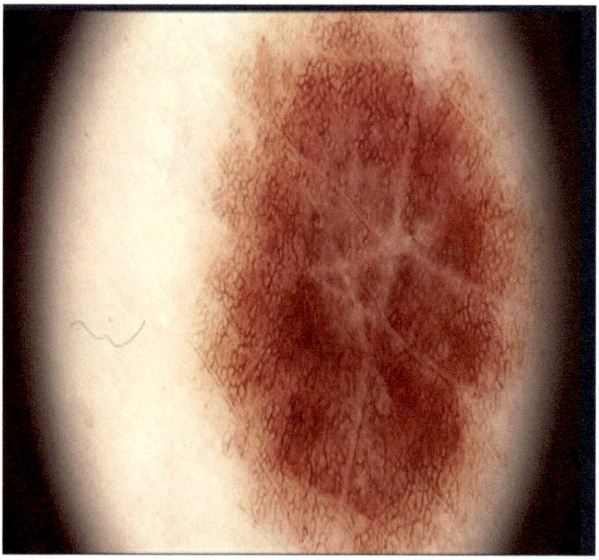

Fig. 7.6 A screenshot of a pigmented lesion. The software provided an AI risk score of 0.1 (any score > 0.5 is considered high risk for malignancy). The lesion imaged in this figure was subsequently excised and confirmed by histopathology as a superficial spreading melanoma with in situ and invasive components

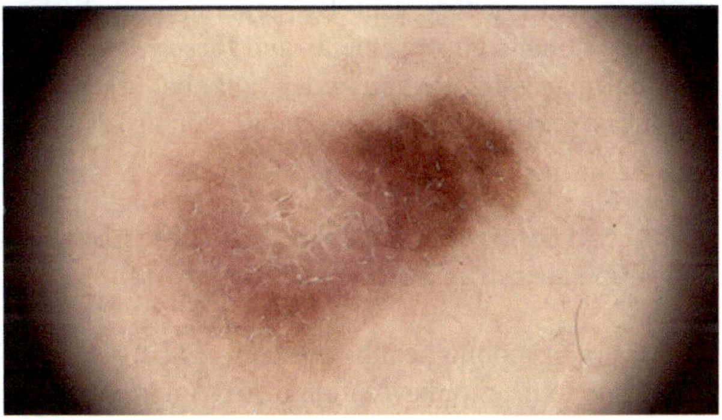

Fig. 7.7 The software provided for the above lesion an AI risk score of 0.85 (any score > 0.5 is considered high risk for malignancy). The lesion imaged in this figure was subsequently excised and confirmed by histopathology as a collision tumor (dermatofibroma and nevus)

above 65% and ROC–AUC values exceeding 0.926 [93]. On the contrary, melanomas that are located at complex anatomical sites, such as subungual (nail) melanomas, the CNN models show declined performance with sensitivity of 53.3%) and ROC–AUC 0.621, indicating a substantial risk of false negatives, while acrolentiginous melanomas (AM) on the skin achieve a reasonable sensitivity (83.3%) and high specificity (91.0%). Considering mucosal melanomas, even though CNNs maintain high sensitivity, their specificity drops to 38%, data that possibly reflect overdiagnosis concerns [93]. Based on these results, it is evident that improvements are urgently needed for rare and site-specific melanomas that are often underrepresented in training datasets.

7.2.3 Bias and Potential Limitations of Current AI Systems

Another topic of concern is potential bias in AI models regarding sex-specific factors, such as differences in skin anatomy and melanoma biology. In a recent study, a market-approved CNN was studied for sex-related diagnostic performance across 1549 dermoscopic images [99]. Despite an imbalance in training data favoring male patients (60% male vs 40% female images), no significant sex-related differences were observed in diagnostic performance. Images from male and female patients had comparable sensitivities, specificities, and AUC values, indicating that, at least for the analyzed CNN, sex-related diagnostic bias was minimal. Nevertheless, essential remain the ongoing vigilance and structured audits of AI systems for sex-related biases.

Last but not least, skin tone represents a critical axis of disparity in dermatology AI applications. The lack of skin tone diversity in dermatological datasets is a well-documented limitation, as the datasets used to train AI models include predominantly fair-skinned patients, limiting CNN generalizability to darker skin types or less represented ethnics such as Latinos [100]. Studies have shown that CNNs trained on such datasets perform poorly on images of darker-skinned individuals [101, 102]. Deep learning techniques such as style transfer and deep blending have been utilized to generate realistic images of darker skin tones as part of the efforts made to address this gap. By generating realistic darker-skin images, models achieved notable improvements and these results emphasize that diversification of training images is not merely desirable but essential for equitable AI performance and improvement of physician training on diverse skin tones [102].

7.2.4 AI Smartphone Apps for Melanoma Detection: Democratization or Delusion?

A new era of mobile health applications, particularly for melanoma detection, has begun due to the rapid evolution of AI. Smartphone apps powered by AI promise to democratize access to dermatologic evaluation, allowing users to scan skin lesions and receive instant risk assessments. However, apart from the unprecedented accessibility of this technology, critical questions about its reliability, regulatory oversight, and real-world impact are raised. The global increase in skin cancer incidence combined with the widespread presence of smartphones is skyrocketing the growth of AI-assisted dermatology apps [103]. Studies show that while some AI models perform comparably to specialists under controlled conditions, they often demonstrate inconsistent accuracy in real-world clinical settings. Some of the limitations that undermine the performance of these tools include poor image quality, device variability, and lack of contextual patient information [104]. Alarmingly, many current apps fail to meet essential labeling and transparency standards, making it difficult for users to understand the capabilities and limitations of this technology [105].

Even though regulatory bodies, such as the therapeutic goods administration (TGA) in Australia and European health authorities, have already responding by emphasizing the need for standardized labeling and rigorous validation, however, most apps that are already directly available to consumers have not undergone robust clinical validation [103, 105]. False reassurance or unnecessary anxiety are the two major ethical concerns that are raised, both of which can have serious consequences for users. At the same time, while from a patient-centered care perspective, mobile apps have the potential to empower individuals and support early melanoma detection, particularly in regions with limited access to dermatologists, on the other hand, experts stress that apps should complement, not replace, professional medical advice [106, 107].

In order to reduce these risks, we should consider some critical steps to ensure these apps benefit rather than harm patients. These include multidisciplinary collaboration, ongoing app monitoring, clearer communication of AI limitations, and user education. Moreover, AI applications must be transparently labeled as providing risk assessments rather than definitive diagnoses, with clear recommendations for follow-up by qualified healthcare providers. It is important to understand that, while AI-powered smartphone apps for melanoma detection embody the promise of democratizing healthcare, without rigorous validation, regulation, and transparency, they risk becoming a dangerous delusion. The future success of these technologies relies on carefully balancing innovation with patient safety, ensuring that the tools genuinely assist in the fight against skin cancer [103, 105, 107].

7.2.5 Explainable AI in Melanoma Diagnosis: A Necessary Evolution

As mentioned previously, in recent years, AI and particularly, deep learning models like CNNs, are being used in melanoma diagnosis through dermoscopic images, demonstrating remarkable performance in diagnosing melanoma. However, despite achieving high accuracy, these models often don't provide insights into their decision-making processes, operating as "black boxes". This lack of transparency has driven the development of explainable artificial intelligence (XAI) to make AI-based melanoma diagnosis both accurate and interpretable [108–110].

A number of visual XAI are now being integrated into algorithms, such as gradient-weighted class activation mapping (Grad-CAM) and local interpretable model-agnostic explanations (LIME). Powerful CNN architectures are combined with XAI methods by models like SmartSkin-XAI and SkinSage XAI to highlight key regions of skin lesions that contribute to a melanoma diagnosis [111, 112]. Proving these explanations help dermatologists understand AI outputs better and build trust in AI-assisted diagnostic support. Furthermore, a study by Chanda et al. showed the critical role of explainability in clinical adoption by proving that dermatologist-like XAI systems improve diagnostic accuracy and increase significantly clinicians' confidence and willingness to rely on AI tools [113]. The technical advancements in XAI-driven melanoma diagnosis go beyond simple visualizations. Researchers like Shah et al. have developed more complex pipelines that integrate optimized deep learning models with feature selection techniques such as particle swarm optimization, ensuring both computational efficiency and clinical interpretability [114]. Their framework, which achieved accuracy levels as high as 98.5% on major skin lesion datasets, incorporated Grad-CAM, LIME, and occlusion sensitivity to make the decision-making process transparent to users.

In conclusion, XAI represents a major leap forward in melanoma diagnosis, offering a bridge between high AI performance and clinical trust. Notably, various XAI techniques are suited to different clinical situations. For instance, Grad-CAM is ideal for offering a quick, intuitive visual summary to support rapid decision-making, whereas methods like LIME and Occlusion Sensitivity are better suited for thorough validation and detailed examination of individual cases. The diverse diagnostic styles and preferences of healthcare professionals can now be adapted thanks to the flexibility of XAI framework [114]. As the field evolves, the focus will increasingly shift toward building inherently interpretable models that mirror dermatologists' reasoning processes. To ensure that AI tools become trusted allies in the early detection and treatment of melanoma further research is needed to assess their impact on diagnostic decision-making [110].

7.2.6 The New Frontier: Multimodal and Generative AI

Multimodal artificial intelligence (MAI) has been introduced as a transformative approach to melanoma diagnosis. Traditional unimodal models, rely solely on dermoscopic or clinical images, often encountering limitations due to data scarcity and intrinsic variability of skin presentations across diverse populations. On the contrary, MAI integrates diverse data sources like dermoscopic images, clinical photographs, patient metadata, and textual clinical notes in a way that real-world dermatological assessment is represented more accurately and offers a richer contextual understanding [115, 116]. The fusion of dermoscopic and clinical images alongside clinical metadata via deep learning outperforms the unimodal models significantly and improves diagnostic metrics such as AUC, sensitivity, and specificity [115–117]. For instance, if we incorporate the clinically validated diagnostic aid of "7-point checklist" into a constrained classifier chain within a multimodal deep network, it will achieve a remarkable diagnostic accuracy of 81.3% [115]. Moreover, novel systems such as SkinGPT-4, offer in-depth analyses, increase accessibility to dermatologic care and generate patient-friendly reports by illustrating the potential to combine large language models (LLMs) with vision transformers to autonomously diagnose skin conditions [118]. At the same time, models like GPT-4 vision have shown improved recognition of melanoma features across a range of skin tones, highlighting their utility in addressing dermatological health disparities [119]. However, challenges such as dataset bias, particularly underrepresentation of darker skin types, and the need for transparent, interpretable models remain key limitations to clinical implementation [120].

Generative artificial intelligence (GAI) enables the simulation, augmentation, and enhancement of dermoscopic image datasets and has emerged as a powerful tool in melanoma diagnostics. In order to model the progression of benign nevi into malignant melanoma, techniques such as cycle-consistent adversarial networks (Cycle-GANs) have been used and provide clinicians and patients with visualizations that help and enrich the understanding of lesion evolution in alignment with the ABCDE criteria [121]. Substantial improvements in the performance of deep learning classifiers have been made by generative models like GANs and ESRGANs that address data scarcity and imbalance by synthetically enlarging training datasets. Additionally, models incorporating hybrid approaches, such as combining VGG19 networks with SVM, have achieved impressive diagnostic accuracies up to 96% [122]. The integration of LLMs with GAI further enhances diagnostic workflows by producing pre-diagnostic textual explanations, supporting clinician decision-making with more interpretable AI outputs [123]. Concerns associated with the fidelity of generated images, bias in training data, and clinical validation of outputs must be addressed before widespread adoption, even if GAI holds significant promise for early detection, simulation-based education, and data augmentation [121, 122].

7.2.7 Practical Realities: Lessons from Clinical Experience

7.2.7.1 False Negative AI Diagnosis of Melanoma

An otherwise healthy 77-year-old female patient presented to the dermatologic clinic in order to check an asymptomatic pigmented lesion on her right lower abdomen. Her son died of metastatic melanoma. Upon clinical examination, an 8 mm, slightly asymmetric, pigmented lesion was seen. No other suspicious lesions were detected. The lesion was imaged dermoscopically by a high-resolution dermoscopic camera and underwent assessment by the FotoFinder Moleanalyzer Pro (FotoFinder, Bad Birnbach, Germany) (Fig. 7.7). This algorithm provided a malignancy risk score of 0.1 on a scale from 0 to 1. The image analysis included structural features such as: symmetry of shape and color, homogeneity of pigment network and absence of blue-whitish veil, atypical vessels, or regression structures. According to the algorithm's risk stratification threshold (typically >0.5 for further action), this score was interpreted as low risk, suggesting a benign melanocytic lesion and subsequently, no further action was recommended by the AI algorithm.

Despite the low malignancy score, the experienced dermatologist given the presence of irregular pigmentation in one quadrant of the lesion and also taking into consideration the patient's age and family history of melanoma. Based on these findings and clinical intuition, the dermatologist recommended excision of the lesion for histopathological evaluation. Histopathology revealed a malignant melanoma with both in situ and invasive components, with a Breslow depth of 0.2 mm., without ulceration, and a low mitotic rate ($<1/mm^2$). The patient underwent a wide local excision with clear margins. The lesion was classified as stage pT1a melanoma under the AJCC eighth edition staging system. This case highlights a false negative diagnosis by an AI system, where a melanoma was misclassified as benign due to its subtle presentation and not taking into consideration the age and clinical history of the patient (metadata).

It is important to keep in mind that AI tools like FotoFinder are trained primarily on pattern recognition and may underperform when subtle visual cues exist without robust context/ melanomas that lack strong dermoscopic hallmarks. Additionally, the algorithm does not integrate clinical history, in our case, the strong familial predisposition, which would have significantly raised the pretest probability of melanoma. This case highlights the importance of clinical assessment using multiple inputs besides dermoscopy and integrating the medical history into diagnosis.

7.2.7.2 False Positive AI Diagnosis of Melanoma

A 59-year-old male patient with dysplastic nevus syndrome (DNS) and a significant personal oncologic history of multiple primary melanomas (one with Breslow thickness of 2.1 mm and positive sentinel lymph node) presented to the dermatologic clinic for his routine follow-up visit. The patient was initially under adjuvant anti-PD-1 immunotherapy, which was later switched to BRAF–MEK inhibitors due to disease progression. During total body dermoscopic imaging, a new pigmented lesion on the left thigh measuring approximately 3.7 mm in diameter was flagged by the Fotofinder's Moleanalyzer pro AI system for further evaluation (Fig. 7.7). The asymmetry in shape, borders, and pigmentation, as well as the pink color in combination with the structureless areas were highlighted by AI-based dermoscopic analysis. The Moleanalyzer pro's score for this lesion was 0.85 on a scale from 0 to 1, classifying it as highly suspicious for melanoma. Given the lesion's appearance and high-risk score, the AI strongly indicated the need for excision.

The dermoscopic image of the lesion was reviewed by an experienced dermatologist with a differential diagnosis that included dysplastic nevi, collision tumor (dermatofibroma and nevi), and melanoma. However, given this particular clinical context, the decision was to excise the lesion. The histopathologic analysis revealed a benign collision tumor, composed of a compound melanocytic nevus, without atypia with an adjacent dermatofibroma, with typical storiform spindle cell proliferation and overlying epidermal hyperplasia. No evidence of melanoma or dysplasia was found, and no further treatment was needed.

In this case the diagnostic complexities that clinicians encounter when using AI in high-risk melanoma patients is highlighted, particularly in patients with a history of locoregional disease and ongoing systematic therapy. In this case a few key interpretive challenges for AI assessment can be identified. Firstly, collision tumors consist a common pitfall in melanoma diagnosis as they can mimic melanoma dermoscopically due to their mixed structural features. AI algorithms are trained on standard lesion morphologies and collision tumors are infrequent. Lastly, the AI algorithm's lack of contextual integration as it is not able to incorporate patient history and therapeutic background which are critical in high-risk patients. Nevertheless, in patients with a significant melanoma burden, a low threshold for excision remains clinically appropriate, as the potential consequences of missing a true recurrence or a new primary tumor outweigh the risks of unnecessary removal.

7.3 AI in Melanoma Diagnosis: Reflectance Confocal Microscopy

Reflectance Confocal Microscopy (RCM) is a noninvasive imaging modality that captures cellular-level imaging of the skin and plays a critical role in the early diagnosis of melanoma. One of the first attempts to automate melanoma diagnosis with RCM was based on classical ML techniques [124]. *Koller* et al., developed a classification tree algorithm based on wavelet-transformed features from 16,269 RCM images, achieving high intra-set classification accuracies of 93.6% for melanoma and 90.4% for nevi. However, the generalization in independent datasets was moderate, with malignant classification rates around 55% in melanomas and 47% in benign lesions, highlighting the limitations of feature-engineering approaches and the need for more reliable, generalized models and datasets with standardized image acquisition. A similar approach was presented in the study by *Gareau* et al. as a computer vision algorithm that quantified the presence of pagetoid melanocytes and dermal–epidermal junction (DEJ) disarray, two key features for melanoma diagnosis [125]. These foundational works demonstrated the technical feasibility but also highlighted limitations of early feature-based approaches.

With the introduction of deep learning and particularly CNNs, RCM image analysis was significantly enhanced. *Wodzinski* et al. developed a ResNet-based CNN classifier that categorized RCM mosaics into melanoma, basal cell carcinoma (BCC), and benign nevi with an accuracy reaching 87%, which was higher than the accuracy achieved by medical confocal users [126]. Remarkably, deep networks have the ability to learn complex, hierarchical features directly from image data and eliminate the need for manual feature engineering consequently outperforming traditional methods. Furthermore, *Mandal* et al. in their study, addressed the complexity of 3D RCM stacks by introducing local z-projection (LZP), a method that compresses 3D information into a 2D plane. This innovation allowed efficient CNN-based classification of difficult-to-distinguish lesions such as lentigo maligna from atypical intraepidermal melanocytic proliferation [127, 128].

A recent systematic review by *Patel* et al. presented findings from various AI models applied to noninvasive imaging modalities, including RCM. They reported a mean diagnostic accuracy of 82.72% for AI models based on RCM, slightly lower than that achieved with dermoscopic images but still clinically significant. Notably, studies showed that the performance of human dermatologists when interpreting RCM data were often matched or exceeded by AI models, particularly when integrated with optimized DL architectures [129]. Furthermore, new methods, including a multitask cycle GAN model named DermoGAN, have been proposed for automated cell segmentation in RCM images. The success of unsupervised learning models like DermoGAN—although initially designed for keratinocyte identification rather than melanoma detection—underscores the expanding potential for advanced AI architectures in RCM data interpretation [130].

7.4 AI in Melanoma Diagnosis: Pathology

The combination of the increasing incidence of skin cancer and the shortage of dermatopathologists has led to heavier workloads in pathology departments worldwide. Traditionally, the histopathological evaluation of melanoma, is based largely on hematoxylin and eosin (H&E) stained sections and immunohistochemistry (IHC). This protocol remains the gold standard; however, it is laborious, subjective, and time-consuming. The foundation for applying AI in digital pathology is provided by whole-slide imaging (WSI). By integrating digital slides into the pathology workflow, advanced algorithms and computer-aided diagnostic tools expand the frontiers of the pathologist's view beyond the traditional microscopic slide and allow access to broader knowledge beyond human limits and boundaries. Studies have already proven that AI systems trained on digitized WSI can demonstrate high diagnostic accuracy, sensitivity, and specificity, closely matching or even surpassing the performance of human experts [131]. For instance, accuracy rates exceeding 95% are achieved by CNN models successfully trained to distinguish between healthy tissue and melanoma, significantly reducing interobserver variability. These models work by autonomously learning and recognizing complex patterns in tissue architecture that may be imperceptible to the human eye, thus enhancing the objectivity and efficiency of melanoma diagnosis [132]. Digital pathology and AI offer significant potential for advancing dermatooncology and precision medicine, as they can help automate and standardize many tasks that are currently manual and subjective [133]. AI is rapidly transforming dermatopathology by enhancing the precision, efficiency, and reproducibility of melanoma diagnosis, staging and prognostic prediction.

Despite the transformative potential of AI in dermatopathology and especially melanoma diagnosis, significant challenges remain and include dataset biases, transparency, and generalizability. More specifically, the datasets on which the training of AI models is based often lack diversity, include small sample sizes and lack consistency regarding imaging techniques. Furthermore, the "black box" nature of deep learning algorithms like CNNs makes it difficult for clinicians to interpret or trust the AI's decision-making processes, posing a challenge for its adoption in clinical practice. Possible solutions might be considered the integration of explainable AI, the development of larger and more inclusive standardized datasets, as well as the clinical validation and utility of the AI dermatopathology models [134, 135].

7.4.1 AI-Based Detection of Melanoma Metastasis in Lymph Nodes

Melanoma staging relies on the evaluation of sentinel lymph nodes (SLNs) for micrometastases. Recently, *Shaker* et al. presented their study in which an AI-driven model was trained on 53 H&E-stained WSIs to identify melanoma metastases without the aid of additional immunohistochemical staining [136]. The results showed that the AI algorithm demonstrated a specificity of 0.91 and a sensitivity of 0.74 in effectively distinguishing between tumor deposits larger than 0.1 mm and those exceeding 1 mm, which are critical thresholds for clinical management, while also reaching high agreement with the pathologist's classification. A similar approach had been followed a few years prior by *Jansen* et al. [137] In their study, they applied deep learning across multicenter cohorts to detect metastasis in SLNs, achieving AUC values of 0.9630 and 0.9856 on two test cohorts from different laboratories. Their model was capable of classifying metastasis by size, in line with staging requirements, while at the same time significantly reducing the need for supplementary IHC staining. Finally, *Siarov* et al., developed a deep learning model able to identify and differentiate nodal metastasis in sentinel node biopsies (SNB) from intranodal nevus (INN), further demonstrating that AI models could reach dermatologist-level performance, achieving an AUC of 0.965 [138].

Accurate SNB status is a crucial part of melanoma staging as the number of metastatic lymph nodes a patient's significantly affects prognosis and appropriate management [139]. The accurate distinction between nodal metastasis of melanoma and INN is particularly important to avoid misdiagnosis and inappropriate clinical management. From the studies mentioned, it is obvious that AI has the potential to automate the laborious process of slide review, standardize measurement of metastasis size, and streamline prognostic evaluations without compromising diagnostic accuracy. However, further validation is needed.

7.4.2 AI Models for Prognostic Prediction

The prognostic prediction for melanoma is slowly being transformed, particularly through analysis of dermatopathology slides with AI tools. One of the first deep learning models combining convolutional and recurrent neural networks to predict distant metastatic recurrence (DMR) and disease-specific survival (DSS) based solely on H&E-stained slides of primary melanomas was developed by *Kulkarni* et al. [140] This model was trained across 108 patients and validated on two independent cohorts, achieving AUCs of 0.905 and 0.880, respectively. It focused on tumor morphology, immune cell distribution, and regional interactions within the tumor microenvironment, in order to stratify patients into high- and low-risk groups, offering a noninvasive and practical alternative to the current molecular assays. However, the retrospective design, the small number of patients and the specific tissue quality requirements were some of the limitations of the study preventing its immediate application in clinical practice. Following a similar trajectory, *Comes* et al. *(2022)* explored deep learning applications for predicting disease-free survival (DFS) at 1 year in cutaneous melanoma patients [141]. Nonetheless, this study—like other developed AI models exploring digital slide analysis to provide accurate predictions for melanoma patients prognosis—did not reach performance accurate enough to be applied in clinical settings [140, 142, 143].

Building on their earlier research, *Comes* et al. (2024) further refined AI-based prognostic models by focusing specifically on negative sentinel lymph node (SLN-) melanoma patients [144]. In this study, two distinct models analyzing manually annotated tumor regions with and without immune cell infiltration, were developed finding that regions containing tumor cells alone were more predictive. Their best model, trained on 71 patients and externally validated on 23 patients. It managed to reach an AUC of 79.1% in the investigational cohort and 76.5% in the validation cohort. In this particular study explainable AI techniques were incorporated to highlight image areas most critical for prediction, facilitating clinical interpretability. Finally, in another remarkable study, researchers developed and validated an AI-assisted model to predict metastasis risk and overall survival in patients with nodular melanoma [145] *Xu* et al. used data from 4727 patients in the SEER database and tested multiple machine learning algorithms, with the multilayer perceptron (MLP) model achieving the best performance with an AUC of 0.932, accuracy of 0.856, and sensitivity of 0.878. Independent risk factors for metastasis and prognosis included age, marital status, gender, primary tumor site, surgery, radiation, chemotherapy, and N stage. To predict 1-, 3-, and 5-year survival rates, a prognostic nomogram was constructed, offering better individualized risk stratification than traditional staging methods. The results from both studies present a major step toward noninvasive, accurate risk assessment of recurrence and metastasis in melanoma patients, and they provide valuable assistance in clinical decision-making [144, 145].

7.4.3 Deep Learning for Tumor Microenvironment Analysis

It is well-established that the tumor microenvironment, particularly the presence of tumor-infiltrating lymphocytes (TILs), plays a pivotal role in melanoma outcomes [146]. In routine diagnostic practice, TILs in primary melanoma are classified according to their distribution and intensity as brisk/non-brisk,/absent, or alternatively based on the density as absent/mild/moderate/marked and distribution as absent/focal/multifocal/diffuse of the immune infiltrate [147, 148]. In the study by *Ugolini* et al., a CNN recognizing lymphocytic density within the tumor area from the H&E WSI and automatically extracting a TIL score in primary melanomas was developed [149]. Remarkably, the AI-derived TIL score demonstrated very high sensitivity and specificity and correlated strongly with clinical outcomes, outperforming manual assessments in reproducibility. The quantification of TILs by AI offers a standardized prognostic biomarker and could refine patient stratification for immunotherapy, a cornerstone in modern melanoma treatment.

Moreover, *Zormpas-Petridis* et al. introduced superpixel-based conditional random fields (SuperCRF), a new deep learning framework that improves cell classification in melanoma histopathology images by combining detailed local (individual cell) and global (tissue region) information [150]. While traditional deep learning models focus mostly on the shape of single cell nuclei, SuperCRF is developed to mimic how pathologists consider surrounding tissue structure by using a multi-resolution method. More specifically, the first step of this method is to detect cells with a CNN and then in the second step, to refine these predictions by applying a machine learning (ML)-based regional classification using superpixels at lower image resolutions. By modeling relationships between neighboring cells and regional tissue types with a conditional random field (CRF), SuperCRF boosts classification accuracy by about 12% compared to deep learning alone. Importantly, this study proves that a higher ratio of stromal cells and certain lymphocyte distributions correlates with poorer patient survival, offering a better way to predict outcomes in melanoma.

7.5 AI in Melanoma Treatment

Beyond melanoma diagnosis, AI has emerged as a valuable tool in the management of melanoma patients by personalizing treatment strategies based on tumor characteristics and predicting patient prognosis relying on genetic mutations, response to immunotherapy and other factors. AI technologies hold the promise of improving diagnostic speed, reducing human error, and enabling more personalized therapeutic approaches with the goal to enhance patient outcomes in melanoma care.

7.5.1 AI and Immunotherapy Response Prediction

Immunotherapy has significantly improved melanoma patients' survival by revolutionizing the treatment of advanced melanoma [151–153]. However, there is a variability in response to immune checkpoint inhibitors (ICI), like anti-PD1 or anti-CTLA4 drugs, with some patients being nonresponders. Considering this, together with the potentially life-threatening adverse events that patients undergoing ICI treatment could suffer, the prediction of a patient's immunotherapy response consists of clinical priority [154]. Current tools rely mostly on stratifying patients based on the levels of predictive biomarkers like PD-L1 expression, tumor mutational burden (TMB) and immune-related RNA signatures. Even though this method has remarkable success in some patients, it is not accurate enough to guide treatment decisions as the majority still fail to respond to ICI effectively [155]. A better solution for this critical gap in precision medicine might be offered by tailored, built AI models using ML techniques to identify and combine many different types of data, such as gene activity, mutations, and immune-related signals, to estimate the likelihood of a good response to ICI [156, 157]. There are several published studies demonstrating ML models for ICI outcomes prediction based on non-NGS features like clinical biomarkers, blood tests, or tissue samples, while some integrated genomic or transcriptomic data. Although a pan-cancer multi-omics ML model has been developed, no multi-omics models tailored to specific cancer types exist yet, and different algorithms like random forests, logistic regression, XGBoost, and neural networks have been used [158–164].

Recently, *Gschwind* et al. introduced an ML model based on the least absolute shrinkage and selection operator (LASSO) regression, trained on a meta-cohort of 449 melanoma patients for the prediction of anti-PD1 response [165]. This model captured somatic and germline properties as well as resistance mechanisms and transcriptomic immune signatures by integrating 49 biomarkers, which derived from whole-exome sequencing (WES) and RNA sequencing. The outcome was recorded as a RECIST score, and when compared to nonsynonymous tumor mutation burden (nsTMB) alone, the model substantially improved the prediction of anti-PD1 outcomes achieving an area under the receiver operating characteristic curve (AUC) of 0.70 in the training set and 0.64 in the test set. Notably, a layer of patient-level interpretability was introduced with the use of Shapley additive explanations (SHAP), which allowed clinicians to understand which biomarkers were driving each individual prediction. T-cell receptor entropy, the interferon-gamma to immunosuppression ratio, and mutations in genes such as B2M and CTNNB1 are some of the additional features that were included. However, paired WES and RNA-seq data are not routinely used in clinical settings, leading to limitations in incorporating this model into everyday clinical practice.

A deep learning model based on a modified transformer architecture was developed by *Wang* et al., integrating multimodal data, including TMB, PD-L1 expression, single-cell RNA sequencing-derived immune profiles, and somatic copy number alterations (SCNA) [166]. The model's dynamic attention mechanisms allowed it to adjust feature importance depending on the cancer type, achieving an

Table 7.3 Some of the recently proposed models for ICI response prediction in melanoma patients

Criteria	Gschwind et al. [165]	Wang et al. [166]	Ye et al. [167]
Model type	LASSO regression	Transformer (DL)	Graph neural network (GNN)
Data types	Genomics + Transcriptomics	Multi-omics + scRNA-seq	Transcriptomics + Pathways
Explainability	SHAP + permutation	Attention layers	Integrated gradients
Performance (melanoma)	AUC 0.64–0.70	AUC 0.71	AUC 0.854
Clinical suitability	High (simple and transparent)	Moderate (complex)	Moderate-high (biological alignment)
Novelty	Patient-level SHAP explanation	Attention for omics fusion	Pathway-guided GNN with lab validation

Even though they aim to be biologically accurate and make strong predictions, there is a variability in their performance, explainability and clinical suitability. The best way to move forward might be by combining all three, leading to a superpowerful, explainable, and flexible immunotherapy prediction system

AUC of 0.71 in melanoma and even higher values in other cancers such as non-small cell lung cancer (NSCLC). Remarkably, even though this model is complex and has lower interpretability compared to classical methods making it difficult to be implemented in daily clinical settings, it has demonstrated impressive cross-cancer generalizability.

Another innovative approach to predict melanoma response to immune checkpoint inhibitors, including CTLA-4 and PD-1 therapies, was reported by *Ye* et al. [167] In this study, graph neural networks (GNNs) were employed to map transcriptomic data onto biological pathways derived from Reactome databases. GNNs are particularly superior over CNNs and other ML methods when processing graphical data, owing to their enhanced performance and interpret ability. Via this model, the responseScore was developed, achieving exceptionally high predictive performance, with an AUC of 0.854 in training and 0.824 in testing datasets. Furthermore, 13 genes that show promise as potential tumor markers or therapeutic targets were identified in this study and functional experiments validated the biological role of PSMB6, one of the key genes identified, in modulating anti-tumor immunity. It is worth noting that the use of GNN assisted in bridging the gap between prediction and mechanistic understanding by linking changes in gene expression to alterations in immune-related pathways (Table 7.3).

7.5.2 AI in Peripheral and Microbiome Biomarkers

Apart from tumor-specific characteristics, there are other parameters, such as gut microbiome that are associated with ICI therapy efficacy in melanoma patients. The gut microbiome has emerged as a critical modulator of host immune responses and consequently influences outcomes in cancer immunotherapy [168–170]. Statistical models and ML have been used in recent studies to uncover microbial signatures like *Akkermansia* in order to predict response to therapy, especially in cutaneous melanoma, contributing significantly to advancements in gut microbiome research. In the study by Liang et al., a 16S rRNA sequencing and machine learning were used to identify and prove that bacterial taxa like Akkermansia was linked to better outcomes, achieving at the same time good predictive accuracy [171]. In a newly published study by *Zhou* et al., these findings were expanded by using metagenomics sequencing data of stool samples of melanoma patients before receiving immunotherapy. The results proved a positive correlation between *Akkermansia* and *Rutstroemia* being consistently associated with favorable outcomes across cohorts. The researchers used SHAP (SHapley Additive exPlanations) methodology, which provided an interpretable ML framework that identified key genera—like *Romboutsia, Endomicrobium*—whose increased abundance in responders suggested functional contributions to immune modulation, possibly through short-chain fatty acid (SCFA) production and maintenance of mucosal integrity. Other taxa associated with responders were *Aggregatilinea, Candidatus Moduliflexus, Colwellia, Akkermansia, Mucispirillum,* and *Rutstroemia,* while on the contrary, *Zancudomyces* was linked to nonresponders [172]. Additionally, powered by ML, tools like the Myeloid Index Score (MIS) have been built and validated. MIS quantifies immune cell dysfunction and further personalizes melanoma treatment by stratifying patients based on their systemic immune responses [173].

AI use in gut microbiome-related ICI response appears to be a promising but complex landscape. Its limitations include inter-individual microbiome variability and confounding factors such as antibiotic usage, diet, and tumor heterogeneity. Superior predictive tools might come by integrating functional microbial outputs (e.g., metatranscriptomics and metabolomics) and host immune profiling in future models. Even though we are still in early stages, studies like these lay crucial groundwork for microbiome-informed precision oncology strategies.

7.6 Radiomics and Deep Learning in Treatment Monitoring

Radiomics and artificial intelligence (AI) are revolutionizing melanoma management by enabling noninvasive, image based biomarkers that predict treatment response and survival outcomes using radiological images. Radiomics is an emerging field that intends to extract information from standard of care radiological images, to provide information beyond what can be achieved from human imaging interpretation alone ML models have the ability to extract quantitative imaging features like skewness, kurtosis, metabolic tumor volume (MTV), total lesion glycolysis (TLG), and informational measures of correlation (IMC), achieving high predictive accuracy. Predictive accuracy can be further elevated when clinical variables like lactate dehydrogenase (LDH) levels are combined in the ML model [174, 175]. Regarding metastatic melanoma, CT and MRI imaging from melanoma patients treated with anti-PD-1 and BRAF-targeted therapies were used in studies to characterize organ-specific patterns of disease control and progression. They developed clinically informed AI-driven radiomic models to predict sites of likely progression and were able to distinguish disease control from progression with area under the curve (AUC) values up to 0.85 [174]. Moreover, FDG–PET/CT radiomics, are capable of capturing tumor heterogeneity beyond standardized uptake values (SUV), and textural features extracted from PET images that have been linked to overall survival and treatment resistance, providing valuable prognostic information [175].

Predictive modeling and early identification of resistance are further improved by delta-radiomics. As "delta-radiomics", we refer to a radiomics approach that analyzes changes (deltas "Δ") in imaging features over time, usually before and after a treatment, or during therapy across multiple time points. More specifically, quantitative features like texture, shape, and intensity are extracted in standard radiomics from medical images (CT, MRI, and PET scans) at one time point for the prediction of treatment response, prognosis, or tumor biology. On the other hand, delta radiomics is based on the comparison between the features from two or more imaging studies—for example, baseline vs follow-up—and the examination of these features' evolution [176].

The integration of radiomics and AI in clinical practice is very promising for personalizing melanoma therapies, enabling early adaptation of treatment plans and reducing reliance on invasive biopsies. The combination of imaging biomarkers with clinical and molecular data, like BRAF and NRAS mutation status could further enhance outcome prediction and patient stratification [175, 177]. However, there are still challenges that we need to address such as data standardization across imaging platforms, the biological interpretation of extracted features, and the need for external validation of predictive models [178, 179].

References

1. Malvehy J, Puig S. Follow-up of melanocytic skin lesions with digital total-body photography and digital dermoscopy: a two-step method. Clin Dermatol. 2002;20(3):297–304. https://doi.org/10.1016/s0738-081x(02)00220-1. PMID: 12074871.
2. Vestergaard ME, Macaskill P, Holt PE, Menzies SW. Dermoscopy compared with naked eye examination for the diagnosis of primary melanoma: a meta-analysis of studies performed in a clinical setting. Br J Dermatol. 2008;159:669–76.
3. Salerni G, Terán T, Puig S, Malvehy J, Zalaudek I, Argenziano G, Kittler H. Meta-analysis of digital dermoscopy follow-up of melanocytic skin lesions: a study on behalf of the International Dermoscopy Society. J Eur Acad Dermatol Venereol. 2013;27(7):805–14. https://doi.org/10.1111/jdv.12032. Epub 2012 Nov 26.
4. Nelson KC, Swetter SM, Saboda K, Chen SC, Curiel-Lewandrowski C. Evaluation of the number-needed-to-biopsy metric for the diagnosis of cutaneous melanoma: a systematic review and meta-analysis. JAMA Dermatol. 2019;155(10):1167–74. https://doi.org/10.1001/jamadermatol.2019.1514. PMID: 31290958; PMCID: PMC6624799.
5. Soyer HP, Jayasinghe D, Rodriguez-Acevedo AJ, et al. 3D Total-body photography in patients at high risk for melanoma: a randomized clinical trial. JAMA Dermatol. Published online March 26, 2025. https://doi.org/10.1001/jamadermatol.2025.0211.
6. Lindsay D, Soyer HP, Janda M, et al. Cost-effectiveness analysis of 3D total-body photography for people at high risk of melanoma. JAMA Dermatol. Published online March 26, 2025. https://doi.org/10.1001/jamadermatol.2025.0219.

7. Esteva A, Kuprel B, Novoa RA, et al. Dermatologist-level classification of skin cancer with deep neural networks [published correction appears in Nature. 2017 Jun 28;546(7660):686. doi: 10.1038/nature22985.]. Nature. 2017;542(7639):115–8. https://doi.org/10.1038/nature21056.
8. Tschandl P, Codella N, Akay BN, Argenziano G, Braun RP, Cabo H, et al. Comparison of the accuracy of human readers versus machine learning algorithms for pigmented skin lesion classification: an open, web-based, international, diagnostic study. Lancet Oncol. 2019;20:938e47.
9. Haenssle HA, Fink C, Schneiderbauer R, Toberer F, Buhl T, Blum A, Kalloo A, Hassen ABH, Thomas L, Enk A, Uhlmann L, Reader study level-I and level-II Groups, Alt C, Arenbergerova M, Bakos R, Baltzer A, Bertlich I, Blum A, Bokor-Billmann T, Bowling J, Braghiroli N, Braun R, Buder-Bakhaya K, Buhl T, Cabo H, Cabrijan L, Cevic N, Classen A, Deltgen D, Fink C, Georgieva I, Hakim-Meibodi LE, Hanner S, Hartmann F, Hartmann J, Haus G, Hoxha E, Karls R, Koga H, Kreusch J, Lallas A, Majenka P, Marghoob A, Massone C, Mekokishvili L, Mestel D, Meyer V, Neuberger A, Nielsen K, Oliviero M, Pampena R, Paoli J, Pawlik E, Rao B, Rendon A, Russo T, Sadek A, Samhaber K, Schneiderbauer R, Schweizer A, Toberer F, Trennheuser L, Vlahova L, Wald A, Winkler J, Wölbing P, Zalaudek I. Man against machine: diagnostic performance of a deep learning convolutional neural network for dermoscopic melanoma recognition in comparison to 58 dermatologists. Ann Oncol. 2018;29(8):1836–42. https://doi.org/10.1093/annonc/mdy166. PMID: 29846502.
10. Primiero CA, Rezze GG, Caffery LJ, et al. A narrative review: opportunities and challenges in artificial intelligence skin image analyses using total body photography. J Invest Dermatol. 2024;144(6):1200–7. https://doi.org/10.1016/j.jid.2023.11.007.
11. Haenssle HA, Fink C, Toberer F, Winkler J, Stolz W, Deinlein T, Hofmann-Wellenhof R, Lallas A, Emmert S, Buhl T, Zutt M, Blum A, Abassi MS, Thomas L, Tromme I, Tschandl P, Enk A, Rosenberger A, Reader Study Level I and Level II Groups. Man against machine reloaded: performance of a market-approved convolutional neural network in classifying a broad spectrum of skin lesions in comparison with 96 dermatologists working under less artificial conditions. Ann Oncol. 2020;31(1):137–43. https://doi.org/10.1016/j.annonc.2019.10.013.
12. Salinas MP, Sepúlveda J, Hidalgo L, et al. A systematic review and meta-analysis of artificial intelligence versus clinicians for skin cancer diagnosis [published correction appears in NPJ Digit Med. 2024 May 24;7(1):141. doi: 10.1038/s41746-024-01138-0.]. NPJ Digit Med. 2024;7(1):125. Published 2024 May 14. https://doi.org/10.1038/s41746-024-01103-x.
13. Han SS, Navarrete-Dechent C, Liopyris K, et al. The degradation of performance of a state-of-the-art skin image classifier when applied to patient-driven internet search. Sci Rep. 2022;12(1):16260. Published 2022 Sep 28. https://doi.org/10.1038/s41598-022-20632-7.
14. Han SS, Kim YJ, Moon IJ, et al. Evaluation of artificial intelligence-assisted diagnosis of skin neoplasms: a single-center, paralleled, unmasked, randomized controlled trial. J Invest Dermatol. 2022;142(9):2353–2362.e2. https://doi.org/10.1016/j.jid.2022.02.003.
15. Winkler JK, Blum A, Kommoss K, Enk A, Toberer F, Rosenberger A, et al. Assessment of diagnostic performance of dermatologists cooperating with a convolutional neural network in a prospective clinical study: human with machine. JAMA Dermatol. 2023;159:621e7.
16. Goessinger EV, Niederfeilner JC, Cerminara S, et al. Patient and dermatologists' perspectives on augmented intelligence for melanoma screening: a prospective study. J Eur Acad Dermatol Venereol. 2024;38(12):2240–9. https://doi.org/10.1111/jdv.19905.
17. Cerminara SE, Cheng P, Kostner L, et al. Diagnostic performance of augmented intelligence with 2D and 3D total body photography and convolutional neural networks in a high-risk population for melanoma under real-world conditions: a new era of skin cancer screening? Eur J Cancer. 2023;190:112954. https://doi.org/10.1016/j.ejca.2023.112954.
18. Ba W, Wu H, Chen WW, et al. Convolutional neural network assistance significantly improves dermatologists' diagnosis of cutaneous tumours using clinical images. Eur J Cancer. 2022;169:156–65. https://doi.org/10.1016/j.ejca.2022.04.015.
19. Balasubramaniam V. Artificial intelligence algorithm with SVM classification using dermoscopic images for melanoma diagnosis. J Artif Intell Capsule Netw. 2021;3:34–42.

20. Liu Y, Li C, Li F, Lin R, Zhang D, Lian Y. Advances in computer vision and deep learning-facilitated early detection of melanoma. Brief Funct Genomics. 2025;24:elaf002. https://doi.org/10.1093/bfgp/elaf002.
21. Rastgoo M, et al. Classification of melanoma lesions using sparse coded features and random forests. In: Sidibé D, Morel O, editors. Proc. SPIE 9785, Medical Imaging 2016: computer-aided diagnosis, vol. 9785. Bellingham: SPIE; 2016. p. 97850C.
22. Hosny KM, Kassem MA, Fouad MM. Classification of skin lesions into seven classes using transfer learning with AlexNet. J Digit Imaging. 2020;33:1325–34.
23. Hosny KM, Kassem MA, Foaud MM. Classification of skin lesions using transfer learning and augmentation with Alexnet. PLoS One. 2019;14:e0217293.
24. Govindaswamy B, Mallappa M. Detection and segmentation of melanoma skin cancer in dermoscopy images using modified Alexnet convolutional neural network-morphological methodology. Concurrency Comput Pract Exp. 2022;34:e7266.
25. Quishpe-Usca A, Cuenca-Dominguez S, Arias-Viñansaca A, et al. The effect of hair removal and filtering on melanoma detection: a comparative deep learning study with AlexNet CNN. PeerJ Comput Sci. 2024;10:e1953.
26. Yilmaz E, Trocan M. A modified version of GoogLeNet for melanoma diagnosis. J Inf Telecommun. 2021;5:395–405.
27. Rajinikanth V, Kadry S, Damaševičius R, et al. Skin melanoma segmentation using VGG-UNet with Adam/SGD optimizer: a study. In: 2022 Third International Conference on Intelligent Computing Instrumentation and Control Technologies (ICICICT). Piscataway: IEEE; 2022. p. 982–6.
28. Adegun AA, Viriri S. FCN-based DenseNet framework for automated detection and classification of skin lesions in dermoscopy images. IEEE Access. 2020;8:150377–96.
29. Jaworek-Korjakowska J, Kleczek P, Gorgon M. Melanoma thickness prediction based on convolutional neural network with GG-19 model transfer learning. In: Proceedings of the IEEE/CVF conference on computer vision and pattern recognition workshops. Piscataway: IEEE; 2019.
30. Aljohani K, Turki T. Automatic classification of melanoma skin cancer with deep convolutional neural networks. AI. 2022;3:512–25.
31. Tabrizchi H, Parvizpour S, Razmara J. An improved VGG model for skin cancer detection. Neural Process Lett. 2023;55:3715–32.
32. Manasa K, Vishnu MG. Skin cancer detection using VGG16. Eur J Mol Clin Med. 2021;8:1419–27.
33. Zhao C, Shuai R, Ma L, et al. Dermoscopy image classification based on StyleGAN and DenseNet201. IEEE Access. 2021;9:8659–79.
34. Gong A, Yao X, Lin W. Dermoscopy image classification based on StyleGANs and decision fusion. IEEE Access. 2020;8:70640–50.
35. Gu Y, Ge Z, Bonnington CP, et al. Progressive transfer learning and adversarial domain adaptation for cross-domain skin disease classification. IEEE J Biomed Health Inform. 2019;24:1379–93.
36. Baur C, Albarqouni S, Navab N. MelanoGANs: high resolution skin lesion synthesis with GANs. arXiv preprintarXiv:1804.04338. 2018.
37. Yi X, Walia E, Babyn P. Unsupervised and semi-supervised learning with categorical generative adversarial networks assisted by wasserstein distance for dermoscopy image classification. arXiv preprint arXiv:1804.03700. 2018.
38. Acosta MFJ, Tovar LYC, Garcia-Zapirain MB, et al. Melanoma diagnosis using deep learning techniques on dermatoscopic images. BMC Med Imaging. 2021;21:1–11.
39. Bajwa MN, Muta K, Malik MI, et al. Computer-aided diagnosis of skin diseases using deep neural networks. Appl Sci. 2020;10:2488.
40. Lucius M, de All J, de All JA, et al. Deep neural frameworks improve the accuracy of general practitioners in the classification of pigmented skin lesions. Diagnostics. 2020;10:969.
41. Mendes DB, da Silva NC. Skin lesions classification using convolutional neural networks in clinical images. arXiv preprint arXiv:1812.02316 2018.

42. Song J, Li J, Ma S, et al. Melanoma classification in dermoscopy images via ensemble learning on deep neural network. In: 2020 IEEE International Conference on Bioinformatics and Biomedicine (BIBM). Piscataway: IEEE; 2020. p. 751–6.
43. Akram T, Lodhi HMJ, Naqvi SR, et al. A multilevel features selection framework for skin lesion classification. Human-centric Comput Info Sci. 2020;10:1–26.
44. Al-Masni MA, Kim D-H, Kim T-S. Multiple skin lesions diagnostics via integrated deep convolutional networks for segmentation and classification. Comput Methods Prog Biomed. 2020;190:105351.
45. Chaturvedi SS, Tembhurne JV, Diwan T. A multi-class skin cancer classification using deep convolutional neural networks. Multimed Tools Appl. 2020;79:28477–98.
46. Almaraz-Damian J-A, Ponomaryov V, Sadovnychiy S, et al. Melanoma and nevus skin lesion classification using handcraft and deep learning feature fusion via mutual information measures. Entropy. 2020;22:484.
47. Ahmad B, Usama M, Huang C-M, et al. Discriminative feature learning for skin disease classification using deep convolutional neural network. IEEE Access. 2020;8:39025–33.
48. Ichim L, Popescu D. Melanoma detection using an objective system based on multiple connected neural networks. IEEE Access. 2020;8:179189–202.
49. Gouda N, Amudha J. Skin cancer classification using ResNet. In: 2020 IEEE 5th International Conference on Computing Communication and Automation (ICCCA). Piscataway: IEEE; 2020. p. 536–41.
50. Budhiman A, Suyanto S, Arifianto A. Melanoma cancer classification using Resnet with data augmentation. In: 2019 International seminar on research of information technology and intelligent systems (ISRITI). Piscataway: IEEE; 2019. p. 17–20.
51. Demir A, Yilmaz F, Kose O. Early detection of skin cancer using deep learning architectures: resnet-101 and inception-v3. In: 2019 medical technologies congress (TIPTEKNO). Piscataway: IEEE; 2019. p. 1–4.
52. Chen EZ, Dong X, Li X, et al. Lesion attributes segmentation for melanoma detection with multi-task u-net. In: 2019 IEEE 16th International Symposium on Biomedical Imaging (ISBI 2019). Piscataway: IEEE; 2019. p. 485–8.
53. Nazi ZA, Abir TA. Automatic skin lesion segmentation and melanoma detection: transfer learning approach with u-net and dcnn-svm. In: Proceedings of International Joint Conference on Computational Intelligence: IJCCI 2018. Singapore: Springer; 2020. p. 371–81.
54. Liu L, Mou L, Zhu XX, Mandal M. Skin lesion segmentation based on improved u-net. In: 2019 IEEE Canadian conference of electrical and computer engineering (CCECE). Piscataway: IEEE; 2019. p. 1–4.
55. Roja RD, Siva Ranjani S. U-Net based segmentation and multiple feature extraction of dermascopic images for efficient diagnosis of melanoma. In: Computer aided intervention and diagnostics in clinical and medical images. Cham: Springer; 2019. p. 81–101.
56. Alahmadi MD. Multiscale attention U-net for skin lesion segmentation. IEEE Access. 2022;10:59145–54.
57. Naranpanawa DNU, Gu Y, Chandra SS, et al. Slim-yolo: a simplified object detection model for the detection of pigmented iris freckles as a potential biomarker for cutaneous melanoma. In: 2021 Digital Image Computing: Techniques and Applications (DICTA). Piscataway: IEEE; 2021. p. 1–8.
58. Albahli S, Nida N, Irtaza A, et al. Melanoma lesion detection and segmentation using YOLOv4-DarkNet and active contour. IEEE Access. 2020;8:198403–14.
59. Banerjee S, Singh SK, Das A, Bag R. Diagnoses of melanoma lesion using YOLOv3. In: Computational advancement in communication, circuits and systems: proceedings of 3rd ICCACCS 2020. Singapore: Springer; 2022. p. 291–302.
60. Nersisson R, Iyer TJ, Joseph Raj AN, et al. A dermoscopic skin lesion classification technique using YOLO-CNN and traditional feature model. Arab J Sci Eng. 2021;46:9797–808.
61. AlSadhan NA, Alamri SA, Ben Ismail MM, et al. Skin cancer recognition using unified deep convolutional neural networks. Cancer. 2024;16:1246.

62. Albahli S. A robust YOLOv8-based framework for real-time melanoma detection and segmentation with multi-dataset training. Diagnostics (Basel). 2025;15(6):691. Published 2025 Mar 11. https://doi.org/10.3390/diagnostics15060691.
63. Lu X, Zadeh YAFA. Deep learning-based classification for melanoma detection using XceptionNet. J Healthcare Eng. 2022;2022:1–10.
64. Kassani SH, Kassani PH. A comparative study of deep learning architectures on melanoma detection. Tissue Cell. 2019;58:76–83.
65. Perez E, Reyes O, Ventura S. Convolutional neural networks for the automatic diagnosis of melanoma: an extensive experimental study. Med Image Anal. 2021;67:101858.
66. Rasul MF, Dey NK, Hashem MMA. A comparative study of neural network architectures for lesion segmentation and melanoma detection. In: 2020 IEEE Region 10 Symposium (TENSYMP). Piscataway: IEEE; 2020. p. 1572–5.
67. Qureshi MN, Umar MS, Shahab S. A transfer-learning-based novel convolution neural network for melanoma classification. Comput Secur. 2022;11:64.
68. Abbas Q, Gul A. Detection and classification of malignant melanoma using deep features of NASNet. SN Comput Sci. 2022;4:21.
69. Rahman MA, Bazgir E, Hossain SMS, et al. Skin cancer classification using NASNet. Int J Sci Res Arch. 2024;11:775–85.
70. Girdhar N, Sinha A, Gupta S. DenseNet-II: an improved deep convolutional neural network for melanoma cancer detection. Soft Comput. 2023;27:13285–304.
71. Zhang Y, Wang C. SIIM-ISIC melanoma classification with DenseNet. In: 2021 IEEE 2nd International Conference on Big Data, Artificial Intelligence and Internet of Things Engineering (ICBAIE). Piscataway: IEEE; 2021. p. 14–7.
72. Munaf A, Hoque A, Jawwad KA. DenseNet based skin lesion classification and melanoma detection. Dhaka: Diss. Brac University; 2021.
73. Nawaz M, Nazir T, Masood M, et al. Melanoma segmentation: a framework of improved DenseNet77 and UNET convolutional neural network. Int J Imaging Syst Technol. 2022;32:2137–53.
74. Chaturvedi SS, Gupta K, Prasad PS. Skin lesion analyser: an efficient seven-way multi-class skin cancer classification using MobileNet. In: Advanced machine learning technologies and applications: proceedings of AMLTA 2020. Singapore: Springer; 2021. p. 165–76.
75. Indraswari R, Rokhana R, Herulambang W. Melanoma image classification based on MobileNetV2 network. Procedia Comput Sci. 2022;197:198–207.
76. Boulahia SY, Benatia MA, Bouzar A. Att2ResNet: a deep attention-based approach for melanoma skin cancer classification. Int J Imaging Syst Technol. 2022;32:476–89.
77. Cao X, Pan J-S, Wang Z, et al. Application of generated mask method based on mask R-CNN in classification and detection of melanoma. Comput Methods Prog Biomed. 2021;207:106174.
78. Anantharaman R, Velazquez M, Lee Y. Utilizing mask R-CNN for detection and segmentation of oral diseases. In: 2018 IEEE international conference on bioinformatics and biomedicine (BIBM). Piscataway: IEEE; 2018. p. 2197–204.
79. Huang C, Yu A, Wang Y, He H. Skin lesion segmentation based on mask R-CNN. In: 2020 International Conference on Virtual Reality and Visualization (ICVRV). Piscataway: IEEE; 2020. p. 63–7.
80. Khan MA, Akram T, Zhang Y-D, et al. Attributes based skin lesion detection and recognition: a mask RCNN and transfer learning-based deep learning framework. Pattern Recogn Lett. 2021;143:58–66.
81. Bagheri F, Tarokh MJ, Ziaratban M. Skin lesion segmentation from dermoscopic images by using mask R-CNN, retina Deeplab, and graph-based methods. Biomed Signal Process Control. 2021;67:102533.
82. Zou Q, Cheng J, Liang Z. Automatic diagnosis of melanoma based on EfficientNet and patch strategy. Int J Comput Intell Syst. 2023;16:87.
83. Venugopal V, Joseph J, Vipin das M, et al. An EfficientNet based modified sigmoid transform for enhancing dermatological macro-images of melanoma and nevi skin lesions. Comput Methods Prog Biomed. 2022;222:106935.

84. Papiththira S, Kokul T. Melanoma skin cancer detection using EfficientNet and channel attention module. In: 2021 IEEE 16th International Conference on Industrial and Information Systems (ICIIS). Piscataway: IEEE; 2021. p. 227–32.
85. Zhang R. Melanoma detection using convolutional neural network. In: 2021 IEEE International conference on consumer electronics and computer engineering (ICCECE). Piscataway: IEEE; 2021. p. 75–8.
86. Codella NCF, Gutman D, Celebi ME, Helba B, Marchetti MA, Dusza SW, et al. Skin lesion analysis toward melanoma detection: a challenge at the 2017 International symposium on biomedical imaging (ISBI), hosted by the international skin imaging collaboration (ISIC). In: 2018 IEEE 15th international symposium biomedicine imaging (ISBI 2018). New York: IEEE; 2018. p. 168–72.
87. Marchetti MA, Codella NCF, Dusza SW, Gutman DA, Helba B, Kalloo A, et al. Results of the 2016 International Skin Imaging Collaboration International Symposium on Biomedical Imaging challenge: comparison of the accuracy of computer algorithms to dermatologists for the diagnosis of melanoma from dermoscopic images. J Am Acad Dermatol. 2018;78:270–277.e1.
88. Tschandl P, Rinner C, Apalla Z, Argenziano G, Codella N, Halpern A, et al. Human-computer collaboration for skin cancer recognition. Nat Med. 2020;26:1229–34.
89. Combalia M, Codella N, Rotemberg V, Carrera C, Dusza S, Gutman D, et al. Validation of artificial intelligence prediction models for skin cancer diagnosis using dermoscopy images: the 2019 International Skin Imaging Collaboration Grand Challenge. Lancet Digit Health. 2022;4:e330e9.
90. Gonza'lez-Cruz C, Jofre MA, Podlipnik S, Combalia M, Gareau D, Gamboa M, et al. Machine learning in melanoma diagnosis. Limitations about to be overcome. Actas Dermosifiliogr (Engl). 2020;111:313e6.
91. Goyal M, Knackstedt T, Yan S, Hassanpour S. Artificial intelligence-based image classification methods for diagnosis of skin cancer: challenges and opportunities. Comput Biol Med. 2020;127:104065.
92. Kommoss KS, Winkler JK, Mueller-Christmann C, Bardehle F, Toberer F, Stolz W, et al. Observational study investigating the level of support from a convolutional neural network in face and scalp lesions deemed diagnostically 'unclear' by dermatologists. Eur J Cancer. 2023;185:53e60.
93. Winkler JK, Sies K, Fink C, et al. Melanoma recognition by a deep learning convolutional neural network-performance in different melanoma subtypes and localisations. Eur J Cancer. 2020;127:21–9. https://doi.org/10.1016/j.ejca.2019.11.020.
94. D'Alessandro B. Methods and apparatus for identifying skin features of interest, US11164670B2, 2021. Accesses: 01 Nov 2024. [Online]. Available: https://patents.google.com/patent/US11164670B2/en.
95. Betz-Stablein B, D'Alessandro B, Koh U, et al. Reproducible Naevus counts using 3D total body photography and convolutional neural networks. Dermatology. 2022;238(1):4–11. https://doi.org/10.1159/000517218.
96. Marchetti MA, Nazir ZH, Nanda JK, et al. 3D whole-body skin imaging for automated melanoma detection. J Eur Acad Dermatol Venereol. 2023;37(5):945–50. https://doi.org/10.1111/jdv.18924.
97. Kurtansky NR, D'Alessandro BM, Gillis MC, et al. The SLICE-3D dataset: 400,000 skin lesion image crops extracted from 3D TBP for skin cancer detection. Sci Data. 2024;11(1):884. Published 2024 Aug 14. https://doi.org/10.1038/s41597-024-03743-w.
98. Rutjes C, Mothershaw A, D'Alessandro BM, et al. Combining automated lesion risk and change assessment improves melanoma detection: a retrospective accuracy study. J Invest Dermatol. 2025;145(3):703–706.e1. https://doi.org/10.1016/j.jid.2024.07.027.
99. Sies K, Winkler JK, Fink C, et al. Does sex matter? Analysis of sex-related differences in the diagnostic performance of a market-approved convolutional neural network for skin cancer detection. Eur J Cancer. 2022;164:88–94. https://doi.org/10.1016/j.ejca.2021.12.034.

100. Hidalgo L, Salinas MP, Sepúlveda J, Carrasco K, Romero P, Pedro A, et al. Creating a dermatologic database for artificial intelligence, a Chilean experience, and advice from ChatGPT. JEADV Clin Pract. 2024;4(1):296–8.
101. Groh M, Badri O, Daneshjou R, et al. Deep learning-aided decision support for diagnosis of skin disease across skin tones. Nat Med. 2024;30(2):573–83. https://doi.org/10.1038/s41591-023-02728-3.
102. Rezk E, Eltorki M, El-Dakhakhni W. Improving skin color diversity in cancer detection: deep learning approach. JMIR Dermatol. 2022;5(3):e39143. https://doi.org/10.2196/39143. PMID: 39475773; PMCID: PMC10334920.
103. Sangers TE, Kittler H, Blum A, et al. Position statement of the EADV artificial intelligence (AI) task force on AI-assisted smartphone apps and web-based services for skin disease. J Eur Acad Dermatol Venereol. 2024;38(1):22–30. https://doi.org/10.1111/jdv.19521.
104. Menzies SW, Sinz C, Menzies M, et al. Comparison of humans versus mobile phone-powered artificial intelligence for the diagnosis and management of pigmented skin cancer in secondary care: a multicentre, prospective, diagnostic, clinical trial. Lancet Digit Health. 2023;5(10):e679–91. https://doi.org/10.1016/S2589-7500(23)00130-9.
105. Oloruntoba A, Ingvar Å, Sashindranath M, et al. Examining labelling guidelines for AI-based software as a medical device: a review and analysis of dermatology mobile applications in Australia. Australas J Dermatol. 2024;65(5):409–22. https://doi.org/10.1111/ajd.14269.
106. Marsden H, Kemos P, Venzi M, et al. Accuracy of an artificial intelligence as a medical device as part of a UK-based skin cancer teledermatology service. Front Med (Lausanne). 2024;11:1302363. Published 2024 Mar 22. https://doi.org/10.3389/fmed.2024.1302363.
107. Dréno B, Mohr P, Sicard J, et al. Multidisciplinary patient-centered approach to the management of skin cancer. J Eur Acad Dermatol Venereol. 2024;38(Suppl 5):21–5. https://doi.org/10.1111/jdv.19573.
108. European Commision. Ethics guidelines for trustworthy AI. https://digital-strategy.ec.europa.eu/en/library/ethics-guidelines-trustworthy-ai. Last accessed 17-05-2023.
109. Sangers TE, Wakkee M, Moolenburgh FJ, Nijsten T, Lugtenberg M. Towards successful implementation of artificial intelligence in skin cancer care: a qualitative study exploring the views of dermatologists and general practitioners. Arch Dermatol Res. 2023;315(5):1187–95.
110. Hauser K, Kurz A, Haggenmüller S, Maron RC, von Kalle C, Utikal JS, et al. Explainable artificial intelligence in skin cancer recognition: a systematic review. Eur J Cancer. 2022;167:54–69.
111. Hamim SA, Tamim MUI, Mridha MF, Safran M, Che D. SmartSkin-XAI: an interpretable deep learning approach for enhanced skin cancer diagnosis in smart healthcare. Diagnostics (Basel). 2024;15(1):64. Published 2024 Dec 30. https://doi.org/10.3390/diagnostics15010064.
112. Munjal G, Bhardwaj P, Bhargava V, Singh S, Nagpal N. SkinSage XAI: an explainable deep learning solution for skin lesion diagnosis. Health Care Science. 2024;3(6):438–55. Published 2024 Nov 28. https://doi.org/10.1002/hcs2.121.
113. Chanda T, Hauser K, Hobelsberger S, et al. Dermatologist-like explainable AI enhances trust and confidence in diagnosing melanoma. Nat Commun. 2024;15(1):524. Published 2024 Jan 15. https://doi.org/10.1038/s41467-023-43095-4.
114. Shah SAH, Shah STH, Khaled R, et al. Explainable AI-based skin cancer detection using CNN, particle swarm optimization and machine learning. J Imaging. 2024;10(12):332. Published 2024 Dec 22. https://doi.org/10.3390/jimaging10120332.
115. Lucieri A, Bajwa MN, Braun SA, Malik MI, Dengel A, Ahmed S. ExAID: a multimodal explanation framework for computer-aided diagnosis of skin lesions. Comput Methods Prog Biomed. 2022;215:106620. https://doi.org/10.1016/j.cmpb.2022.106620.
116. Yap J, Yolland W, Tschandl P. Multimodal skin lesion classification using deep learning. Exp Dermatol. 2018;27:1261–7.
117. Ou C, et al. A deep learning based multimodal fusion model for skin lesion diagnosis using smartphone collected clinical images and metadata. Front Surg. 2022;9:1029991.

118. Zhou J, He X, Sun L, et al. Pre-trained multimodal large language model enhances dermatological diagnosis using SkinGPT-4. Nat Commun. 2024;15(1):5649. Published 2024 Jul 5. https://doi.org/10.1038/s41467-024-50043-3.
119. Cirone K, Akrout M, Abid L, Oakley A. Assessing the utility of multimodal large language models (GPT-4 vision and large language and vision assistant) in identifying melanoma across different skin tones. JMIR Dermatol. 2024;7:e55508. Published 2024 Mar 13. https://doi.org/10.2196/55508.
120. Kalidindi S. The role of artificial intelligence in the diagnosis of melanoma. Cureus. 2024;16(9):e69818. Published 2024 Sep 20. https://doi.org/10.7759/cureus.69818.
121. Jütte L, González-Villà S, Quintana J, Steven M, Garcia R, Roth B. Integrating generative AI with ABCDE rule analysis for enhanced skin cancer diagnosis, dermatologist training and patient education. Front Med (Lausanne). 2024;11:1445318. Published 2024 Oct 3. https://doi.org/10.3389/fmed.2024.1445318.
122. Saeed M, Naseer A, Masood H, Shafiq ur Rehman, Gruhn V. The power of generative AI to augment for enhanced skin cancer classification: a deep learning approach. IEEE Access. 2023;11:130330–44.
123. Marques AG, Vinicius M, da J, Teixeira C, Mauricio C, Hugo V, et al. New approach generative AI melanoma data fusion for classification in dermoscopic images with large language model 2024;1–6.
124. Koller S, Wiltgen M, Ahlgrimm-Siess V, et al. In vivo reflectance confocal microscopy: automated diagnostic image analysis of melanocytic skin tumours. J Eur Acad Dermatol Venereol. 2011;25(5):554–8. https://doi.org/10.1111/j.1468-3083.2010.03834.x.
125. Gareau D, Hennessy R, Wan E, Pellacani G, Jacques SL. Automated detection of malignant features in confocal microscopy on superficial spreading melanoma versus nevi. J Biomed Opt. 2010;15(6):061713. https://doi.org/10.1117/1.3524301.
126. Wodzinski M, Skalski A, Witkowski A, Pellacani G, Ludzik J. Convolutional neural network approach to classify skin lesions using reflectance confocal microscopy. Annu Int Conf IEEE Eng Med Biol Soc. 2019;2019:4754–7.
127. Mandal A, Priyam S, Chan HH, et al. Computer-aided diagnosis of melanoma subtypes using reflectance confocal images. Cancers (Basel). 2023;15(5):1428. Published 2023 Feb 23. https://doi.org/10.3390/cancers15051428.
128. Campanella G, Navarrete-Dechent C, Liopyris K, Monnier J, Aleissa S, Minhas B, et al. Deep learning for basal cell carcinoma detection for reflectance confocal microscopy. J Invest Dermatol. 2022;142(1):97–103.
129. Patel RH, Foltz EA, Witkowski A, Ludzik J. Analysis of artificial intelligence-based approaches applied to non-invasive imaging for early detection of melanoma: a systematic review. Cancers (Basel). 2023;15(19):4694. Published 2023 Sep 23. https://doi.org/10.3390/cancers15194694.
130. Lboukili I, Stamatas G, Descombes X. DermoGAN: multi-task cycle generative adversarial networks for unsupervised automatic cell identification on in vivo reflectance confocal microscopy images of the human epidermis. J Biomed Opt. 2024;29(8):086003. https://doi.org/10.1117/1.JBO.29.8.086003.
131. Hekler A, Utikal JS, Enk AH, et al. Pathologist-level classification of histopathological melanoma images with deep neural networks. Eur J Cancer. 2019;115:79–83. https://doi.org/10.1016/j.ejca.2019.04.021.
132. De Logu F, Ugolini F, Maio V, et al. Recognition of cutaneous melanoma on digitized histopathological slides via artificial intelligence algorithm. Front Oncologia. 2020;10:1559. Published 2020 Aug 20. https://doi.org/10.3389/fonc.2020.01559.
133. Niazi MKK, Parwani AV, Gurcan MN. Digital pathology and artificial intelligence. Lancet Oncol. 2019;20:e253–61. https://doi.org/10.1016/S1470-2045(19)30154-8.
134. Kamal R, Jehad Feras AlSamhori, Noel A, Qaqish LN, Jaber LA, Rawan Abujudeh, et al. Transforming dermatopathology with AI: addressing bias, enhancing interpretability, and shaping future diagnostics. Dermatol Rev. 2025;6(1)

135. Lalmalani RM, Lim CXY, Oh CC. Artificial intelligence in dermatopathology: a systematic review. Clin Exp Dermatol. 2025;50(2):251–9. https://doi.org/10.1093/ced/llae361.
136. Shaker N, Niu S, Blankenship H, et al. Artificial intelligence and convolutional neural networks-driven detection of micro and macro metastasis of cutaneous melanoma to the lymph nodes. Am J Dermatopathol. 2025;47(5):361–4. https://doi.org/10.1097/DAD.0000000000002954.
137. Jansen P, Baguer DO, Duschner N, et al. Deep learning detection of melanoma metastases in lymph nodes. Eur J Cancer. 2023;188:161–70. https://doi.org/10.1016/j.ejca.2023.04.023.
138. Siarov J, et al. Deep learning model shows pathologist-level detection of sentinel node metastasis of melanoma and intra-nodal nevi. Front Med. 2024;11:1418013.
139. Gershenwald JE, Scolyer RA, Hess KR, Sondak VK, Long GV, Ross MI, et al. Melanoma staging: evidence-based changes in the American Joint Committee on Cancer eighth edition cancer staging manual. CA Cancer J Clin. 2017;67:472–92. https://doi.org/10.3322/caac.21409.
140. Kulkarni PM, Robinson EJ, Pradhan JS, et al. Deep learning based on standard H&E images of primary melanoma tumors identifies patients at risk for visceral recurrence and death. Clin Cancer Res. 2020;26:1126–34. https://doi.org/10.1158/1078-0432.CCR-19-1495.
141. Comes MC, Fucci L, Mele F, et al. A deep learning model based on whole slide images to predict disease-free survival in cutaneous melanoma patients. Sci Rep. 2022;12:20366. https://doi.org/10.1038/s41598-022-24315-1.
142. Adeuyan O, Gordon ER, Kenchappa D, et al. An update on methods for detection of prognostic and predictive biomarkers in melanoma. Front Cell Dev Biol. 2023;11 https://doi.org/10.3389/fcell.2023.1290696.
143. Hu J, Cui C, Yang W, et al. Using deep learning to predict anti-PD-1 response in melanoma and lung cancer patients from histopathology images. Transl Oncol. 2021;14:100921. https://doi.org/10.1016/j.tranon.2020.100921.
144. Comes MC, Fucci L, Strippoli S, et al. An artificial intelligence-based model exploiting H&E images to predict recurrence in negative sentinel lymph-node melanoma patients. J Transl Med. 2024;22(1):838. https://doi.org/10.1186/s12967-024-05629-2.
145. Xu C, Yu X, Ding Z, et al. Artificial intelligence-assisted metastasis and prognosis model for patients with nodular melanoma. PLoS One. 2024;19(8):e0305468. Published 2024 Aug 7. https://doi.org/10.1371/journal.pone.0305468.
146. Maibach F, Sadozai H, Seyed Jafari SM, Hunger RE, Schenk M. Tumor-infiltrating lymphocytes and their prognostic value in cutaneous melanoma. Front Immunol. 2020;11:2105.
147. Azimi F, Scolyer RA, Rumcheva P, Moncrieff M, Murali R, McCarthy SW, Saw RP, Thompson JF. Tumor-infiltrating lymphocyte grade is an independent predictor of sentinel lymph node status and survival in patients with cutaneous melanoma. J Clin Oncol. 2012;30:2678–83.
148. Clark WH, Elder DE, Guerry D, Braitman LE, Trock BJ, Schultz D, Synnestvedt M, Halpern AC. Model predicting survival in stage I melanoma based on tumor progression. J Natl Cancer Inst. 1989;81:1893–904.
149. Ugolini F, et al. Tumor-infiltrating lymphocyte recognition in primary melanoma by deep learning convolutional neural network. Am J Pathol. 2023;193(12):2099–110.
150. Zormpas-Petridis K, Failmezger H, Raza SEA, Roxanis I, Jamin Y, Yuan Y. Superpixel-based conditional random fields (SuperCRF): incorporating global and local context for enhanced deep learning in melanoma histopathology. Front Oncol. 2019;9:1045.
151. Hodi FS, O'Day SJ, McDermott DF, Weber RW, Sosman JA, Haanen JB, Gonzalez R, Robert C, Schadendorf D, Hassel JC, et al. Improved survival with Ipilimumab in patients with metastatic melanoma. N Engl J Med. 2010;363:711–23.
152. Barone A, Hazarika M, Theoret MR, Mishra-Kalyani P, Chen H, He K, Sridhara R, Subramaniam S, Pfuma E, Wang Y, et al. FDA approval summary: pembrolizumab for the treatment of patients with unresectable or metastatic melanoma. Clin Cancer Res. 2017;23:5661–5.

153. Hazarika M, Chuk MK, Theoret MR, Mushti S, He K, Weis SL, Putman AH, Helms WS, Cao X, Li H, et al. U.S. FDA approval summary: Nivolumab for treatment of unresectable or metastatic melanoma following progression on Ipilimumab. Clin Cancer Res. 2017;23:3484–8.
154. Martins F, Sofiya L, Sykiotis GP, Lamine F, Maillard M, Fraga M, Shabafrouz K, Ribi C, Cairoli A, Guex-Crosier Y, et al. Adverse effects of immune-checkpoint inhibitors: epidemiology, management and surveillance. Nat Rev Clin Oncol. 2019;16:563–80.
155. Valero C, Lee M, Hoen D, Zehir A, Berger MF, Seshan VE, Chan TA, Morris LGT. Response rates to anti–PD-1 immunotherapy in microsatellite-stable solid tumors with 10 or more mutations per Megabase. JAMA Oncol. 2021;7:739–43.
156. Prelaj A, Miskovic V, Zanitti M, et al. Artificial intelligence for predictive biomarker discovery in immuno-oncology: a systematic review. Ann Oncol. 2024;35(1):29–65. https://doi.org/10.1016/j.annonc.2023.10.125.
157. Zhang C, Fonseca L d AF, Shi Z, et al. Systematic review of radiomic biomarkers for predicting immune checkpoint inhibitor treatment outcomes. Methods. 2021;188:61–72. https://doi.org/10.1016/j.ymeth.2020.11.005.
158. Yoo S-K, Fitzgerald CW, Cho BA, Fitzgerald BG, Han C, Koh ES, Pandey A, Sfreddo H, Crowley F, Korostin MR, et al. Prediction of checkpoint inhibitor immunotherapy efficacy for cancer using routine blood tests and clinical data. Nat Med. 2025:1–12.
159. Benzekry S, Grangeon M, Karlsen M, Alexa M, Bicalho-Frazeto I, Chaleat S, Tomasini P, Barbolosi D, Barlesi F, Greillier L. Machine learning for prediction of immunotherapy efficacy in non-small cell lung cancer from simple clinical and biological data. Cancer. 2021;13:6210.
160. Johannet P, Coudray N, Donnelly DM, Jour G, Illa-Bochaca I, Xia Y, Johnson DB, Wheless L, Patrinely JR, Nomikou S, et al. Using machine learning algorithms to predict immunotherapy response in patients with advanced melanoma. Clin Cancer Res. 2021;27:131–40.
161. Schina A, Sztupinszki Z, Marie Svane I, Szallasi Z, Jönsson G, Donia M. Intratumoral T-cell and B-cell receptor architecture associates with distinct immune tumor microenvironment features and clinical outcomes of anti-PD-1/L1 immunotherapy. J Immunother Cancer. 2023;11:e006941.
162. Bigelow E, Saria S, Piening B, Curti B, Dowdell A, Weerasinghe R, Bifulco C, Urba W, Finkelstein N, Fertig EJ, et al. A random forest genomic classifier for tumor agnostic prediction of response to anti-PD1 immunotherapy. Cancer Inform. 2022;21:11769351221136081.
163. Chowell D, Yoo S-K, Valero C, Pastore A, Krishna C, Lee M, Hoen D, Shi H, Kelly DW, Patel N, et al. Improved prediction of immune checkpoint blockade efficacy across multiple cancer types. Nat Biotechnol. 2022;40:499–506.
164. Litchfield K, Reading JL, Puttick C, Thakkar K, Abbosh C, Bentham R, Watkins TBK, Rosenthal R, Biswas D, Rowan A, et al. Meta-analysis of tumor- and T cell-intrinsic mechanisms of sensitization to checkpoint inhibition. Cell. 2021;184:596–614.e514.
165. Gschwind A, Ossowski S. AI model for predicting anti-PD1 response in melanoma using multi-omics biomarkers. Cancers (Basel). 2025;17(5):714. Published 2025 Feb 20. https://doi.org/10.3390/cancers17050714.
166. Wang R, Liu Q, You W, Chen Y. A multi-task deep learning model based on comprehensive feature integration and self-attention mechanism for predicting response to anti-PD1/PD-L1. Int Immunopharmacol. 2024;142(Pt A):113099. https://doi.org/10.1016/j.intimp.2024.113099.
167. Ye M, Ren S, Luo H, et al. Integration of graph neural networks and transcriptomics analysis identify key pathways and gene signature for immunotherapy response and prognosis of skin melanoma. BMC Cancer. 2025;25(1):648. Published 2025 Apr 9. https://doi.org/10.1186/s12885-025-13611-4.
168. Liu S, Liu J, Mei Y, Zhang W. Gut microbiota affects PD-L1 therapy and its mechanism in melanoma. Cancer Immunol Immunother. 2025;74(5):169. Published 2025 Apr 11. https://doi.org/10.1007/s00262-025-04018-y.
169. Macandog ADG, Catozzi C, Capone M, et al. Longitudinal analysis of the gut microbiota during anti-PD-1 therapy reveals stable microbial features of response in melanoma patients. Cell Host Microbe. 2024;32(11):2004–2018.e9. https://doi.org/10.1016/j.chom.2024.10.006.

170. Szóstak N, Budnik M, Tomela K, et al. Exploring correlations between gut mycobiome and lymphocytes in melanoma patients undergoing anti-PD-1 therapy. Cancer Immunol Immunother. 2025;74(4):110. Published 2025 Feb 25. https://doi.org/10.1007/s00262-024-03918-9.
171. Liang H, Jo JH, Zhang Z, et al. Predicting cancer immunotherapy response from gut microbiomes using machine learning models. Oncotarget. 2022;13:876–89. https://doi.org/10.18632/oncotarget.28252.
172. Zhou Y, Han W, Feng Y, et al. Revealing gut microbiota biomarkers associated with melanoma immunotherapy response and key bacteria-fungi interaction relationships: evidence from metagenomics, machine learning, and SHAP methodology. Front Immunol. 2025;16:1539653. Published 2025 Mar 18. https://doi.org/10.3389/fimmu.2025.1539653.
173. Huber V, Guardo LD, Lalli L, et al. Back to simplicity: a four-marker blood cell score to quantify prognostically relevant myeloid cells in melanoma patients. J Immunother Cancer. 2021;9(2):e001167. https://doi.org/10.1136/jitc-2020-001167.
174. Tompkins AG, Gray ZN, Dadey RE, et al. Radiomic analysis of patient and interorgan heterogeneity in response to immunotherapies and BRAF-targeted therapy in metastatic melanoma. J Immunother Cancer. 2025;13(2):e009568. Published 2025 Feb 12. https://doi.org/10.1136/jitc-2024-009568.
175. Amrane K, Meur CL, Thuillier P, et al. Review on radiomic analysis in 18F-fluorodeoxyglucose positron emission tomography for prediction of melanoma outcomes. Cancer Imaging. 2024;24(1):87. Published 2024 Jul 5. https://doi.org/10.1186/s40644-024-00732-5.
176. Peisen F, Gerken A, Hering A, et al. Can delta radiomics improve the prediction of best overall response, progression-free survival, and overall survival of melanoma patients treated with immune checkpoint inhibitors? [published correction appears in Cancers (Basel). 2024 Dec 24;17(1):1. doi: 103390/cancers17010001]. Cancers (Basel). 2024;16(15):2669. Published 2024 Jul 26. https://doi.org/10.3390/cancers16152669.
177. Currie G, Hawk KE, Rohren E, Vial A, Klein R. Machine learning and deep learning in medical imaging: intelligent imaging. J Med Imaging Radiat Sci. 2019;50(4):477–87. https://doi.org/10.1016/j.jmir.2019.09.005.
178. Broggi G, Maniaci A, Lentini M, et al. Artificial intelligence in head and neck cancer diagnosis: a comprehensive review with emphasis on radiomics, histopathological, and molecular applications. Cancers (Basel). 2024;16(21):3623. Published 2024 Oct 27. https://doi.org/10.3390/cancers16213623.
179. Semerci ZM, Toru HS, Çobankent Aytekin E, et al. The role of artificial intelligence in early diagnosis and molecular classification of head and neck skin cancers: a multidisciplinary approach. Diagnostics (Basel). 2024;14(14):1477. Published 2024 Jul 10. https://doi.org/10.3390/diagnostics14141477.

Noncancerous Lesions and Artificial Intelligence

8

Marios Papadakis and Dimitra Koumaki

8.1 Introduction

Dermatology skin conditions are among the most common reasons for visiting general practitioners. Diagnostic approaches traditionally involve patient history, clinical examination, dermoscopic imaging, and occasionally histopathology. However, many skin lesions share similar visual features, making accurate diagnosis challenging, even for experienced clinicians.

Due to the shortage of dermatologists, many patients must wait extended periods for evaluation. A significant proportion of these patients present with noncancerous lesions that can resemble malignant ones. Examples include seborrheic keratosis, dermatofibroma, hemangioma, and melanocytic nevi. Differentiating benign from malignant lesions is clinically important to avoid unnecessary surgical procedures and follow-ups.

An even more valuable tool would be a multiclass classification system capable of not only distinguishing between benign and malignant lesions but also aiding in the identification of specific conditions. This could lead to more efficient treatment planning and improved patient outcomes.

8.2 AI Systems Applied in Benign Lesions

Seborrheic keratoses and dermatofibromas are among the most frequently encountered benign skin lesions, making them key targets for AI-based diagnostic tools. Given their prevalence in the benign category across multiple studies, these

M. Papadakis · D. Koumaki (✉)
Department of Surgery II, University of Witten-Herdecke, Herdecke, Germany

Department of Dermatology, University Hospital of Heraklion, Heraklion, Greece

E. Karampinis et al. (eds.), *Artificial Intelligence Applications in Dermatology*,
https://doi.org/10.1007/978-3-032-15614-3_8

conditions offer valuable opportunities for developing and refining AI systems in dermatology.

8.2.1 Seborrheic Keratosis

Seborrheic keratosis (SK) is the most common benign epidermal lesion, particularly prevalent in older adults. These lesions appear as waxy, elevated, wart-like growths and typically develop on areas with high sebaceous gland activity, such as the face, chest, and back [1]. They may also exhibit outward or thickened growth. Due to their clinical variability, SKs are often mistaken for malignant lesions, including melanoma and nonmelanoma skin cancers, leading to unnecessary surgical excisions (Fig. 8.1).

Han et al. evaluated the diagnostic accuracy of an AI model for seborrheic keratosis using two datasets: Asan and Edinburgh. In the Asan dataset, the model achieved 83% sensitivity and 86% specificity, with an area under the curve (AUC) of 0.90. Similar performance was observed with the Edinburgh dataset, showing 80% sensitivity, 83% specificity, and an AUC of 0.89. These results were comparable to those for other benign and malignant lesions in the same study.

Jansen et al. investigated the potential of deep learning algorithms to distinguish seborrheic keratosis from Bowen's disease, a precancerous condition that can occasionally arise within SK lesions. Their model, trained on histopathological slides of

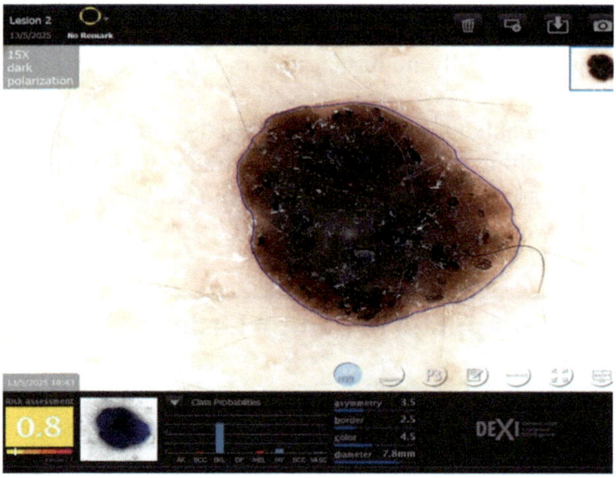

Fig. 8.1 Canfield's DEXI® (dermoscopy explained intelligence) is an AI-based dermoscopic research tool to assist clinicians in the evaluation of skin lesions. DEXI consists of an overall risk assessment score on a scale of 0–10, as well as several explainable components, including a spatial heatmap indicating where DEXI is focusing on, and a probability graph showing individual probabilities for the five benign classes and three malignant classes (melanoma, BCC, and SCC) [6]. According to the AI score system, the most likely diagnosis of the lesion is correctly benign-keratosis like lesion. (Image owned by Professor Dimitrios Sgouros)

Bowen's disease, irritated SK, and non-irritated SK, performed well in differentiating BD from non-irritated SK, achieving 95–99% sensitivity and 97–99% specificity. On external validation data, sensitivity and specificity remained high (95% and 90%, respectively; AUC: 98%). However, distinguishing BD from irritated SK proved more difficult, with a lower specificity of 66% (sensitivity 95%, AUC 92%), likely due to the limited number of irritated SK images. An important feature of this study was the inclusion of "collision tumors," where both SK and BD were present within the same lesion. In such cases, the algorithm prioritized the detection of the precancerous component. While this led to misclassification of some irritated SK areas as BD, the authors argue this is a beneficial feature, alerting pathologists not to overlook a potentially serious finding. They described AI as a "second set of eyes" in both routine and complex diagnoses [2].

In a similar study, Reddy et al. applied a CNN model to differentiate SK from actinic keratosis, another precancerous lesion. The model showed high diagnostic accuracy (99.5%), with a sensitivity of over 99% for actinic keratosis and a reported specificity of 100%. The team also investigated the accuracy of four CNN networks in differentiating between basal cell carcinoma (BCC) and SK and found the CNN model to be superior to the average of the general dermatologists and comparable to the expert dermatologists [1, 3].

Zhu et al. developed a fine-tuned model using the ImageNet dataset, including 13,603 dermoscopic images classified into 14 categories. Among these, 553 images (4%) were of seborrheic keratosis. Their model achieved an overall accuracy of 95%, with 86% sensitivity, and 96% specificity for SK [4].

Liutkus et al. used a YOLO-based multiclass classification model, which showed significantly lower performance for SK compared to other lesions. The model achieved 52% sensitivity and 93% specificity for SK, whereas it performed better for melanoma (88% sensitivity and 87% specificity) and melanocytic nevi (77% sensitivity and 91% specificity). Dermatologists, both experienced and beginner-level, outperformed the model in SK classification (sensitivity/specificity: 89%/99% for experts; 73%/89% for beginners). The reduced AI performance was attributed to automatic region selection, which cropped out key dermoscopic features—such as sharp demarcation and milia-like cysts—typically located at the lesion's edges [5].

A major limitation of these studies is the underrepresentation or absence of seborrheic keratosis subtypes in the training datasets. Notably, SK is not included in several large public datasets, limiting the generalizability and robustness of many AI models targeting these lesions [5].

8.2.2 Dermatofibroma

Dermatofibromas often emerge as small, thickened nodules with a reddish-brown hue, typically growing slowly and measuring under a centimeter, though larger lesions at diagnosis may be more likely to recur. In other cases, they may appear as firm or slightly sunken papules or plaques, either solitary or clustered, and can range in color from yellow and red to various shades of brown or even purple [7]. Dermatofibromas often develop as a reaction to minor skin injuries, such as insect bites or small puncture wounds from objects like glass splinters [8]. Currently, four key histological features are recognized in dermatofibromas: A fine pigmented meshwork at the edges, a central area resembling a white scar, a reticular white pattern, and uniform pigmentation throughout [9] (Fig. 8.2).

The performance of AI systems in detecting dermatofibroma has shown promising results. Han et al. (2023) reported a sensitivity of 81–88% and a specificity of 88–93%, with overall accuracy ranging from 90% to 95% using the Asan and Edinburgh datasets [10]. Zhu et al. achieved even higher performance with a fine-tuned model trained on the ImageNet dataset, reporting 99% accuracy, 100% sensitivity, and 99% specificity for dermatofibroma detection among 14 diagnostic categories, based on 343 dermoscopic images (2.5% of the total 13,603 images) [4]. Another model using the ISIC dataset generalizes well without overfitting and accurately identifies dermatofibroma, nevus pigmentosus, squamous cell carcinoma, and melanoma, achieving 99% accuracy with a minimal loss of 0.0346 The completeness and diagnostic accuracy of chatbot-generated reports have also been evaluated, revealing that dermatofibroma is frequently identified as a likely diagnosis when a peripheral delicate pigment network and a central white patch are present [11].

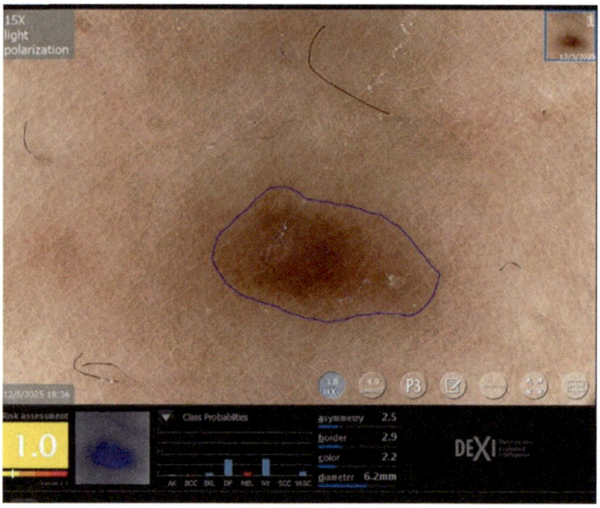

Fig. 8.2 According to Canfield's DEXI®, the lesion presented can be melanocytic nevi or DF, with similar diagnosis percentages. (Image owned by Professor Dimitrios Sgouros)

8.2.3 Hemangioma

Skin hemangiomas are common benign vascular tumors that typically arise from an abnormal proliferation of blood vessels within the skin. They most often appear during infancy or early childhood, though they can also occur in adults. Clinically, hemangiomas present as soft, raised lesions that vary in color from bright red to purplish-blue, depending on their depth and vascular composition.

Dermoscopy enhances the diagnostic accuracy of hemangiomas by revealing characteristic vascular structures. Common dermoscopic features include a red-blue lacunar pattern, consisting of well-demarcated, round or oval vascular lacunae, often separated by whitish septa. These lacunae represent dilated blood-filled vessels and help differentiate hemangiomas from other vascular or pigmented skin lesions

Skin hemangiomas have served as candidates for evaluation by artificial intelligence (AI) systems. Recent CNN-based studies have explored the application of AI models to accurately detect hemangiomas or/and differentiate them from other vascular or pigmented lesions. In the study from Han et al., hemangioma demonstrated with 77% the lowest sensitivity from all 12 skin lesions in the Edinburgh dataset (AUC 0,83), the sensitivity being 82% in the Asan test (AUC 0,89). The specificity of the Edinburgh dataset was 75% the second lowest after intraepithelial carcinoma (70%). The Asan dataset was 84% [10]. Zhu et al. reported a model accuracy of 98%, with sensitivity 98%, and specificity 98% for hemangioma in the finetuned AI model of the ImageNet dataset of 200 dermoscopic images out of a total of 13,603 images (1,5%) [4].

8.3 Conclusions

Artificial intelligence can assist in distinguishing benign from malignant lesions using binary classification systems, and it can also provide specific diagnoses for benign lesions through multiclass systems. AI models, when adequately and correctly trained, have the potential to outperform even experienced dermatologists. The diagnostic accuracy of CNN based AI systems depends on the size of the training datasets; generally, larger datasets result in higher accuracy. Malignant conditions are more frequently misclassified as other malignancies rather than as benign conditions.

References

1. Reddy S, Giri D, Patel R. Artificial intelligence-based distinction of actinic keratosis and seborrheic keratosis. Cureus. 2024; https://doi.org/10.7759/cureus.58692.
2. Jansen P, Baguer DO, Duschner N, Le'Clerc Arrastia J, Schmidt M, Wiepjes B, et al. Evaluation of a deep learning approach to differentiate Bowen's disease and seborrheic keratosis. Cancers (Basel). 2022;14:3518. https://doi.org/10.3390/cancers14143518.

3. Huang K, He X, Jin Z, Wu L, Zhao X, Wu Z, et al. Assistant diagnosis of basal cell carcinoma and seborrheic keratosis in Chinese population using convolutional neural network. J Healthc Eng. 2020;2020:1–8. https://doi.org/10.1155/2020/1713904.
4. Zhu C-Y, Wang Y-K, Chen H-P, Gao K-L, Shu C, Wang J-C, et al. A deep learning based framework for diagnosing multiple skin diseases in a clinical environment. Front Med (Lausanne). 2021;8 https://doi.org/10.3389/fmed.2021.626369.
5. Liutkus J, Kriukas A, Stragyte D, Mazeika E, Raudonis V, Galetzka W, et al. Accuracy of a smartphone-based artificial intelligence application for classification of melanomas, melanocytic nevi, and seborrheic Keratoses. Diagnostics. 2023;13:2139. https://doi.org/10.3390/diagnostics13132139.
6. Cerminara SE, Cheng P, Kostner L, Huber S, Kunz M, Maul J-T, et al. Diagnostic performance of augmented intelligence with 2D and 3D total body photography and convolutional neural networks in a high-risk population for melanoma under real-world conditions: a new era of skin cancer screening? Eur J Cancer. 2023;190:112954. https://doi.org/10.1016/j.ejca.2023.112954.
7. Orzan OA, Dorobanțu AM, Gurău CD, Ali S, Mihai MM, Popa LG, et al. Challenging patterns of atypical dermatofibromas and promising diagnostic tools for differential diagnosis of malignant lesions. Diagnostics. 2023;13:671. https://doi.org/10.3390/diagnostics13040671.
8. Fu'adah YN, Pratiwi NC, Pramudito MA, Ibrahim N. Convolutional neural network (CNN) for automatic skin cancer classification system. IOP Conf Ser Mater Sci Eng. 2020;982:012005. https://doi.org/10.1088/1757-899X/982/1/012005.
9. Kormos NF, Paval ID, Baican AL. Factors contributing to the false diagnosis of misleading dermatofibromas. Cancer Rep. 2025;8 https://doi.org/10.1002/cnr2.70164.
10. Han SS, Kim MS, Lim W, Park GH, Park I, Chang SE. Classification of the clinical images for benign and malignant cutaneous tumors using a deep learning algorithm. J Invest Dermatol. 2018;138:1529–38. https://doi.org/10.1016/j.jid.2018.01.028.
11. Karampinis E, Toli O, Georgopoulou K-E, Kampra E, Spyridonidou C, Roussaki Schulze A-V, et al. Can artificial intelligence "hold" a Dermoscope?—the evaluation of an artificial intelligence chatbot to translate the dermoscopic language. Diagnostics. 2024;14:1165. https://doi.org/10.3390/diagnostics14111165.

Part III

Artificial Intelligence in Inflammatory Dermatoses

Psoriasis and Artificial Intelligence

9

Efterpi Zafiriou and Natalia Rompoti

9.1 Introduction

Psoriasis is a chronic, immune-mediated skin disease, affecting approximately 2–3% of the general population, with a prevalence ranging from 0.3% to 0.6%. In recent years, deeper knowledge of psoriasis pathogenesis and its impact on the patient's quality of life has led to a better understanding of the cumulative life course impairment associated with this inflammatory skin disorder. This is not limited to the direct effect of psoriatic disease on the patient himself, but also includes its correlation with several comorbidities, such as cardiovascular, metabolic, and psychiatric diseases. Identifying patients who are most likely to benefit from timely and effective therapeutic intervention is of critical importance. Ideally, such an approach would embrace the principles of personalized medicine, tailoring treatment to each individual with psoriasis. By taking into account both patient- and disease-specific characteristics, it aims to distinguish cases in which early intervention could not only modify the course of the disease but also help prevent or positively influence the onset of various comorbidities [1].

Therefore, the management of psoriasis should extend beyond the initiation of medical treatment. It should encompass a comprehensive approach that includes accurate diagnosis of this inflammation-mediated skin disorder, assessment of involvement in special anatomical sites, identification of potential comorbidities, and evaluation for the presence of coexisting psoriatic arthritis. Educating the

E. Zafiriou (✉)
Department of Dermatology, Faculty of Medicine, School of Health Sciences, University General Hospital of Larissa, University of Thessaly, Larissa, Greece

N. Rompoti
1st Department of Dermatology-Venereology, Medical School, National and Kapodistrian University of Athens, "A. Sygros" Hospital for Skin and Venereal Diseases, Athens, Greece

E. Karampinis et al. (eds.), *Artificial Intelligence Applications in Dermatology*,
https://doi.org/10.1007/978-3-032-15614-3_9

patient and his social environment is also part of disease management, along with evaluating disease severity, and making an effort therapeutically to apply precision medicine.

Artificial intelligence (AI) could revolutionize how psoriasis is approached in terms of diagnosis, treatment, and management.

AI programs in psoriasis could be implemented in the education of both physicians and patients. Providing numerous and accurate data concerning several aspects of this inflammatory skin disease could lead to continuous education that optimizes the management of psoriasis. Moreover, AI could support the differential diagnosis of psoriasis from normal skin or other skin disorders, which could be beneficial in cases where access to a specialized clinician is limited or a skin biopsy is not an option. Furthermore, the objective quantification of psoriasis characteristics—such as disease severity—could enhance the consistency of disease assessment by providing a more standardized language. This approach may prove valuable both in routine clinical practice and in randomized controlled trials (RCTs). Processing through AI all available information concerning pathogenesis, therapeutic options, and response to treatment could lead to the development of biomarkers of prognostic and monitoring value for psoriasis management. Finally, AI could be used ideally to support the clinician in applying personalized medicine, thus finding the optimal treatment for each patient [2].

When properly implemented, AI could serve as a valuable ally to both patients and dermatologists, helping to bridge knowledge gaps and enhance the potential for a more holistic and optimized approach to psoriasis management. Clinicians should keep in mind, however, that AI systems analyze imported data, making unbiased access to information crucial. Therefore, accuracy refinement as a result of a representative dataset could enhance AI precision in the future, making it a clinical decision support tool for the holistic approach of the psoriatic disease.

9.2 Prevention of Psoriasis Proposed by AI

Identifying risk factors that may exacerbate psoriasis or contribute to comorbidities, such as the development of psoriatic arthritis (PsA), is crucial for recognizing patients who could benefit most from early intervention. Proactive management can significantly reduce the cumulative life course impairment in these individuals (CLCI). AI can analyze imported patient data and lifestyle parameters to predict potential psoriasis exacerbation before it occurs. This could allow patients to take preventive measures, such as adjusting medications or avoiding known trigger factors, to minimize the risk of flare-ups. A step further would be to use AI-based primary prevention methods to identify patients at risk for developing psoriasis [1].

On that basis, Guo et al. pioneered in 2014 the development of an AI program designed to predict psoriasis. Their innovative system employed three feature selection algorithms to analyze gene expression profiles derived from two microarray data sets, successfully identifying 21 features located in 18 genes associated with psoriasis. The results provided were instrumental in constructing a classification model that employed only three features from two different genes, IGFL1 and C10orf99. This method achieved an impressive average overall accuracy of 99.8% across three different validation strategies, resulting in a novel psoriasis prediction model [3]. Moreover, researchers published in 2021 a strong predictive model for psoriasis using only demographic parameters and standard hospital test data from 466 psoriasis patients and 520 healthy controls. They applied the Boruta feature selection method to determine the most pertinent features, which were then used to build a Random Forest model. Overall, 26 different key features were identified as predictive factors, and the developed classification model achieved an average accuracy of 86.9% in predicting psoriatic disease [4]. In the same year, data from another study model for predicting psoriasis risk were published. The model processed genetic and genomic data involving 1462 individuals with PsA and 1132 psoriasis patients. Seven different supervised AI algorithms were included, highlighting two known human leukocyte antigen (HLA) genes, HLA_C_06 and HLA_B_27, as potentially the most significant genetic factors associated with psoriasis development [5].

Concerning the risk of comorbidities in the form of cardiovascular disorders, metabolic diseases, or psychiatric disorders, and the development of PsA, AI techniques have been leveraged in studies focusing on the early detection of risk factors. Advanced machine learning (ML) algorithms are used to identify characteristics that correlate with an increased risk of comorbidities in this population. For instance, by incorporating natural language processing (NLP) and genetic data from electronic medical records, researchers identified, with the use of 31 variants, predictors related to the development of PsA [5]. Additionally, Patrick and colleagues used ML techniques to identify, with the assistance of genetic data alone, nine new loci for psoriasis and psoriasis subtypes [6]. Furthermore, research has developed ML models based on blood immune profiling and serum proteomics to differentiate between psoriasis patients with and without joint involvement. These models led to the development of a predictive algorithm for minimal disease activity in psoriasis. Variables such as global pain, the psoriatic arthritis impact of disease (PsAID), patient global disease assessment, and physical function (measured by the Health Assessment Questionnaire-Disability Index) exhibited the highest predictive power [4].

Another study examined the prognostic value of red blood cell distribution width (RDW) and mean platelet volume (MPV) for predicting major cardiovascular events in patients with psoriatic arthritis (PsA), analyzing a comprehensive dataset exceeding 50 million patient records. Findings indicated that elevated levels of these parameters beyond defined thresholds correlated with a heightened cardiovascular risk and diminished response to therapy. Specifically, the incidence of myocardial infarction, atrial fibrillation, and chronic heart failure was highest among patients exhibiting elevated levels of both RDW and MPV, particularly among patients suffering from skin psoriasis. The incidence of these cardiovascular disorders was also increased with elevated RDW in patients with PsA. Among patients treated with various systemic and biologic agents, a decrease in elevated RDW from baseline during one year of follow-up was linked to ongoing therapeutic success [7].

9.3 AI-Based Diagnosis of Psoriasis

In recent years, significant efforts have been directed toward applying AI in the diagnosis and differential diagnosis of psoriatic disease. Specifically, through a machine learning process and evaluation of skin images, psoriasis could be distinguished from clinically healthy skin and diagnosed over other inflammatory skin diseases.

In 2011, Mashaly and colleagues pioneered the involvement of AI in psoriasis diagnosis. In their study, four different AI techniques (rough sets, topological derivate, K-means clustering, and watershed images) were utilized to evaluate six erythrosquamous disorders. Data were collected from the dermatologic image dataset of a university hospital and dermatologic image atlases. Fifty skin images from each skin condition, including psoriasis, were processed. Rough set-based segmentation demonstrated superior accuracy and sensitivity compared to alternative approaches [8].

A few years later, Shirvastava and his colleagues used principal component analysis (PCA) and support vector machine (SVM) to analyze 270 images of psoriatic skin and compare them to an equal number of clinically healthy skin. The objective was to develop and assess the reliability of a computer-aided diagnostic (CAD) system that analyzes grayscale, color, redness, and chaoticness features. This AI-based algorithm was capable of differentiating lesional from non-lesional skin with a classification accuracy exceeding 99% [9].

Although clinicians typically do not face difficulty in identifying psoriatic lesions versus healthy skin, accurately diagnosing psoriasis among other papulosquamous disorders can sometimes prove challenging. Aggarwal et al. (2019) used deep convolutional neural network (DCNN) analysis with data augmentation of 280 open-source psoriatic lesions to differentially diagnose psoriasis from other inflammatory skin diseases, such as atopic dermatitis, impetigo contagiosa, acne, and rosacea. The study demonstrated that data augmentation can improve ML image identification in every studied skin condition, including psoriasis [10].

DCNN models have also been used in a Chinese study, where 8021 images of skin lesions were collected from a single hospital. The images belonged to different skin conditions—psoriasis, eczema, lichen planus, pemphigus, lupus erythematosus, seborrheic keratosis, basal cell carcinoma, squamous cell carcinoma—and data processing was conducted with a two-stage deep neural network algorithm, designed and developed to identify psoriasis. In the first phase, a multilabel classifier was trained to learn the visual patterns for each skin disorder. In the second phase, the results of the initial stage were used to differentiate psoriasis from other non-psoriatic skin lesions. The accuracy of this AI analysis system was higher than that of 25 Chinese dermatologists, with a missed diagnosis rate of 0.03 vs 0.19, respectively, and a misdiagnosis rate of 0.04 vs 0.10, respectively [11]. Similarly, Wu et al. assessed the diagnostic performance of an artificial intelligence dermatology diagnosis assistant (AIDDA) in accurately differentiating among three inflammatory skin conditions—psoriasis, atopic dermatitis, and eczema—by analyzing 4770 macroscopic images collected from a single center. Psoriasis could be diagnosed using this AI algorithm with an accuracy of 89.46%, compared to 92.57% for atopic dermatitis and eczema [12].

In 2021, two of the largest and most diverse dermatological databases from hospitals in Peking and Xiangya were processed using CNN algorithms. In Peking Union Medical College Hospital, Zhu et al. developed a new framework utilizing deep learning process to categorize 14 different skin conditions, including psoriasis. Information gathered from 13,603 macroscopic pictures of 2538 patients was evaluated and the outcome emphasized the high accuracy of AI in identifying diverse inflammatory and non-inflammatory lesions (lichen planus, rosacea, viral warts, acne vulgaris, keloid and hypertrophic scar, eczema and dermatitis, dermatofibroma, seborrheic dermatitis, seborrheic keratosis, melanocytic nevus, hemangioma, psoriasis, port wine stain, and basal cell carcinoma) [13]. Huang et al. published information on an AI network called Xy-SkinNet, which processed 150,000 clinical pictures of 571 different skin disorders, from which more than 60,000 were psoriatic lesions. The AI model demonstrated a higher accuracy rate than clinicians/dermatologists (84.77% vs 78.15%) [11].

Even in challenging areas for diagnosis and treatment, like the scalp, deep learning methods have proven effective for differentiating psoriasis from seborrheic dermatitis. Specifically, a smartphone-based multispectral imaging system with an external CMOS camera was used for the evaluation of 60 patients with psoriasis, seborrheic dermatitis or no skin condition of the scalp. Macroscopic images were assessed after a training process with 18,000 spectra signatures obtained from skin with scalp psoriasis or seborrheic dermatitis and 2000 spectral signatures for testing using SVM, logi, and MLP algorithms. This AI-based approach demonstrated high sensitivity and specificity in identifying psoriatic lesions and outperformed conventional diagnostic methods (ED and SAM) [14].

Furthermore, a DL model has been developed to facilitate the differential diagnosis of these two conditions on the scalp using dermoscopic imaging (Fig. 9.1). Specifically, 1624 dermoscopic pictures were processed from 735 patients, that led to the development of an AI instrument with high sensitivity and specificity. This model enhanced the diagnostic capabilities of healthcare professionals without specialized training in dermatology, thereby supporting more accurate assessments in clinical practice [15].

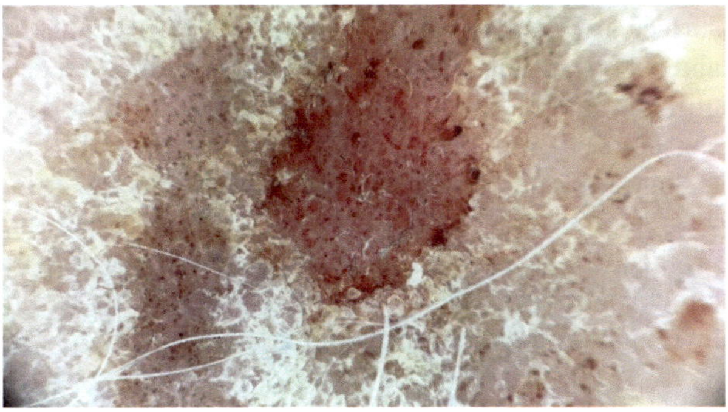

Fig. 9.1 Dermoscopic manifestations of psoriasis vulgaris (red-dotted/vessels and white scales)

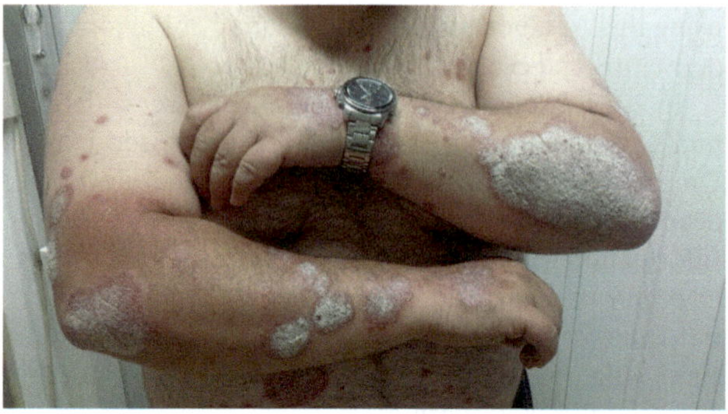

Fig. 9.2 Plaque psoriasis patient presenting with red plaques and silver scales

AI models have also been used to process histopathological features. For instance, 366 histopathology images of 35 patients with either psoriasis, seborrheic dermatitis, lichen planus, pityriasis rosea, chronic dermatitis, or pityriasis rubra pilaris were analyzed in an Indian study. The development of a machine learning process with classification and regression trees (CART), SVM, DT, RF, and gradient boosted decision trees (GBDT) methodology, enabled the identification of these skin conditions with 98.64% accuracy [16].

Diagnosing different types of psoriatic disease—such as plaque (Fig. 9.2), guttate, erythrodermic, pustular, or inverse psoriasis—is a routine process for the dermatologist. In the past years, several AI algorithms have been used to identify different subtypes of this skin disease and explore the method with the best sensitivity and specificity. For instance, convolutional neural networks (CNNs) and long short-term memories (LSTMs) have both been used to assess psoriasis subtypes. Specifically, Aijaz et al. engaged both DL algorithms to develop classification models and proved a high accuracy rate of 84.2% and 72.3%, respectively [17].

9.4 AI-Powered Psoriasis Assessment

AI can also be applied to the segmentation of psoriatic lesions from surrounding healthy skin, enabling more accurate assessment of lesion size and disease severity. The use of automated AI algorithms in image segmentation is of great importance, as it facilitates the performance of more advanced tasks, such as automated body surface area (BSA), psoriasis area and severity index (PASI), and skin biopsy. Taur and colleagues introduced an automated method for segmenting psoriasis images by utilizing neuro-fuzzy classifiers along with orthogonal subspace classifiers. This can be used in a therapy evaluation system [18]. Following this, a segmentation technique based on feed-forward skin features and artificial neural networks (ANNs) was employed to process images of psoriasis and other skin conditions, yielding promising outcomes during the training and generalization phases of the ANNs. The effectiveness of psoriasis image segmentation was further enhanced by a method involving k-means clustering integrated with morphological processing techniques.

In their 2012 study, Bogo et al. employed a two-step algorithm combining color analysis for initial lesion detection with geometric active contours technique for detailed segmentation of psoriatic plaque. The variation in segmentation results between the algorithm and human evaluators is comparable to the variation observed among different human assessments. One year later, Ma and colleagues published results from another visual depiction method for precise plaque segmentation. Specifically, they utilized a new hybrid evolutionary optimiser that combines two swarm-intelligence methods (artificial bee colony (ABC) and the seeker optimization algorithm (SOA)). This hybrid algorithm obtains data from two conventional, local-clustering approaches, fuzzy c-means, and k-means, processing a total of 720 psoriasis images. The study results revealed that this novel AI-assisted method outperforms other swarm-intelligence techniques as well as traditional clustering methods [19].

In the same year, Lu et al. developed a new approach to support psoriasis assessment with image segmentation in a reliable manner. An algorithm that segments scaling in 2D digital photographs was developed. The scaling segmentation issue was approached as a classification and parameter problem. Specifically, a support-vector machine (SVM) assigns an initial, pixel-level label using features drawn from color and scaling texture, and a Markov random field (MRF) subsequently smooths the result. The algorithm has a reliable performance even in varied lighting conditions, skin types, and psoriasis subtypes [20].

Over the past years, subsequent automatic lesion segmentation methods have significantly improved performance by utilizing multiscale superpixels, k-means clustering, and a combination of SVM and Fisher discriminant ratio. Classical, non-deep methods, using super-pixels in combination with clustering or graph-cuts, seem to achieve their task with around 87% accuracy and ≤80% specificity on small cohorts. Moreover, psoriasis lesions can be automatically segmented into RGB color images using an advanced CNN. An example of this use is the modified U-net (PsLSNet), trained on 5241 skin images from 1026 psoriasis patients. This model overcame previous limitations in segmentation, including the presence of artefacts or poor acquisition conditions, thus achieving an accuracy of 94.8%, with 89.6% sensitivity and 97.6% specificity [21].

Although these are preliminary data, the field of segmentation in psoriasis skin lesions is rapidly evolving, leading to higher accuracy and reproducible results. Additionally, automatic methods have been developed for the precise segmentation of skin biopsy images to overcome the challenges faced by pathologists. Histopathological evaluation is known to be subject to considerable inter-observer variability due to the absence of standardized quantitative metrics. Consequently, the development of an automated system is warranted to address these limitations and enhance diagnostic consistency in psoriasis. Pal and colleagues employed deep neural architectures to segment psoriasis skin biopsy images. By employing deep learning models to classify super-pixels generated through simple linear iterative clustering (SLIC), the researchers achieved superior segmentation performance compared to conventional approaches relying on hand-crafted features [22].

9.5 Treatment Plan Tailored by AI Programs

9.5.1 Biomarker-Driven Response to Treatment

The use of ML to predict long-term response to biologic agents is of great importance. Various models, including generalized linear models (GLM), support vector machines (SVM), decision trees, random forests, gradient-boosted trees, and deep learning (DL), have been compared for this purpose. Among these, the GLM proved to be the most accurate and computationally efficient in predicting long-term biologic responses in psoriasis.

AI can be used to assist in biomarker-driven prediction of biologic efficacy, which includes proteomic signatures, transcriptomic clustering, and peripheral blood markers. A study published in 2020 utilized statistical and machine-learning methodologies to forecast drug efficacy in psoriasis patients. They developed a classifier capable of predicting whether a patient would achieve a PASI 75 response after 12 weeks of treatment with either tofacitinib or etanercept. This prediction was based on analyzing patient blood samples for 92 proteins linked to systemic inflammation and 65 associated with cardiovascular disease [23]. In the same year, Damiani et al. created a predictive model using artificial neural networks (ANNs) to identify 'fast responders' in psoriasis. This model predicts whether those treated with secukinumab will achieve at least PASI 75 by the end of the induction phase, based on initial blood count and clinical examination data. Following a training and testing protocol, the model achieved an overall accuracy of 91.9%, correctly predicting 90% of responders and 93.8% of non-responders [24].

9.5.2 Dose-Optimization and Regimen Selection

Other research groups have also explored numerous predictive factors that could gauge treatment effectiveness, including disease characteristics. Through ML methodology, they discovered that a 300 mg dosage of secukinumab offers greater benefits than 150 mg for patients who are anti-tumor necrosis factor (TNF)-naïve, have been treated with one prior anti-TNF agent, are not on methotrexate, have enthesitis at baseline, or have a shorter duration of PsA and display higher baseline PASI [25]. Large-scale modelling of registry data has yielded complementary insights. Gradient-boosted decision-trees trained on the Danish DERMBIO cohort, for example, achieved an area under the curve of 0.85 for predicting biologic discontinuation, highlighting baseline disease severity, sex and prior biologic exposure as dominant features [26].

9.5.3 Drug-Repurposing Pipelines

AI programs are also currently used to analyze the genome involved in psoriatic disease and identify active substances (new or already existing) with a potential therapeutic role in psoriasis. This can lead to a reduction in the time and cost of developing pharmaceuticals and increase the success rate of clinical trials. For instance, a Japanese study team created in 2019 a Python-based software tool called Genome for REPositioning drugs (GREP), designed to quantify the enrichment of a user-selected gene set within the targets of clinical categories. This tool facilitates the identification of potential therapeutic agents across various conditions. It successfully mapped extensive genomic data related to psoriasis to the clinical indication categories of currently used medications. The results encompassed many drugs already approved for psoriasis treatment, alongside the discovery of novel candidate therapies. Further validation of these newly identified drugs could substantially enhance future psoriasis management strategies [27].

In the context of investigating the possible therapeutic role of drugs with no formal indication for psoriasis, Patrick et al. utilized NLP and word embedding techniques to distill information from over 20 million drug-related articles and applied ML to model relationships between drugs and diseases. This method successfully predicted the potential use of budesonide and hydroxychloroquine in treating psoriasis. Importantly, the predicted drug targets were validated by a large-scale RNA sequencing cohort, showing significant enrichment among genes differentially expressed in psoriatic lesional skin. Additionally, to further expand the therapeutic quiver, genome-wide association data (>80 psoriasis loci) were integrated with the GREP software to reveal clinically approved drugs whose target profiles overlap psoriasis-risk genes. Overall, this approach provides an effective means of identifying potential drug candidates for psoriasis treatment through the combined use of natural language processing and machine learning techniques [28].

9.6 AI-Assisted Monitoring and Management of Psoriasis

The use of mobile phone applications or AI-assisted telemedicine has contributed to the management of psoriatic disease, better communication with the patient and their guidance.

9.6.1 AI Tools in Smart Phones and Psoriasis Disease

Early feasibility work by Koller et al. (2011) demonstrated that weekly smartphone-based assessments in 20 patients initiating biologic therapy yielded tele-PASI scores statistically indistinguishable from in-clinic PASI determinations, despite 76.7% overall compliance and ≥ "sufficient" image quality in 95% of transmissions; 88% of participants rated the approach "very good," and 94% would recommend it to peers [29].

In recent years, a smartphone application was developed to support the long-term management of patients receiving biological therapy for psoriasis. This innovative tool aims to optimize patient care by potentially substituting certain routine follow-up visits, thereby minimizing the necessity for frequent clinic attendance. Such an approach not only saves patients valuable time but also facilitates timely and efficient responses to their healthcare needs.

Pangti et al. published the first extensive feasibility evaluation of an AI-driven dermatology app in a population with richly pigmented skin. The application integrates a convolutional neural network classifier covering 40 common dermatoses and was prospectively validated on > 5000 consecutive dermatology outpatients in India. For psoriasis, the model achieved a sensitivity of 68.0% and a specificity of 99.2%, indicating high rule-in accuracy and positioning the tool as a practical diagnostic adjunct in resource-constrained settings [30].

In recent developments, a new study has been initiated to explore the capabilities of a cutting-edge smartphone application designed to monitor the progression of psoriasis (87). Over 12 months, patients participating in the study input various data points, including quality of life assessments, stress questionnaires, self-evaluated psoriasis area and severity index (self-PASI), and lifestyle factors. This information was then compared with data collected by dermatologists to ensure accuracy and reliability. An intriguing feature of this application is its ability to identify lifestyle changes that may occur before noticeable shifts in the PASI score. By doing so, the app can function as an early warning system, alerting patients to potential issues such as rising stress levels or weight gain. This proactive approach allows patients to address these factors before they lead to a psoriasis flare-up, thereby enhancing their overall management of the condition [31].

Physicians also monitor the disease course of psoriasis with the aid of AI. The most popular application is that of patient-reported outcome measures (PROMs) for the evaluation of patients' quality of life, mainly in RCTs, but also in the real-world setting. Electronic patient-reported outcome measures (ePROMs) have revolutionized the way patient data is collected by replacing traditional paper-based methods with an electronic system. This transition has made the process more convenient and appealing for both patients and healthcare providers. ePROMs facilitate the swift collection and reporting of real-time patient symptoms and disease progression. This capability allows physicians to perform remote assessments and manage treatments without the need for in person visits. For example, studies in the literature have highlighted the effectiveness of ePROMs in various fields, such as oncology, where they have been used to monitor symptoms and treatment side effects remotely. In rheumatology, ePROMs have enabled continuous monitoring of disease activity, improving patient outcomes by allowing timely interventions. Similarly, in the field of dermatology, ePROMs have been employed to track skin conditions and treatment responses, providing valuable insights for personalized care. These examples underscore the versatility and value of ePROMs in modern healthcare, making them an integral part of patient management strategies [32].

9.6.2 AI-Assisted Teledermatology

Teledermatology is another field where AI-assisted medicine could be applied. This includes diagnosing and treating patients with psoriasis.

Several studies have repeatedly confirmed the diagnostic reliability of image-based severity scoring. Singh et al. first showed that automated color/texture extraction could supply reliable PASI inputs. In a 12-patient case series, Singh et al. (2011) reported good agreement between remote and face-to-face PASI assessments, while a 10-patient pilot by Frühauf et al. achieved near-perfect concordance for palmoplantar psoriasis and documented high acceptance among both patients ($\approx$ 82%) and teledermatologists (74%) [33].

Randomized trials extend these findings to routine management. An RCT conducted by Armstrong et al. (2018) in 296 patients showed non-inferiority of online consultations versus traditional visits over 12 months (Δ PASI = −0.27; Δ BSA = −0.05%) with a slightly greater DLQI improvement in the telehealth cohort (−1.64 vs −1.18). (92) A parallel analysis by Young et al. (2023) confirmed equivalent reductions in functional impairment and depressive symptoms between modalities [34]. Another study explored a multimedia application designed to evaluate the feasibility and effectiveness of a cloud-based system for interactive management of psoriasis between patients and physicians. The app featured daily skin photographs to monitor changes, a visual analogue scale for assessing itching or pain from lesions, an anxiety and depression scale for psychological evaluation, and comprehensive psoriasis-related content, including images, texts, and videos. The study concluded that this interactive patient–physician management approach, facilitated by the application, led to improved treatment outcomes for individuals with psoriasis [35].

9.7 Psoriasis—AI Informing and Supporting the Patient

e-Health technology in dermatology, including mobile and desktop applications as well as AI-assisted telemedicine, enhances access to information and services that could support better education, management of several skin diseases, communication with the patient, and personalized guidance. In terms of psoriasis, AI-derived technology has been increasingly supporting both dermatologists and patients over the past years in the field of providing information for psoriasis, assisting with the diagnosis, enabling an evaluation of response to treatment, and making patient-specific recommendations. As early as 2013, Banu et al. introduced a mobile and desktop application that employed six classification algorithms to differentiate psoriatic from non-psoriatic lesions (23).

In 2021, Pangti and colleagues developed a CNN-based algorithm to create a mobile health app capable of diagnosing 40 different skin conditions, including psoriasis. Data extracted from this large-scale feasibility study supported the use of AI in enabling patients to recognize common skin conditions at home [30].

In the field of psoriasis, another smartphone application, known as MDi-Psoriasis, was utilized to provide treatment advice for patients with moderate-to-severe psoriasis. This app employs an algorithm that takes into consideration 60 different variables, including information about patient demographics, personal medical history, and disease-specific characteristics. The results of its use indicated that the treatment recommendations generated by the application were comparable to those provided by medical experts. Therefore, the system may prove beneficial as a supplementary aid in the clinical decision-making process [36].

Building on AI-assisted supporting applications for patients with moderate-to-severe psoriasis, Trettin et al. published in 2021 data on the use of a smartphone application to support long-term management of patients under biologic treatment. Alongside analyzing clinical and demographic variables, the system also considered patients' treatment preferences and doctors' perspectives on prior therapeutic outcomes [37].In the same year, a German study conducted in psoriasis patients demonstrated that the use of an AI-assisted smartphone application can support self-assessment of disease severity and its impact on quality of life, in a manner comparable to clinical evaluation by a dermatologist. The app could also correlate lifestyle changes with PASI alteration and identify risk factors for psoriasis flare, such as increasing stress levels or weight gain. This technology could ultimately serve as a supportive tool in patients' daily lives, enabling both self-monitoring and the identification of lifestyle-related risk factors that may contribute to psoriasis exacerbation [38].

9.8 Practical Examples with AI Programs in Psoriasis

AI is a fundamental part of several smartphone applications, including but not limited to:

- DermAssist: An AI-powered mobile application that allows users to take photos of their skin lesions. The app uses a trained model to analyze images and provide preliminary assessments of psoriasis. It helps users understand their condition and encourages them to seek professional medical advice.
- SkinVision: This app employs AI to analyze skin lesions. While primarily focused on skin cancer, it also includes features for recognizing various skin conditions, including psoriasis. Users can upload images, and the app provides risk assessments based on AI analysis.
- SkinTeller: This smartphone app assists in the calculation of PASI with high accuracy.

Moreover, automated total body mapping integrates AI tools into clinical dermatology and offers promising ways for semi-automated assessment of psoriasis severity, particularly through the calculation of PASI. The following commercially available systems currently facilitate standardized photographic documentation, lesion segmentation, and semi-automated PASI estimation [39].

(i) 2D automated total body mapping (ATBM): The FotoFinder ATBM® system (FotoFinder Systems GmbH, Germany) demonstrates a dynamic imaging setup using a high-resolution, cross-polarized xenon-flash camera to generate standardized, full-body 2D images of patients in various anatomical positions. With the PASIscan® software, automated segmentation of psoriatic lesions is performed across defined body regions (head, arms, trunk, and legs), and preliminary PASI parameters—erythema, plaque thickness, and scaling—are generated. These prescores can be manually altered by clinicians, particularly in regions obscured by hair or clothing (e.g., scalp and genital area). Longitudinal image comparison enables quantification of therapeutic response using PASI 50/75/90/100 evaluation tools [40].

(ii) 3D Total Body Photography (3D-TBP): Canfield's DEXI® (Dermoscopy Explained Intelligence) is an AI-based dermoscopic research tool to assist clinicians in the evaluation of skin lesions. It is integrated into Canfield's imaging platforms, such as the DermaGraphix IntelliStudio® (2D) and VECTRA® WB360 (3D) systems, enhancing capabilities like lesion change detection through markerless tracking and AI algorithms. The VECTRA® WB360 system (Canfield Scientific, USA) captures synchronized images from 92 cameras in a single pose, reconstructing a 3D digital avatar of the patient's skin surface. A newly developed algorithm is responsible for an automated lesion segmentation by anatomical region (head and neck, arms, trunk, and legs), while erythema, induration, and scaling must be manually scored to compute the PASI. This approach simplifies and accelerates the imaging process and has been positively received by patients in melanoma screening contexts due to increased efficiency [41] (Fig. 9.3).

Despite the high precision offered by total body photography, several limitations remain. These include substantial setup costs, physical challenges for some patients—particularly the elderly—in assuming required imaging positions, and the labor-intensive nature of image acquisition. Moreover, the current lack of automated

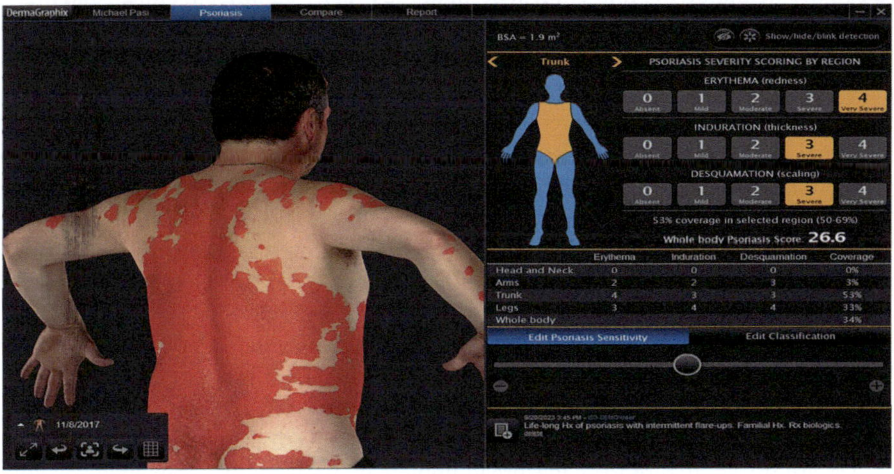

Fig. 9.3 Canfield's DEXI® (dermoscopy explained intelligence) evaluation of psoriatic lesions. (Image reproduced with permission from Canfield © All rights retained)

classification for psoriasis subtypes, along with the need for manual assessment in certain anatomical regions such as the scalp and soles, hinders the possibility of fully automated disease scoring.

9.9 Future Directions and Challenges in AI-Assisted Psoriasis Care

Artificial intelligence (AI) has increasingly become a transformative force in dermatology, offering new avenues for diagnosis, disease monitoring, and personalized treatment strategies, particularly in chronic inflammatory conditions such as psoriasis. Emerging AI-based tools hold significant potential to improve clinical decision-making by analyzing a broad range of inputs—ranging from medical imaging and self-reported patient data to molecular biomarkers. While significant advancements have been achieved, several limitations and challenges remain that must be addressed before AI systems can be reliably and seamlessly incorporated into everyday clinical workflows.

Despite technological advancements, several unmet needs remain. One of the major hurdles in AI applications for dermatology is the lack of diverse datasets. Many AI systems are trained primarily on images of lighter skin tones, making them less reliable in diagnosing conditions across different ethnic backgrounds. This limitation can lead to misdiagnoses and disparities in patient care. Another issue is the inconsistency in image capture and annotation methods across different medical institutions. Without standardized protocols, AI models can produce varying results, making it difficult for clinicians to rely on them consistently. Additionally, AI tools are not yet fully integrated into electronic health record (EHR) systems, limiting their accessibility and use during consultations. In addition to technical limitations, the implementation of AI in clinical dermatology raises significant ethical and logistical concerns. Ensuring the protection of sensitive personal health data—including genetic and biometric information—is critical. For AI systems to be trusted by healthcare providers, transparency and the ability to explain algorithmic decisions must be prioritized. Moreover, disparities in technological infrastructure and resource availability could exacerbate existing inequalities in care access, particularly in underserved regions. Broad adoption will also require targeted educational initiatives to equip healthcare professionals with the skills needed to effectively utilize AI-assisted tools. Interdisciplinary collaboration among healthcare providers, AI developers, and regulatory authorities will be essential to navigate these complex challenges.

AI continues to reshape the landscape of dermatological care, with a particularly strong influence on the management of chronic conditions such as psoriasis. However, its full adoption will require collaborative efforts between researchers, clinicians, and policymakers to address biases, improve transparency, and build the necessary infrastructure for widespread implementation. With responsible development and ethical application, AI can significantly enhance dermatological care, supporting clinicians, and improving patient outcomes in psoriasis and beyond.

References

1. Daugaard C, Iversen L, Hjuler KF. Comorbidity in adult psoriasis: considerations for the clinician. Psoriasis Targets Ther. 2022;12:139–50. https://doi.org/10.2147/PTT.S328572.
2. Liu Z, Wang X, Ma Y, Lin Y, Wang G. Artificial intelligence in psoriasis: where we are and where we are going. Exp Dermatol. 2023;32:1884–99. https://doi.org/10.1111/exd.14938.
3. Guo P, Luo Y, Mai G, Zhang M, Wang G, Zhao M, et al. Gene expression profile based classification models of psoriasis. Genomics. 2014;103:48–55. https://doi.org/10.1016/j.ygeno.2013.11.001.
4. Zhou J, Li Y, Guo X. Predicting psoriasis using routine laboratory tests with random forest. PLoS One. 2021;16:e0258768. https://doi.org/10.1371/journal.pone.0258768.
5. Laborde CM, Larzabal L, González-Cantero Á, Castro-Santos P, Díaz-Peña R. Advances of genomic medicine in psoriatic arthritis. J Pers Med. 2022;12:35. https://doi.org/10.3390/jpm12010035.
6. Patrick MT, Stuart PE, Raja K, Gudjonsson JE, Tejasvi T, Yang J, et al. Genetic signature to provide robust risk assessment of psoriatic arthritis development in psoriasis patients. Nat Commun. 2018;9:4178. https://doi.org/10.1038/s41467-018-06672-6.
7. Conic RR, Damiani G, Schrom KP, Ramser AE, Zheng C, Xu R, et al. Psoriasis and psoriatic arthritis cardiovascular disease endotypes identified by red blood cell distribution width and mean platelet volume. J Clin Med. 2020;9:186. https://doi.org/10.3390/jcm9010186.
8. Mashaly HM, Masood NA, Mohamed ASA. Classification of Papulo-squamous skin diseases using image analysis. Skin Res Technol. 2012;18:36–44. https://doi.org/10.1111/j.1600-0846.2011.00511.x.
9. Umapathy S, Sampath M, Nelufer, Srivastava S. Automated segmentation and classification of psoriasis hand thermal images using machine learning algorithm, 2022, 487–496. https://doi.org/10.1007/978-981-16-2123-9_37.
10. Aggarwal st LtP. Data augmentation in dermatology image recognition using machine learning. Skin Res Technol. 2019;25:815–20. https://doi.org/10.1111/srt.12726.
11. Huang K, Jiang Z, Li Y, Wu Z, Wu X, Zhu W, et al. The classification of six common skin diseases based on Xiangya-Derm: development of a Chinese database for artificial intelligence. J Med Internet Res. 2021;23:e26025. https://doi.org/10.2196/26025.
12. Wu H, Yin H, Chen H, Sun M, Liu X, Yu Y, et al. A deep learning, image based approach for automated diagnosis for inflammatory skin diseases. Ann Transl Med. 2020;8:581. https://doi.org/10.21037/atm.2020.04.39.
13. Zhu C-Y, Wang Y-K, Chen H-P, Gao K-L, Shu C, Wang J-C, et al. A deep learning based framework for diagnosing multiple skin diseases in a clinical environment. Front Med (Lausanne). 2021;8 https://doi.org/10.3389/fmed.2021.626369.
14. Kim S, Kim J, Hwang M, Kim M, Jin Jo S, Je M, et al. Smartphone-based multispectral imaging and machine learning based analysis for discrimination between seborrheic dermatitis and psoriasis on the scalp. Biomed Opt Express. 2019;10:879. https://doi.org/10.1364/BOE.10.000879.
15. Olayah F, Senan EM, Ahmed IA, Awaji B. AI techniques of dermoscopy image analysis for the early detection of skin lesions based on combined CNN features. Diagnostics. 2023;13:1314. https://doi.org/10.3390/diagnostics13071314.
16. Yu K, Syed MN, Bernardis E, Gelfand JM. Machine learning applications in the evaluation and Management of Psoriasis: a systematic review. J Psoriasis Psoriatic Arthritis. 2020;5:147–59. https://doi.org/10.1177/2475530320950267.
17. Aijaz SF, Khan SJ, Azim F, Shakeel CS, Hassan U. Deep learning application for effective classification of different types of psoriasis. J Healthc Eng. 2022;2022:1–12. https://doi.org/10.1155/2022/7541583.
18. Taur JS, Lee GH, Tao CW, Chen CC, Yang CW. Segmentation of psoriasis vulgaris images using multiresolution-based orthogonal subspace techniques. IEEE Trans Syst Man Cybern B Cybern. 2006;36:390–402. https://doi.org/10.1109/TSMCB.2005.859935.

19. Ma G, He B, Yang W, Shu C. Easy-interactive and quick psoriasis lesion segmentation. In: Lin X, Zheng J, editors., 2013, p. 90450T. https://doi.org/10.1117/12.2038065.
20. Lu J, Kazmierczak E, Manton JH, Sinclair R. Automatic segmentation of scaling in 2-D psoriasis skin images. IEEE Trans Med Imaging. 2013;32:719–30. https://doi.org/10.1109/TMI.2012.2236349.
21. Dash M, Londhe ND, Ghosh S, Semwal A, Sonawane RS. PsLSNet: automated psoriasis skin lesion segmentation using modified U-net-based fully convolutional network. Biomed Signal Process Control. 2019;52:226–37. https://doi.org/10.1016/j.bspc.2019.04.002.
22. Kim K-S, Zhang D, Kang M-C, Ko S-J. Improved simple linear iterative clustering superpixels. 2013 IEEE International Symposium on Consumer Electronics (ISCE). IEEE; 2013. p. 259–60. https://doi.org/10.1109/ISCE.2013.6570216.
23. Tomalin LE, Kim J, Correa da Rosa J, Lee J, Fitz LJ, Berstein G, et al. Early quantification of systemic inflammatory proteins predicts long-term treatment response to Tofacitinib and Etanercept. J Invest Dermatol. 2020;140:1026–34. https://doi.org/10.1016/j.jid.2019.09.023.
24. Damiani G, Conic R, Pigatto P, Carrera C, Franchi C, Cattaneo A, et al. Predicting Secukinumab fast-responder profile in psoriatic patients: advanced application of artificial-neural-networks (ANNs). J Drugs Dermatol. 2020;19:1241–6. https://doi.org/10.36849/JDD.2020.5006.
25. Gottlieb AB, Mease PJ, Kirkham B, Nash P, Balsa AC, Combe B, et al. Secukinumab efficacy in psoriatic arthritis. JCR: J Clin Rheumatol. 2021;27:239–47. https://doi.org/10.1097/RHU.0000000000001302.
26. Egeberg A, Rosenø NAL, Thein D, Lørup EH, Nielsen M-L, Nymand L, et al. Drug survival of biologics and novel immunomodulators for rheumatoid arthritis, axial spondyloarthritis, psoriatic arthritis, and psoriasis—a nationwide cohort study from the DANBIO and DERMBIO registries. Semin Arthritis Rheum. 2022;53:151979. https://doi.org/10.1016/j.semarthrit.2022.151979.
27. Zhang J, Lin Z, Zhang Y, Gu H, Li W. Bioinformatics-based drug repositioning and prediction of the main active ingredients and potential mechanisms of action for the efficacy of Dan-Lou tablet. Sci Rep. 2024;14:23297. https://doi.org/10.1038/s41598-024-74243-5.
28. Federico A, Pavel A, Möbus L, McKean D, del Giudice G, Fortino V, et al. The integration of large-scale public data and network analysis uncovers molecular characteristics of psoriasis. Hum Genomics. 2022;16:62. https://doi.org/10.1186/s40246-022-00431-x.
29. Koller S, Hofmann-Wellenhof R, Hayn D, Weger W, Kastner P, Schreier G, et al. Teledermatological monitoring of psoriasis patients on biologic therapy. Acta Dermato Venereologica. 2011;91:680–5. https://doi.org/10.2340/00015555-1148.
30. Pangti R, Mathur J, Chouhan V, Kumar S, Rajput L, Shah S, et al. A machine learning-based, decision support, mobile phone application for diagnosis of common dermatological diseases. J Eur Acad Dermatol Venereol. 2021;35:536–45. https://doi.org/10.1111/jdv.16967.
31. Huang K, Wu X, Li Y, Lv C, Yan Y, Wu Z, et al. Artificial intelligence–based psoriasis severity assessment: real-world study and application. J Med Internet Res. 2023;25:e44932. https://doi.org/10.2196/44932.
32. Mercadal-Orfila G, López Sánchez P, Pou Alonso A, Ibarra-Barrueta O, Monte-Boquet E, Borrás Blasco J, et al. TELEPROM psoriasis: enhancing patient-centered care and health-related quality of life (HRQoL) in moderate-to-severe plaque psoriasis. Front Med (Lausanne). 2024;11 https://doi.org/10.3389/fmed.2024.1465725.
33. Singh P, Soyer HP, Wu J, Salmhofer W, Gilmore S. Tele-assessment of psoriasis area and severity index: a study of the accuracy of digital image capture. Australas J Dermatol. 2011;52:259–63. https://doi.org/10.1111/j.1440-0960.2011.00800.x.
34. Armstrong AW, Chambers CJ, Maverakis E, Cheng MY, Dunnick CA, Chren M-M, et al. Effectiveness of online vs in-person care for adults with psoriasis. JAMA Netw Open. 2018;1:e183062. https://doi.org/10.1001/jamanetworkopen.2018.3062.
35. Zhu B, Wang Y, Zhou X, Cao C, Zong Y, Zhao X, et al. A controlled study of the feasibility and efficacy of a cloud-based interactive management program between patients with psoriasis and physicians. Med Sci Monit. 2019;25:970–6. https://doi.org/10.12659/MSM.913304.

36. Moreno-Ramírez D, Herrerías-Esteban JM, Ojeda-Vila T, Carrascosa JM, Carretero G, de la Cueva P, et al. Fiabilidad de una aplicación de ayuda a la toma de decisiones terapéuticas en el paciente con psoriasis (MDi Psoriasis ®). Actas Dermo-Sifiliogr. 2017;108:650–6. https://doi.org/10.1016/j.ad.2017.02.009.
37. Trettin B, Feldman S, Andersen F, Danbjørg DB, Agerskov H. Improving management of psoriasis patients receiving biological treatment: a qualitative approach. Nurs Open. 2021;8:1283–91. https://doi.org/10.1002/nop2.745.
38. Brandl LC, Liebram C, Schramm W, Pobiruchin M. A German smartphone-based self-management tool for psoriasis: community-driven development and evaluation of quality-of-life effects. JMIR Form Res. 2022;6:e32593. https://doi.org/10.2196/32593.
39. Goessinger EV, Gottfrois P, Mueller AM, Cerminara SE, Navarini AA. Image-based artificial intelligence in psoriasis assessment: the beginning of a new diagnostic era? Am J Clin Dermatol. 2024;25:861–72. https://doi.org/10.1007/s40257-024-00883-y.
40. https://www.fotofinder.de/en/technology/psoriasis/psoriasis. Accessed on 25 May 2025
41. O'Neal D. Demo psoriasis assessment and vitiligo assessment tools: VECTRA WB360 user group meeting presentation. San Diego: Canfield Scientific, 2024 AAD Annual Meeting; 2023 n.d.

Atopic Dermatitis and Artificial Intelligence

10

Efstratios Vakirlis, Iasonas Dermitzakis, and Elena Sotiriou

10.1 General Principles of Atopic Dermatitis

Atopic dermatitis (AD), often referred to as atopic eczema, is recognized as the most prevalent chronic inflammatory skin condition in developed countries. The disorder commonly presents in early childhood, with about 80% of cases manifesting during infancy or childhood, although it can also emerge in adulthood. The point prevalence of AD varies significantly, ranging from 2.7% to 20.1% among children, depending on the region, and from 2.1% to 4.9% in adults. AD is characterized by a high degree of clinical heterogeneity, making its natural progression sometimes unpredictable. Globally, AD was ranked as the 15th most burdensome nonfatal condition between 1990 and 2017, and it is at the forefront of skin-related diseases in terms of disability-adjusted life years (DALYs). Effective management of AD necessitates regular medical evaluations and adherence to treatment regimens, underscoring the importance of a comprehensive approach to care [1]. All key applications of AI discussed are summarized in Fig. 10.1.

E. Vakirlis (✉) · I. Dermitzakis · E. Sotiriou
First Department of Dermatology, School of Medicine, Faculty of Health Sciences, Aristotle University, Thessaloniki, Greece
e-mail: svakirlis@auth.gr; iasonasd@auth.gr; epsotiri@auth.gr

E. Karampinis et al. (eds.), *Artificial Intelligence Applications in Dermatology*,
https://doi.org/10.1007/978-3-032-15614-3_10

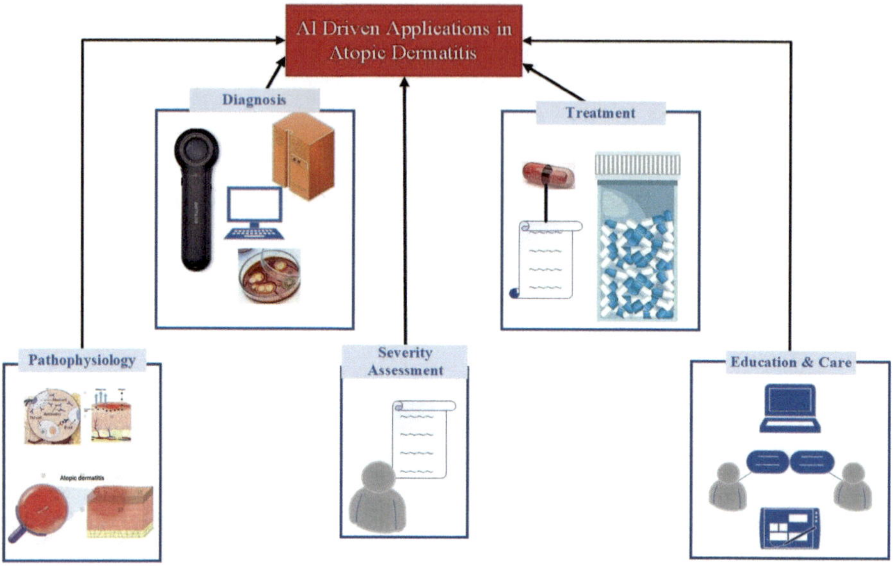

Fig. 10.1 Applications of artificial intelligence in atopic dermatitis

10.2 AI-Enhanced Diagnostics in Atopic Dermatitis

10.2.1 Clinical-Based Diagnostics in AD

One notable advancement is the development of the AI dermatology diagnosis assistant (AIDDA), which leverages the EfficientNet-B4 convolutional neural network (CNN) model [2]. Trained on a comprehensive dataset of 4740 clinical images, AIDDA demonstrated exceptional performance in diagnosing inflammatory skin conditions, including psoriasis and AD. For AD, the model achieved an impressive diagnostic accuracy of 92.57%, with a sensitivity of 94.56% and a specificity of 94.41%. Overall, AIDDA achieved an accuracy of 95.80% across all conditions, reflecting its robustness and reliability. Building on these advancements, another study focused on using the DeepLabv3+ CNN model to enhance image segmentation for dermatological conditions, particularly AD [3]. The DeepLabv3+ model demonstrated sensitivity and specificity rates of approximately 90% when distinguishing AD from other conditions, such as mycosis fungoides, impetigo, and herpesvirus infections. Notably, the model's performance surpassed that of unmodified datasets and was comparable to manually cropped images, highlighting the effectiveness of automated segmentation in reducing reliance on manual annotation. This innovation enhances diagnostic efficiency and has significant potential to improve clinical outcomes for AD patients.

Furthermore, a study investigated the use of the single shot multibox detector (SSD) model, a cutting-edge AI algorithm, for diagnosing skin conditions such as mycosis fungoides, psoriasis, and AD [4]. The SSD model achieved a diagnostic accuracy rate of

93% across 292 test images, correctly classifying 273 cases. Sensitivity rates varied by condition, with mycosis fungoides exhibiting the highest sensitivity at 96%, followed by 94% for psoriasis and 80% for AD. The exceptional performance in detecting mycosis fungoides is attributed to the larger and more distinct lesion characteristics typical of cancer spread. However, the model faced challenges in diagnosing AD due to the subtle features and smaller lesion sizes often located around joints, such as the elbows and arms. Despite these limitations, the SSD model offers a rapid, consistent, and objective method for diagnosing dermatological conditions.

Advancements in AI for dermatological diagnostics were also observed in a study assessing the impact of data augmentation on machine learning image recognition for skin diseases, including acne, atopic dermatitis, rosacea, psoriasis, and impetigo [5]. This research, which focused on open-source dermatological images, utilized the TensorFlow Inception version-3 model to evaluate the effects of data augmentation on model performance. Both augmented and non-augmented datasets were analyzed using statistical tools, including R software, to compare sensitivity, specificity, positive predictive value, and other key performance metrics. The findings demonstrated that incorporating data augmentation significantly enhanced model performance. Improvements were observed across all metrics, including sensitivity, specificity, and the Matthews correlation coefficient (MCC), indicating more robust diagnostic capabilities. These enhancements are particularly valuable for conditions like AD, where visual characteristics can be subtle and variable. The study concluded that deep learning methods, bolstered by data augmentation, offer a promising approach to improving the accuracy of dermatological image differentiation. Evolving from single-model approaches, researchers introduced a multi-model, multi-level system employing artificial neural networks (ANN) to detect AD [6]. Unlike traditional single-model frameworks, this system tailors multiple models to specific input characteristics and integrates their outputs through a decision layer to calculate the probability of an eczema diagnosis. The multi-model architecture demonstrated an improved average confidence level of 68.37%, compared to 63.01% achieved by single-model systems. Additionally, the design minimized overfitting during training, resulting in more robust and stable models. By leveraging advanced ANN architectures, this system provides a scalable and efficient tool for automated dermatological diagnostics. It highlights AI's ability to enhance diagnostic precision and reliability, particularly for challenging conditions like AD.

Expanding beyond clinical-based diagnostics, another study explored the application of AI to improve the detection of AD within routinely collected health data. Researchers utilized the electronic medical record primary care database (EMRPC) in Ontario, Canada, integrating it with the province's health administrative data. Both simple rules-based algorithms and machine learning models were evaluated for their effectiveness in identifying AD. The results revealed that rules-based algorithms achieved a higher positive predictive value (PPV), while the machine learning model—specifically logistic regression—demonstrated greater sensitivity. The rules-based algorithms yielded a high PPV, closely aligning with similar methods used in the United Kingdom and British Columbia [7, 8]. However, health administrative data alone proved insufficient for reliable AD detection. Combining EMRPC with administrative data provided a more robust solution, enabling effective epidemiological research and improved health services planning for AD. This study highlights the broader applicability of AI in leveraging existing health data to enhance the understanding and management of atopic dermatitis.

10.2.2 Imaging-Based Diagnostics in AD

A groundbreaking effort employed CNNs to classify high-frequency ultrasound (HFUS) images of skin, focusing on inflammatory conditions such as atopic dermatitis, psoriasis, and other lesions. Utilizing a comprehensive database of 631 images, encompassing both healthy and pathological skin, the researchers developed a sophisticated framework centered on segmenting the epidermal layer with DeepLab v3+ models [9]. By leveraging transfer learning, the study aimed to refine the model for two primary purposes: extracting regions of interest for classification and generating skin layer maps to assess classification reliability. Key innovations of this approach included the introduction of classification confidence metrics, which evaluate the model's reliability by integrating skin layer maps with Grad-CAM-generated heatmaps, indicating the focus areas of the model's decision-making process. Through multi-criteria evaluation, DenseNet-201 emerged as the most effective model for achieving accurate and reliable classification. This study underscores the efficacy of CNNs in HFUS imaging, offering substantial advantages in terms of accuracy and diagnostic reliability.

Enhancing the use of HFUS imaging, another study developed an advanced, automated methodology for segmenting skin layers, with a specific focus on atopic dermatitis and psoriasis [9, 10]. This approach utilized a U-shaped CNN combined with fuzzy c-means clustering to address the challenges of manual segmentation, particularly in delineating the epidermis and the subepidermal low echogenic band (SLEB). The integration of batch normalization layers within the CNN framework enhanced segmentation robustness, achieving Dice coefficients of 0.87 for the epidermis and 0.83 for the SLEB. Further advancing the application of AI in dermatology, a fully automated framework was introduced to segment the epidermal layer in a variety of skin conditions using 75 MHz HFUS imaging [11]. The framework employed two cascaded DeepLab v3+ models with a ResNet-50 backbone, pre-trained on the ImageNet dataset and fine-tuned with a database of 580 HFUS images. The first model identified the region of interest, while the second executed detailed segmentation. Achieving a Dice index of 0.919 overall and exceeding 0.93 in inflammatory conditions, this methodology demonstrated superior performance compared to existing techniques. The above frameworks' success highlights the critical role of AI in refining the precision of epidermal segmentation and its broader implications for diagnosing and monitoring conditions like atopic dermatitis.

In addition to HFUS imaging, the integration of AI with multiphoton tomography (MPT) for diagnosing AD has also been explored. Researchers utilized CNNs to develop a fully automated method for analyzing MPT data [12]. The application of AI enabled the efficient analysis of 3663 MPT images, encompassing both morphological and metabolic data from AD patients and healthy subjects. This approach achieved remarkable diagnostic accuracy for AD, with a success rate of 97.0%, sensitivity of 0.966, specificity of 0.977, and an F-score of 0.964. The use of deep Taylor decomposition further enhanced the model's interpretability by identifying critical image features influencing the classification process. This innovative methodology highlights the potential of combining MPT with AI to improve diagnostic accuracy and efficiency in dermatology, offering a robust framework for the automated diagnosis of skin disorders. Similarly, raster-scanning optoacoustic mesoscopy (RSOM) was integrated with advanced machine learning models to classify healthy individuals and AD patients while further stratifying AD severity [13]. Three machine learning approaches: random forest (RF), support vector machine (SVM), and convolutional neural networks (CNN), were evaluated. Among these, the CNN model demonstrated outstanding performance, achieving 97% accuracy in distinguishing healthy individuals from AD patients. Recent research has also explored the integration of AI with hyperspectral imaging to enhance lesion classification [14]. This approach has shown promise in distinguishing Mycosis fungoides from clinically similar conditions such as psoriasis and AD, using a dataset comprising 1659 hyperspectral skin images.

10.2.3 Laboratory and Genetic Diagnostics in AD

Advanced machine learning techniques have significantly contributed to understanding the complex interplay between biomarkers and allergic diseases, including AD. A notable study utilizing data from a general population of 161 six-year-old children in the Japan Environment and Children's Study (JECS) revealed that children with AD symptoms had elevated levels of the diagnostic markers CCL17 and CCL27 [15]. Interestingly, higher plasma levels of CCL22 were specifically observed in children with visible flexural eczema, assessed simultaneously with blood sampling. These findings highlight the diagnostic potential of cytokine and chemokine profiling in identifying and understanding AD, offering new avenues for targeted interventions. Complementing the cytokine and chemokine analyses, another study assessed critical skin chemical biomarkers in AD patients using confocal Raman micro-spectroscopy combined with advanced machine learning techniques [16]. This method allowed researchers to effectively differentiate between eczema patients and healthy controls with high diagnostic accuracy. Raman spectra collected from the lower volar forearm revealed key biomarkers, such as proteins and lipids in the stratum corneum. Utilizing partial least squares discriminant analysis, the study achieved a classification sensitivity of 0.94 and specificity of 0.85, validated through a stratified ten-fold cross-validation.

Following recent advancements in laboratory diagnostics for AD through AI, significant progress has been achieved in understanding the genetic underpinnings of the disease. One notable study utilized AI-driven gene expression analysis to explore the genetic framework of AD [17]. Researchers analyzed data from five distinct microarray studies, covering 127 samples and over 250,000 transcripts, to identify genes differentially expressed in AD compared to normal skin. Despite variability in reported differentially expressed genes (DEGs) across studies, they identified 89 consistent AD gene expression signatures, referred to as '89ADGES,' including the FLG gene. By applying a support vector machine (SVM), the study demonstrated that '89ADGES' could differentiate AD from normal skin with an impressive predictive accuracy of 98%. Another study advanced the use of machine learning in AD diagnostics by focusing on pyroptosis-related biological markers (PRBMs) [18]. Using datasets from the gene expression omnibus (GEO) database, researchers conducted an extensive analysis to identify significant pyroptosis-related genes (PRGs) and examined immune cell infiltration, revealing notable differences between AD patients and healthy individuals. Consistent clustering and weighted gene correlation network analysis (WGCNA) identified key PRGs, with the turquoise module emerging as particularly significant. Multiple machine learning algorithms were evaluated, with the extreme gradient boosting model proving the most effective. This facilitated the development of a predictive nomogram incorporating five key PRBMs—HDAC1, GPALPP1, LGALS3, SLC29A1, and RWDD3—substantially improving diagnostic accuracy for AD.

Furthermore, the integration of transcriptomic and microbiota data introduces a novel dimension to AD diagnostics. AI was employed to develop a machine learning classifier capable of predicting AD risk by analyzing data from 161 individuals, both with and without AD [19]. The classifier successfully distinguished AD patients from healthy controls, identifying 35 genes and 50 microbiota features critical for AD prediction. Among these, three genes (*GRP1, CCL22*, and *TTC27*) and three microorganisms (*Akkermanisia, Verrucomicrobia*, and *Propionibacterium*) demonstrated direct or indirect associations with the disease. While further validation is required, this innovative approach underscores the potential of combining transcriptomic and microbiota data to identify new biological markers for AD, offering a more holistic diagnostic framework. The diagnosis of AD often relies on the clinician's subjective evaluation, which can lead to missed or incorrect assessments. To address this challenge, a novel medical prediction model—referred to as bSRWPSO-FKNN—was introduced, integrating an improved particle swarm optimization algorithm (SRWPSO) with fuzzy K-nearest neighbor (FKNN) classification [20]. This model was applied to a dataset comprising clinical and immunological data from patients diagnosed with AD. Through rigorous evaluation using 10 × 10-fold cross-validation, the bSRWPSO-FKNN framework effectively identified key diagnostic features associated with AD, including lymphocyte levels, specific allergen sensitivities (e.g., cat dander, milk, *Dermatophagoides pteronyssinus*/farinae, ragweed, and cod), and total IgE concentration. These findings underscore the potential of the bSRWPSO-FKNN model as a reliable and objective tool to support clinical diagnosis and feature extraction in AD.

10.3 AI Applications in AD Severity and Risk Assessment

10.3.1 Severity Assessment Utilizing Clinical Features

AI has emerged as a transformative tool in assessing AD severity, offering solutions to the challenges posed by traditional methods. For instance, the eczema area and severity index (EASI), commonly used to evaluate AD severity, often struggles with achieving consistency and objectivity due to its reliance on subjective assessments. A study explored the application of CNNs to measure key EASI components—erythema, papulation, excoriation, and lichenification—from clinical images [21]. Using a dataset of 8000 clinical AD images scored by dermatologists, four CNN architectures (ResNet V1, ResNet V2, GoogLeNet, and VGG-Net) were trained and evaluated. These CNNs achieved remarkable accuracy, including 99.17% for erythema and 97.17% for lichenification, even under varying lighting conditions. Similarly, the SCORing Atopic Dermatitis (SCORAD) tool, another widely used clinical evaluation method, presents challenges such as time-intensive processes and interobserver variability. To address these issues, researchers introduced Automatic SCORAD, an AI-driven system that employs CNNs to analyze skin lesion images and automatically assess AD severity [22]. The system provides a rapid, objective alternative to traditional SCORAD, delivering results consistent with expert dermatologists while reducing inconsistencies across evaluations. Complementing these advances, a machine learning analysis based on data from a large international web-based survey of individuals with AD underscored the value of patient-reported outcomes [23]. Interestingly, the findings highlight the critical importance of incorporating patient perspectives into the evaluation of disease severity, beyond clinical or visual assessments alone.

Further advancements in AI-based AD severity assessment have been demonstrated using CNNs trained on large-scale datasets. One study graded AD severity using 9192 clinical images with ground truth labels provided by five board-certified dermatologists based on the investigator's global assessment (IGA) and six clinical signs of AD [24]. Various training approaches, including ensemble versus integration, hard-label versus soft-label methods, and train-set pruning, were tested. This study demonstrated that CNN-based models can objectively assess AD severity. The ensemble-soft-label-pruning CNN model emerged as the most effective. Given the variability among human evaluators and the time-intensive nature of clinical scoring, integrating soft-labeling with train-set pruning offers a faster, standardized alternative. These findings emphasize that CNN models trained with multi-evaluator datasets outperform those trained on individual evaluator datasets, particularly when assessments are highly concordant among dermatologists. Moreover, the adaptability of AI in diverse patient populations was highlighted in a study evaluating deep learning models for automated AD severity scoring in Acehnese patients from Indonesia [25]. This dataset comprised images taken using a 12-megapixel smartphone camera under dermatologist supervision. Five pre-trained CNN architectures—ResNet50, VGGNet19, MobileNetV3, MnasNet, and EfficientNetB0—were assessed. Among them, ResNet50 demonstrated superior performance with an accuracy of 89.8%, precision of 90.0%, sensitivity of 89.8%, specificity of 96.6%, and an F1-score of 89.85%. These findings underscore AI's versatility and precision in assessing AD severity, even within specific ethnic populations or settings with resource constraints.

10.3.2 Advanced Imaging and Biochemical Profiling for Severity Assessment

Recent advances in AI have significantly enhanced methods for assessing the severity of AD. An innovative AI-driven method addresses the challenges of quantifying inflammation in AD. Conventional diagnostic approaches, such as skin biopsies, are invasive and fail to capture the underlying cellular processes contributing to disease progression. To overcome these limitations, researchers employed coherent anti-Stokes Raman scattering and stimulated Raman scattering imaging, coupled with deep learning, to analyze cellular-level inflammation in an AD mouse model [26]. This approach provided high-resolution, time-specific disease scores derived from morphological and physiological data. The AI algorithms enabled precise quantification of inflammatory states without invasive procedures, offering new insights into disease progression and severity. The integration of raster-scanning optoacoustic mesoscopy (RSOM) with machine learning represents another significant advancement in AD. RSOM, a noninvasive imaging technique, was utilized alongside three machine learning approaches—random forest (RF), support vector machine (SVM), and CNN—to stratify AD severity. Among these, RF achieved the highest accuracy at 65% for distinguishing between mild and moderate-to-severe AD conditions. This stratification is critical for tailoring treatment strategies and improving patient outcomes.

Additionally, handheld confocal Raman spectroscopy (CRS) systems have emerged as practical, portable tools for evaluating AD severity through skin biochemical profiles. By leveraging advanced AI methodologies, specifically an SVM model, researchers classified and staged AD based on measurements of transepidermal water loss, skin surface moisture, and key biochemical constituents such as water, ceramides, and urocanic acid [27]. In a prospective study involving 30 AD patients and 14 healthy participants, the SVM model demonstrated strong performance with a cross-validated area under the curve (AUC) of 0.857 and an accuracy of 0.841. Moreover, the study introduced the eczema biochemical index (EBI), a novel metric correlating strongly with the SCORAD severity assessment. The handheld CRS system provides a noninvasive, user-friendly solution for assessing AD severity across various body regions. By integrating AI-driven analysis with practical usability, this innovation improves the accuracy and efficiency of AD severity assessment, facilitates personalized treatment planning, and provides substantial value for both clinical decision-making and research in disease monitoring.

Building upon these advancements in noninvasive imaging and AI integration, hyperspectral imaging has also emerged as a promising modality for severity assessment in AD. A parameter-based transfer learning approach was employed to classify the severity of AD using hyperspectral imaging data [28]. In this framework, datasets related to psoriasis, skin cancer, eczema, and AD were utilized as source domains, while the hyperspectral image set served as the target domain for wavelength-specific classification of AD. The highest classification accuracy, reaching 83%, was attained when ResNet50 was initially trained on an augmented psoriasis dataset, and the learned parameters were subsequently transferred to train the model on the target dataset in the Near-infrared (NIR) spectrum. A slightly lower but still notable accuracy of 81% was achieved when ResNet50 was trained on the non-augmented psoriasis dataset, followed by fine-tuning on the target dataset in the red (R) spectral range. These results highlight the adaptability of ResNet50 across different domains and underscore the psoriasis dataset's value as a robust source for pretraining in hyperspectral AD classification tasks.

10.4 AI in Predicting Severity and Progression of AD

The integration of AI into the study of AD has provided groundbreaking insights into disease prediction. A comprehensive study utilized advanced machine learning techniques, particularly gradient boosting, to analyze factors influencing AD severity [29]. The dataset included 367 individuals, both adolescents and adults with active AD, examining 130 potential severity-associated factors. The machine learning model demonstrated a slightly higher predictive accuracy compared to traditional multinomial logistic regression. The analysis revealed significant associations between severe AD and specific demographic and clinical factors, such as age groups 12–21 years and above 52 years, late onset of AD, elevated serum immunoglobulin E levels, higher eosinophil counts, the presence of atopic stigmata, male gender, infrequent exercise, smoking history, and comorbid alopecia areata. To further personalize AD management, researchers have developed a mechanistic machine learning model using Bayesian inference to predict daily changes in AD severity at the individual level [30]. The model was trained on longitudinal data from two clinical studies, encompassing daily severity scores and treatment details for 393 pediatric AD patients over periods of 16 weeks and 6 months. Validation using a forward-chaining framework demonstrated the model's ability to forecast future severity scores with a 60% improvement over chance predictions. This innovation addresses the unpredictable nature of AD flares and variable therapy responses, offering a practical tool for tailored treatment strategies.

The transformative role of AI in advancing the understanding of AD progression continues to grow, with new studies leveraging advanced computational techniques to unravel the complexities of this chronic condition. One such investigation utilized the partitioning around medoids algorithm on data from the pediatric eczema elective registry to analyze phenotypically distinct subgroups of children with AD [31]. This unsupervised clustering approach, applied to a dataset of over 8000 children, identified significant variations in long-term AD outcomes among these subgroups. The study underscores the value of early phenotypic characteristics as predictors of disease progression, highlighting how hypothesis-independent statistical techniques can uncover nuanced insights into AD's trajectory. Building on this foundation, a longitudinal cohort study in Taiwan examined the increasing incidence of childhood AD and allergic rhinitis through the lens of AI [32]. Researchers analyzed data from 1439 mother-infant pairs across nine maternity hospitals, integrating variables such as demographics, socioeconomic status, lifestyle, medical history, and environmental exposures. Employing tree-based machine learning models, the study achieved impressive predictive accuracies. A critical finding was the influence of prenatal air quality, particularly nitrogen dioxide (NO_2) exposure, on allergic disease prediction. These results highlight AI's ability to synthesize heterogeneous datasets and deliver superior sensitivity and specificity in predicting complex health conditions.

The impact of environmental factors on AD has further been investigated. Epidemiological evidence suggests that air pollution and climate changes significantly contribute to the development and exacerbation of AD. A study conducted in Southern Italy monitored 60 patients over 18 months to evaluate the effects of atmospheric and environmental factors on AD severity, using the SCORAD index for clinical assessments [33]. Environmental variables such as temperature, humidity, particulate matter with a diameter of 10 mm or less (PM10), NO_2, tropospheric ozone (O_3), and total pollen count (TPC) were analyzed through an artificial neural network (ANN). The ANN achieved a strong predictive performance for disease severity based on pollution data, identifying air pollutants as significant contributors to symptom exacerbation. Factors such as temperature, humidity, PM10, NO_2, O_3, and TPC exhibited positive correlations with increased AD severity, whereas weather-related factors had comparatively less predictive power. These findings highlight the utility of AI, particularly ANN, in uncovering environmental triggers of AD and enabling the development of predictive alerts for severity assessment.

Expanding these insights, machine learning has significantly improved the analysis of environmental and maternal factors influencing childhood AD. A study analyzing data from 1151 mother–child pairs in two multi-ethnic Asian birth cohorts employed advanced algorithms such as XGBoost, genetic algorithms, and logistic regression to investigate preconception and antenatal exposures [34]. Key maternal risk factors, including preconception alcohol consumption and depressive symptoms during pregnancy, were identified as significant contributors to increased risks of eczema and rhinitis in children. Additionally, mechanistic modeling revealed protective effects of higher maternal blood neopterin and child blood dimethylglycine against wheeze, while early-life infections were linked to the onset of eczema and rhinitis. These findings emphasize the role of inflammatory pathways in disease programming and highlight modifiable maternal exposures as potential targets for intervention.

10.5 Therapeutic Target Identification and Drug Discovery

Significant innovations have also been made in leveraging AI for therapeutic advancements in AD. A groundbreaking contribution is the introduction of DRAGONET, an advanced computational framework that utilizes deep learning to design drug candidate molecules based on patient-specific gene expression profiles [35]. DRAGONET employs a transformer-based variational autoencoder to create a latent space representing molecular structures. By integrating substructures from disease-correlated molecules, this model generates compounds capable of counteracting disease-specific gene expression patterns. Applied to AD, gastric cancer, and

Alzheimer's disease, DRAGONET successfully identified molecular candidates chemically similar to registered therapies. This demonstrates AI's transformative role in precision medicine, particularly for diseases lacking well-defined therapeutic targets. By harnessing patient-specific data, DRAGONET offers a novel and efficient pathway for de novo drug discovery, accelerating the development of targeted treatments for complex diseases such as AD.

Complementing this effort, another study focused on keratinocyte gene expression in AD and other inflammatory skin conditions using machine learning and in silico transcriptomic deconvolution [36]. Analyzing seven datasets comprising 406 samples, researchers identified three distinct keratinocyte transcriptomic profiles—KC1, KC2, and KC17—each associated with specific immune signals driven by T helper (Th) cells. Cross-validation across different disease stages revealed that keratinocyte responses are therapy-dependent. For instance, broad-spectrum treatments like ciclosporin normalized the KC17 response in AD lesions, restoring them to a nonlesional profile, whereas the Th2-specific therapy dupilumab primarily reversed the KC2 profile without affecting KC17. This analysis emphasizes that targeting a single immune axis may be insufficient to resolve keratinocyte abnormalities entirely. By uncovering therapy-specific transcriptomic shifts, the study highlights AI's capability to unravel complex disease mechanisms, guiding the development of more personalized and effective treatment strategies for AD.

In addition to these computational advances, another study combined network analysis, deep learning, and molecular simulation to identify and validate potential multi-target drugs for AD. Researchers used the TCM Taiwan database to pinpoint caffeoyl malic acid (CMA) as a small molecule capable of inhibiting key AD therapeutic targets, TNFα and IL-4. A deep learning model based on a CNN confirmed CMA's efficacy as a potent TNFα inhibitors [37]. Molecular simulations further revealed that CMA binds stably to TNFα and IL-4, inducing structural changes that disrupt protein–receptor interactions. Specifically, CMA increased the distance between chains A and C of TNFα and narrowed the gap between IL-4's α helices, effectively hindering their complex formation and signaling activity. This integrative approach highlights CMA's potential as a dual inhibitor for TNFα/IL-4 pathways in AD treatment. The application of advanced computational techniques not only accelerates drug discovery but also paves the way for targeted multi-pathway therapeutic interventions in AD management.

Systemic therapies like dupilumab have revolutionized the treatment landscape for AD. Despite its demonstrated efficacy, a significant subset of patients experiences suboptimal responses to dupilumab. A study utilized machine learning to analyze electronic health records and insurance claims data from 419 AD patients aged 12 years and older who initiated dupilumab treatment between April 2017 and June 2019 [38]. Nonresponse indicators included treatment discontinuation, additional systemic or phototherapy usage, high-potency topical corticosteroid application, AD-related hospital or emergency visits, and incident skin infections. Among these patients, 35% exhibited at least one nonresponse indicator within 6 months, with dupilumab discontinuation being the most common. Additionally, key predictors of nonresponse were identified, including the use of ibuprofen and a Quan-Charlson Comorbidity Index score of 3–4.

While dupilumab is highly effective in alleviating pruritus and improving sleep for many AD patients, its sleep-related adverse-drug reactions (ADRs) are poorly understood, particularly in real-world settings. Using the World Health Organization's global pharmacovigilance database, VigiBase™, researchers investigated patterns of sleep-related ADRs associated with dupilumab through disproportionality analysis with the Bayesian confidence propagation neural network (BCPNN) [38]. The analysis revealed significant associations for sleep deficit, generic sleep disorders, nocturnal dyspnea, and middle insomnia. However, rarer ADRs, including restless leg syndrome, narcolepsy, and bruxism, did not reach statistical significance. These findings emphasize the importance of monitoring sleep-related outcomes in patients treated with dupilumab. Facial erythema is another notable complication associated with dupilumab treatment, underscoring the need for effective stratification to address heterogeneous patient responses. A study employed AI-driven techniques to analyze factors influencing the severity of facial erythema and develop a predictive model for drug response [39]. The model achieved an accuracy of 89.10%, identifying eight significant predictors: age, sex, lactate dehydrogenase, immunoglobulin E, eosinophil count, white blood cell count, and allergies to Alnus and cedar. By integrating demographic and clinical data, this AI-powered approach supports personalized treatment strategies for dupilumab-treated patients, enhancing the ability to predict and mitigate adverse responses such as facial erythema.

In the same context, a post hoc analysis of the Phase 3 BREEZE-AD7 trial assessed predictors of response to baricitinib 4 mg in combination with topical corticosteroids in adults with moderate-to-severe AD [40]. Classification and regression tree analysis identified baseline body surface area (BSA) involvement as the strongest predictor of clinical response at Week 16. Through machine learning techniques, researchers concluded that patients with BSA between 10% and 40% and an Itch Numerical Rating Scale (Itch NRS) score ≥ 7 demonstrated the highest response rates. Among these patients, 69% attained at least a 75% improvement in the Eczema Area and Severity Index (EASI75), and 58% experienced an Itch NRS $\geq$ 4-point improvement following 16 weeks of treatment. These findings underscore AI's potential in uncovering critical factors influencing therapeutic outcomes. By identifying significant predictors, this approach provides valuable insights into optimizing systemic therapies for AD, allowing clinicians to personalize treatment plans and mitigate risks of nonresponse.

With respect to imaging technologies and AI, line-field confocal optical coherence tomography (LC-OCT) has been demonstrated as a powerful tool for investigating AD [41]. By integrating LC-OCT with AI algorithms, researchers achieved real-time, noninvasive imaging of skin during AD flare-ups and remission periods under topical steroid treatment. Quantitative analyses included parameters such as epidermal and stratum corneum (SC) thickness, dermo-epidermal junction (DEJ) morphology, and keratinocyte nuclei characteristics. A novel AI-derived metric, "nuclei atypia," effectively quantified abnormalities in epidermal renewal and highlighted disrupted keratinocyte maturation. Findings revealed that chronic AD lesions exhibited greater nuclei atypia compared to acute lesions. Furthermore, in comparison to healthy skin, AD lesions demonstrated a thicker epidermis and SC, undulated DEJ, and larger, less compact keratinocyte nuclei. Remarkably, these abnormalities normalized within 2 weeks of treatment, coinciding with clinical improvements. This study highlights the transformative potential of AI-enhanced LC-OCT imaging in providing detailed and objective assessments of AD. By accurately quantifying epidermal renewal and lesion severity, this approach offers significant advancements in monitoring therapeutic responses.

10.6 AI in Patient Education and Care

10.6.1 Patient Education

Recent studies have explored the utility and limitations of large language models (LLMs) like ChatGPT in dermatological care, particularly in patient education. One study assessed the accuracy and comprehensiveness of ChatGPT's responses to common patient inquiries about AD and acne vulgaris, highlighting its potential as an educational tool [42]. ChatGPT demonstrated greater accuracy in addressing AD-related inquiries compared to those about acne. However, it was noted that the use of advanced terminology, such as "meta-analysis," could confuse patients, pointing to the challenges of providing nuanced, patient-specific guidance for complex conditions like AD and acne. Building on this, another study evaluated the performance of LLMs, including GPT-4, ChatGPT-3.5, DermGPT, and DocsGPT, in generating patient education materials (PEMs) for dermatologic conditions [42, 43]. The study emphasized the importance of producing PEMs at specified Flesch-Kincaid reading levels (FKRLs) to enhance accessibility and comprehension. Among these, GPT-4 consistently excelled at generating fifth-grade PEMs for both common and rare conditions, outperforming ChatGPT-3.5, DermGPT, and DocsGPT. However, at the seventh-grade FKRL, ChatGPT-3.5 and DocsGPT surpassed GPT-4 for rare conditions, while performance across models was comparable for common conditions. DermGPT ranked highest in readability and patient understanding for common conditions, while GPT-4 excelled in rare conditions. Overall, LLM-generated PEMs were found to be accurate, readable, and comprehensible, meeting desired FKRLs and demonstrating significant potential to improve health literacy in dermatology.

A recent study compared the readability and comprehensibility of information on atopic dermatitis (AD) provided by AI chatbots—ChatGPT, Gemini, and Claude—with the top Google search results for "atopic dermatitis" [44]. The chatbots were tasked with explaining AD in general terms and simplifying the language for low-literacy audiences. While AI-generated responses demonstrated promise, they often failed to meet the readability standards required for lower-literacy patients. Conversely, Google search results were marginally more accessible to a broader audience. However, both sources fell short in achieving the comprehensibility necessary for most patients. Limitations included the scoring methods used, which did not consider visuals, layout, cultural sensitivity, or patient-specific factors such as anxiety and motivation. In a separate investigation, researchers assessed the reliability and quality of ChatGPT-4's responses to 99 frequently asked questions from AD patients [45]. Dermatologists from an international group contributed questions addressing the etiology, management, and consequences of AD. A panel of dermatology experts specializing in therapeutic patient education evaluated ChatGPT-4's responses, which consistently provided comprehensive and high-quality answers without requiring specific prompts or additional context. This research underscores the potential of AI as a supplementary resource for addressing patient queries, particularly amid increasing demands on clinicians. As patients increasingly rely on AI for medical information, ensuring the reliability of tools like ChatGPT-4 is essential for enhancing patient education and supporting informed healthcare decisions.

Another perspective investigated the impact of ChatGPT on anxiety levels among parents of children with AD [46]. While ChatGPT offers temporary reassurance and accessible information, its inability to verify references or provide professional-level guidance poses risks of misinformation. This can lead to unnecessary concerns or misinformed decisions, such as adopting restrictive diets without medical evidence. The platform itself acknowledges these limitations, explicitly advising users to seek professional medical advice. Clinicians play a pivotal role in addressing these challenges by staying informed about ChatGPT's capabilities and limitations and guiding parents toward reliable, evidence-based resources such as the Society of Pediatric Dermatology, the American Academy of Dermatology (AAD), and the National Eczema Association. By integrating AI tools with professional oversight, the benefits of accessible, AI-generated information can be maximized while minimizing potential harms, supporting informed and confident disease management for families managing AD occurring in children or/amd adults (Fig. 10.2).

10.6.2 Management of AD Care

AI has demonstrated remarkable potential in advancing personalized healthcare strategies by integrating data from personal devices and sensors. This capability is particularly significant for chronic skin conditions like AD, where continuous

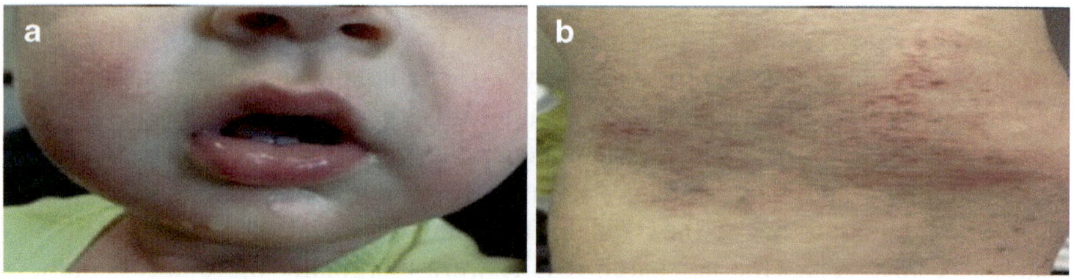

Fig. 10.2 Images (**a** and **b**) presenting AD manifestations at different ages

monitoring and individualized care are essential. In this context, the Atopic App serves as an example of how digital innovation can revolutionize AD care [47]. This mobile health platform incorporates an AI model to assess AD severity based on the eczema area and severity index, offering actionable insights into treatment plans, flare-up triggers, and disease dynamics. Follow-up assessments showed a significant reduction in AD severity, as measured by the patient-oriented eczema measure. These findings illustrate the potential of AI-powered tools to support disease monitoring, improve adherence to management plans, and enhance caregiver involvement, ultimately fostering better health outcomes.

In addition to AI-driven monitoring and diagnostics, digital psychological self-care interventions are emerging as promising tools for managing AD. Recent developments have introduced self-guided digital programs based on cognitive behavioral therapy (CBT), designed to support patients in managing symptoms such as itching, stress, and impaired quality of life [48]. One 8-week self-management CBT intervention, supplemented with brief pre- and post-intervention telephone interviews, demonstrated feasibility and promising preliminary effects on dermatological quality of life and psychological well-being. Furthermore, comparisons of newly developed digital self-care tools—including those targeting insomnia, alcohol use, and AD—with their therapist-guided counterparts revealed similar within-group effect sizes and clinical response rates, despite significantly reduced clinician involvement and participant reading load [49]. These findings suggest that some guided Internet-based interventions may be effectively adapted into self-guided digital formats. However, further randomized trials are necessary to assess their comparative efficacy and to determine which patient groups may benefit more from guided support.

AI has also been instrumental in improving the measurement and analysis of AD-specific behaviors, such as nocturnal scratching, which is a critical indicator of disease activity. A study introduced an advanced algorithm utilizing high-resolution wrist actigraphy data to detect scratching events during sleep [50]. The system employs three-dimensional accelerometer sensors sampled at ≥20 Hz, processing data in two steps: motion segmentation (classifying "no motion," "single-handed motion," and "both-handed motion") and motion classification (differentiating scratching from other movements) using a bidirectional recurrent neural network (RNN) classifier. When compared to manually scored infrared video data from 24 participants (18 AD patients and six healthy controls), the algorithm achieved an F1 score of 0.68 and a rank correlation of 0.945, significantly outperforming a previously published method (F1 score of 0.09, rank correlation of 0.466). This AI-driven approach provides a precise, noninvasive measurement of scratching behavior, supporting better monitoring of disease activity.

Beyond patient-level interventions, AI plays a crucial role in addressing broader environmental and systemic challenges in AD management. The integration of AI in dermatology enables advanced diagnostics, predictive modeling, and personalized treatment strategies that can mitigate the impact of environmental factors, such as climate change, on AD [51]. By enhancing the precision, efficiency, and accessibility of AD care, AI offers opportunities to improve global healthcare outcomes. However, realizing the full potential of AI requires overcoming challenges such as data governance, algorithmic bias, and the need for professional education.

Addressing these hurdles is essential to foster a future of more effective and patient-centered dermatological care. Together, these developments illustrate how AI can enhance multiple facets of AD management, from personalized care and behavior monitoring to addressing systemic and environmental challenges.

10.7 AI in Action: Clinical Scenarios of AI

The integration of AI in dermatology is revolutionizing the management of AD. Below are specific examples of real-world and experimental AI applications, accompanied by an interpretation of their outcomes:

10.7.1 Case 1: Automated Severity Scoring Using Clinical Images

Scenario A 32-year-old patient presents with chronic atopic dermatitis affecting the hands, face, and neck. Dermatologists evaluate the condition's severity using the EASI, but discrepancies arise in their assessments. To resolve this, AI-based tools such as the automatic SCORAD system are applied to the patient's clinical images.

AI Application The automatic SCORAD, powered by convolutional neural networks (CNNs), analyzes the images to score erythema, excoriation, and lichenification objectively. By cross-referencing AI-derived scores with dermatologist evaluations, consistency is improved. The AI system identifies erythema as moderate (2/3), excoriation as severe (3/3), and lichenification as mild (1/3). The final severity score aligns closely with consensus dermatologist evaluations but removes interobserver variability, demonstrating the tool's reliability and efficiency in clinical practice.

10.7.2 Case 2: Predicting Treatment Response

Scenario A 45-year-old male patient with moderate-to-severe AD starts dupilumab treatment but experiences persistent facial erythema despite improvement in other symptoms. Clinicians suspect a heterogeneous treatment response and use AI-powered predictive models to stratify the patient's phenotype.

AI Application The AI system, using LightGBM gradient boosting algorithms, analyzes patient-specific clinical and demographic factors, including IgE levels, eosinophil counts, and allergy profiles. It classifies the patient into a "persistent residual erythema" cluster. The model suggests that facial erythema in this phenotype is associated with elevated IgE levels and Alnus pollen allergy. Recommendations include adjunctive topical corticosteroids for facial erythema, improving symptom control. This example highlights AI's role in tailoring treatment to individual patient profiles.

10.7.3 Case 3: Identifying Comorbidities and Endotypes

Scenario A 10-year-old boy with atopic dermatitis presents with asthma and seasonal allergies. The clinicians suspect underlying immune dysfunction but face challenges in determining the dominant inflammatory pathways driving the disease.

AI Application Machine learning algorithms analyze the child's cytokine and chemokine profiles, classifying them into distinct clusters based on random forest dissimilarity analysis. Elevated IL-33 and CCL27 levels are identified as key markers of his endotype. The AI model indicates a Th2-driven inflammatory response, recommending dupilumab as a systemic therapy to target IL-4 and IL-13 pathways. Additionally, it predicts a high likelihood of comorbid food allergies, prompting dietary evaluation. This case demonstrates AI's potential to personalize treatment and manage comorbidities effectively.

10.7.4 Case 4: Genomic Studies Using AI-Enhanced EHR Mining

Scenario Researchers aim to include 500 patients with AD in a genome-wide association study (GWAS) to identify novel genetic markers. Accurate phenotyping of patients from electronic health records (EHRs) is challenging due to inconsistent coding.

AI Application Natural language processing (NLP) algorithms extract clinical notes and coded data to identify eligible AD cases. Lasso logistic regression models refine case definitions with high sensitivity and specificity. The AI system increases the study's inclusion rate by 30%, ensuring robust genomic analysis. Novel markers associated with skin barrier dysfunction are identified, highlighting AI's transformative potential in precision medicine.

10.8 Conclusions

AD is a clinically and immunologically heterogeneous inflammatory skin disease, presenting significant challenges in diagnosis, classification, and personalized management. The emergence of AI offers promising avenues to address these complexities. Leveraging machine learning algorithms, deep learning architectures, and integrative data analysis, AI is increasingly demonstrating its capacity to revolutionize dermatological research and practice. Applications of AI in AD span a wide spectrum, from non-invasive imaging and automated lesion assessment to the identification of molecular signatures and prediction of therapeutic responses. These innovations have the potential to enhance diagnostic precision, uncover novel pathogenic pathways, and enable individualized treatment strategies. As such, AI is poised to reshape the landscape of AD care toward a more efficient and patient-centered paradigm. However, the integration of AI into clinical practice must be approached with caution and critical oversight. AI should be regarded as an augmentative tool that supports, rather than replaces, clinical expertise. Importantly, the performance and fairness of AI systems are intrinsically tied to the quality and diversity of the data on which they are trained. Presently, many models are developed using datasets disproportionately composed of individuals with lighter skin tones, which limits their generalizability and risks perpetuating diagnostic inaccuracies and healthcare disparities for people with skin of color. To ensure equitable benefit, future AI development must prioritize the inclusion of diverse and representative patient populations. Moreover, ethical considerations, such as algorithmic transparency, data privacy, and accountability, must be embedded throughout the design and implementation process. Clinician trust and patient understanding are equally vital; the mechanisms and limitations of AI tools should be communicated clearly to support informed, confident use in real-world settings. Successful deployment of AI in AD care will depend not only on technological innovation but also on broader efforts to improve digital literacy and healthcare access. As we move from proof-of-concept studies to routine clinical application, multidisciplinary collaboration will be essential to refine and validate AI models across varied clinical environments and populations. Ultimately, the future of AD management lies in harnessing AI to enable more precise, equitable, and responsive care. When thoughtfully integrated, AI can become a transformative force that enhances physician capabilities, bridges research gaps, and improves outcomes for all individuals affected by atopic dermatitis.

References

1. Fasseeh AN, Elezbawy B, Korra N, Tannira M, Dalle H, Aderian S, et al. Burden of atopic dermatitis in adults and adolescents: a systematic literature review. Dermatol Ther (Heidelb). 2022;12:2653–68. https://doi.org/10.1007/s13555-022-00819-6.
2. Wu H, Yin H, Chen H, Sun M, Liu X, Yu Y, et al. A deep learning, image based approach for automated diagnosis for inflammatory skin diseases. Ann Transl Med. 2020;8:581. https://doi.org/10.21037/atm.2020.04.39.
3. Yanagisawa Y, Shido K, Kojima K, Yamasaki K. Convolutional neural network-based skin image segmentation model to improve classification of skin diseases in conventional and non-standardized picture images. J Dermatol Sci. 2023;109:30–6. https://doi.org/10.1016/j.jdermsci.2023.01.005.
4. Hsiao Y-P, Chiu C-W, Lu C-W, Nguyen HT, Tseng YS, Hsieh S-C, et al. Identification of skin lesions by using single-step multiframe detector. J Clin Med. 2021;10:144. https://doi.org/10.3390/jcm10010144.
5. Aggarwal SLP. Data augmentation in dermatology image recognition using machine learning. Skin Res Technol. 2019;25:815–20. https://doi.org/10.1111/srt.12726.
6. Abdalla M, Chen B, Santiago R, Young J, Eder L, Chan A-W, et al. Accuracy of algorithms to identify people with atopic dermatitis in Ontario routinely collected health databases. J Invest Dermatol. 2021;141:1840–3. https://doi.org/10.1016/j.jid.2021.01.009.
7. Zhang T, Lee TK, Lui H, Dutz J, Dawes M, Lee A, et al. Health insurance claim- and prescription record-based algorithms as a population-based method for eczema ascertainment. J Eur Acad Dermatol Venereol. 2020;34 https://doi.org/10.1111/jdv.16315.

8. Abuabara K, Magyari AM, Hoffstad O, Jabbar-Lopez ZK, Smeeth L, Williams HC, et al. Development and validation of an algorithm to accurately identify atopic eczema patients in primary care electronic health records from the UK. J Invest Dermatol. 2017;137:1655–62. https://doi.org/10.1016/j.jid.2017.03.029.
9. Czajkowska J, Badura P, Korzekwa S, Płatkowska-Szczerek A, Słowińska M. Deep learning-based high-frequency ultrasound skin image classification with multicriteria model evaluation. Sensors. 2021;21:5846. https://doi.org/10.3390/s21175846.
10. Czajkowska J, Badura P, Korzekwa S, Płatkowska-Szczerek A. Deep learning approach to skin layers segmentation in inflammatory dermatoses. Ultrasonics. 2021;114:106412. https://doi.org/10.1016/j.ultras.2021.106412.
11. Czajkowska J, Badura P, Korzekwa S, Płatkowska-Szczerek A. Automated segmentation of epidermis in high-frequency ultrasound of pathological skin using a cascade of DeepLab v3+ networks and fuzzy connectedness. Comput Med Imaging Graph. 2022;95:102023. https://doi.org/10.1016/j.compmedimag.2021.102023.
12. Guimarães P, Batista A, Zieger M, Kaatz M, Koenig K. Artificial intelligence in multiphoton tomography: atopic dermatitis diagnosis. Sci Rep. 2020;10:7968. https://doi.org/10.1038/s41598-020-64937-x.
13. Park S, Saw SN, Li X, Paknezhad M, Coppola D, Dinish US, et al. Model learning analysis of 3D optoacoustic mesoscopy images for the classification of atopic dermatitis. Biomed Opt Express. 2021;12:3671. https://doi.org/10.1364/BOE.415105.
14. Huang H-Y, Nguyen H-T, Lin T-L, Saenprasarn P, Liu P-H, Wang H-C. Identification of skin lesions by snapshot hyperspectral imaging. Cancers (Basel). 2024;16:217. https://doi.org/10.3390/cancers16010217.
15. Yamamoto-Hanada K, Kawakami E, Saito-Abe M, Sato M, Mitsubuchi H, Oda M, et al. Exploratory analysis of plasma cytokine/chemokine levels in 6-year-old children from a birth cohort study. Cytokine. 2020;130:155051. https://doi.org/10.1016/j.cyto.2020.155051.
16. Dev K, Ho CJH, Bi R, Yew YW, Dinish SU, Attia ABE, et al. Machine learning assisted handheld confocal Raman micro-spectroscopy for identification of clinically relevant atopic eczema biomarkers. Sensors (Basel). 2022;22:4674. https://doi.org/10.3390/s22134674.
17. Ghosh D, Ding L, Sivaprasad U, Geh E, Biagini Myers J, Bernstein JA, et al. Multiple transcriptome data analysis reveals biologically relevant atopic dermatitis signature genes and pathways. PLoS One. 2015;10:e0144316. https://doi.org/10.1371/journal.pone.0144316.
18. Wu W, Chen G, Zhang Z, He M, Li H, Yan F. Construction and verification of atopic dermatitis diagnostic model based on pyroptosis related biological markers using machine learning methods. BMC Med Genet. 2023;16:138. https://doi.org/10.1186/s12920-023-01552-5.
19. Jiang Z, Li J, Kong N, Kim J-H, Kim B-S, Lee M-J, et al. Accurate diagnosis of atopic dermatitis by combining transcriptome and microbiota data with supervised machine learning. Sci Rep. 2022;12:290. https://doi.org/10.1038/s41598-021-04373-7.
20. Li Y, Zhao D, Xu Z, Heidari AA, Chen H, Jiang X, et al. bSRWPSO-FKNN: a boosted PSO with fuzzy K-nearest neighbor classifier for predicting atopic dermatitis disease. Front Neuroinform. 2023;16 https://doi.org/10.3389/fninf.2022.1063048.
21. Bang CH, Yoon JW, Ryu JY, Chun JH, Han JH, Lee YB, et al. Automated severity scoring of atopic dermatitis patients by a deep neural network. Sci Rep. 2021;11:6049. https://doi.org/10.1038/s41598-021-85489-8.
22. Medela A, Mac Carthy T, Aguilar Robles SA, Chiesa-Estomba CM, Grimalt R. Automatic SCOring of atopic dermatitis using deep learning: a pilot study. JID Innov. 2022;2:100107. https://doi.org/10.1016/j.xjidi.2022.100107.
23. Paul C, Griffiths CEM, Costanzo A, Herranz P, Grond S, Mert C, et al. Factors predicting quality of life impairment in adult patients with atopic dermatitis: results from a patient survey and machine learning analysis. Dermatol Ther (Heidelb). 2023;13:981–95. https://doi.org/10.1007/s13555-023-00897-0.
24. Cho SI, Lee D, Han B, Lee JS, Hong JY, Chung JH, et al. Practical training approaches for discordant atopic dermatitis severity datasets: merging methods with soft-label and

train-set pruning. IEEE J Biomed Health Inform. 2023;27:166–75. https://doi.org/10.1109/JBHI.2022.3218166.
25. Maulana A, Noviandy TR, Suhendra R, Earlia N, Bulqiah M, Idroes GM, et al. Evaluation of atopic dermatitis severity using artificial intelligence. Narra J. 2023;3:e511. https://doi.org/10.52225/narra.v3i3.511.
26. Greenfield DA, Feizpour A, Evans CL. Quantifying inflammatory response and drug-aided resolution in an atopic dermatitis model with deep learning. J Invest Dermatol. 2023;143:1430–1438.e4. https://doi.org/10.1016/j.jid.2023.01.026.
27. Ho CJH, Yew YW, Dinish US, Kuan AHY, Wong MKW, Bi R, et al. Handheld confocal Raman spectroscopy (CRS) for objective assessment of skin barrier function and stratification of severity in atopic dermatitis (AD) patients. J Dermatol Sci. 2020;98:20–5. https://doi.org/10.1016/j.jdermsci.2020.02.001.
28. Kim EB, Baek YS, Lee O. Parameter-based transfer learning for severity classification of atopic dermatitis using hyperspectral imaging. Skin Res Technol. 2024;30 https://doi.org/10.1111/srt.13704.
29. Maintz L, Welchowski T, Herrmann N, Brauer J, Kläschen AS, Fimmers R, et al. Machine learning–based deep phenotyping of atopic dermatitis. JAMA Dermatol. 2021;157:1414. https://doi.org/10.1001/jamadermatol.2021.3668.
30. Hurault G, Domínguez-Hüttinger E, Langan SM, Williams HC, Tanaka RJ. Personalized prediction of daily eczema severity scores using a mechanistic machine learning model. Clin Exp Allergy. 2020;50:1258–66. https://doi.org/10.1111/cea.13717.
31. Berna R, Mitra N, Hoffstad O, Wan J, Margolis DJ. Identifying phenotypes of atopic dermatitis in a longitudinal United States cohort using unbiased statistical clustering. J Invest Dermatol. 2020;140:477–9. https://doi.org/10.1016/j.jid.2019.08.432.
32. Huang Y, Wen H-J, Guo Y-LL, Wei T-Y, Wang W-C, Tsai S-F, et al. Prenatal exposure to air pollutants and childhood atopic dermatitis and allergic rhinitis adopting machine learning approaches: 14-year follow-up birth cohort study. Sci Total Environ. 2021;777:145982. https://doi.org/10.1016/j.scitotenv.2021.145982.
33. Patella V, Florio G, Palmieri M, Bousquet J, Tonacci A, Giuliano A, et al. Atopic dermatitis severity during exposure to air pollutants and weather changes with an Artificial Neural Network (ANN) analysis. Pediatr Allergy Immunol. 2020;31:938–45. https://doi.org/10.1111/pai.13314.
34. Dong Y, Lau HX, Suaini NHA, Kee MZL, Ooi DSQ, Shek LP, et al. A machine-learning exploration of the exposome from preconception in early childhood atopic eczema, rhinitis and wheeze development. Environ Res. 2024;250:118523. https://doi.org/10.1016/j.envres.2024.118523.
35. Yamanaka C, Uki S, Kaitoh K, Iwata M, Yamanishi Y. De novo drug design based on patient gene expression profiles via deep learning. Mol Inform. 2023;42 https://doi.org/10.1002/minf.202300064.
36. Clayton K, Vallejo A, Sirvent S, Davies J, Porter G, Reading IC, et al. Machine learning applied to atopic dermatitis transcriptome reveals distinct therapy-dependent modification of the keratinocyte immunophenotype*. Br J Dermatol. 2021;184:913–22. https://doi.org/10.1111/bjd.19431.
37. Wang Y, Qin D, Jin L, Liang G. Caffeoyl malic acid is a potential dual inhibitor targeting TNFα/IL-4 evaluated by a combination strategy of network analysis-deep learning-molecular simulation. Comput Biol Med. 2022;145:105410. https://doi.org/10.1016/j.compbiomed.2022.105410.
38. Wu JJ, Hong C, Merola JF, Gruben D, Güler E, Feeney C, et al. Predictors of nonresponse to dupilumab in patients with atopic dermatitis. Ann Allergy Asthma Immunol. 2022;129:354–359.e5. https://doi.org/10.1016/j.anai.2022.05.025.
39. Ashizaki K, Ishikawa T, Nomura Y. Residual facial erythema in atopic dermatitis patients treated with dupilumab stratified by machine learning. J Eur Acad Dermatol Venereol. 2024;38:2286–94. https://doi.org/10.1111/jdv.19909.

40. Thyssen JP, de Bruin-Weller M, Costanzo A, Grond S, Schuster C, Liu C, et al. Baseline body surface area and itch severity define response to Baricitinib in patients with moderate-to-severe atopic dermatitis at week 16. Adv Ther. 2023;40:3574–87. https://doi.org/10.1007/s12325-023-02528-8.
41. Le Blay H, Raynaud E, Bouayadi S, Rieux E, Rolland G, Saussine A, et al. Epidermal renewal during the treatment of atopic dermatitis lesions: a study coupling line-field confocal optical coherence tomography with artificial intelligence quantifications. Skin Res Technol. 2024;30 https://doi.org/10.1111/srt.13891.
42. Lambert R, Choo Z-Y, Gradwohl K, Schroedl L, Ruiz De Luzuriaga A. Assessing the application of large language models in generating dermatologic patient education materials according to reading level: qualitative study. JMIR Dermatol. 2024;7:e55898. https://doi.org/10.2196/55898.
43. Lakdawala N, Channa L, Gronbeck C, Lakdawala N, Weston G, Sloan B, et al. Assessing the accuracy and comprehensiveness of ChatGPT in offering clinical guidance for atopic dermatitis and acne vulgaris. JMIR Dermatol. 2023;6:e50409. https://doi.org/10.2196/50409.
44. Ahuja K, Lio P. Readability of patient materials on atopic dermatitis: the possible role of artificial intelligence. Pediatr Dermatol. 2024;41:1251–2. https://doi.org/10.1111/pde.15674.
45. Sulejmani P, Negris O, Aoki V, Chu C, Eichenfield L, Misery L, et al. A large language model artificial intelligence for patient queries in atopic dermatitis. J Eur Acad Dermatol Venereol. 2024;38 https://doi.org/10.1111/jdv.19737.
46. Ahuja K, DeSena G, Laageide L, El-Feghaly J, Lio P. From eczema to anxiety: how artificial intelligence shapes parental perspectives. Pediatr Dermatol. 2023;40:964–5. https://doi.org/10.1111/pde.15417.
47. Zvulunov A, Lenevich S, Migacheva N. A mobile health app for facilitating disease management in children with atopic dermatitis: feasibility and impact study. JMIR Dermatol. 2023;6:e49278. https://doi.org/10.2196/49278.
48. Kern D, Ljótsson B, Lönndahl L, Hedman-Lagerlöf E, Bradley M, Lindefors N, et al. A digital self-help intervention for atopic dermatitis: analysis of secondary outcomes from a feasibility study. JMIR Dermatol. 2023;6:e42360. https://doi.org/10.2196/42360.
49. Kraepelien M, Hentati A, Kern D, Sundström C, Jernelöv S, Lindefors N. Transforming guided internet interventions into simplified and self-guided digital tools—experiences from three recent projects. Internet Interv. 2023;34:100693. https://doi.org/10.1016/j.invent.2023.100693.
50. Moreau A, Anderer P, Ross M, Cerny A, Almazan TH, Peterson B. Detection of nocturnal scratching movements in patients with atopic dermatitis using accelerometers and recurrent neural networks. IEEE J Biomed Health Inform. 2018;22:1011–8. https://doi.org/10.1109/JBHI.2017.2710798.
51. Goldust M, Grant-Kels JM. Using AI to help address skin health challenges caused by climate change. Int J Dermatol. 2024;63 https://doi.org/10.1111/ijd.17222.

AI-Powered Approach to Acne

11

Panagiota Tanga, Emmanouil Karampinis, and Markos Papakonstantis

11.1 Key Elements of Acne

Acne vulgaris is one of the most widespread skin conditions globally, affecting around 85% of teenagers and young adults, although it can also continue into later life. Besides the physical appearance of acne, it can cause significant emotional and psychological distress, including feelings of embarrassment, anxiety, and even depression, all of which can seriously impact a person's quality of life. Acne commonly appears in areas rich in sebaceous (oil) glands—such as the face, chest, and back. There are several types of acne, including acne conglobata, rosacea, fulminans, cosmetica, excoriée (also called picker's acne), acne medicamentosa, acne chloracne, and acne mechanica. However, the most common form—making up 99% of cases—is acne vulgaris [1]. This type includes two main kinds of lesions: noninflammatory (like blackheads and whiteheads) and inflammatory (like papules, pustules, nodules, and cysts). Blackheads, or open comedones, form when oil and dead skin clog hair follicles but remain open at the surface, giving them a dark color. These lesions are typically mild and found on the face, back, shoulders, arms, and chest. Whiteheads, or closed comedones, happen when similar blockages close off the follicle opening, creating small, white bumps. These are especially common in the T-zone—forehead, nose, and chin [2]. Papules are red, swollen bumps caused by inflammation from bacteria, oil buildup, and hormonal activity. They are considered a link between noninflammatory and inflammatory acne and are typically under

P. Tanga · M. Papakonstantis (✉)
Clinic of Dermatology, 401 General Military Hospital of Athens, Athens, Greece

E. Karampinis
Second Dermatology Department, School of Health Sciences, Aristotle University of Thessaloniki, Thessaloniki, Greece

Department of Dermatology, Faculty of Medicine, School of Health Sciences, University General Hospital of Larissa, University of Thessaly, Larissa, Greece

E. Karampinis et al. (eds.), *Artificial Intelligence Applications in Dermatology*,
https://doi.org/10.1007/978-3-032-15614-3_11

5 mm in size, without pus. Pustules, on the other hand, are pus-filled bumps surrounded by red, irritated skin and tend to show up in similar areas as papules. Nodular acne is more severe and occurs when clogged pores become inflamed, forming large, painful lumps beneath the skin—often along the jawline and chin. These lesions do not respond well to over-the-counter treatments and can last for weeks or even months [3]. Cystic acne is the most severe type, involving deep, painful, pus-filled lumps under the skin. It is common in people with oily skin and can lead to scarring. Like nodules, cysts can appear on the face, neck, back, chest, shoulders, and arms, and people often have a mix of both inflammatory and noninflammatory lesions [4]. Traditional acne treatment options include topical therapies (e.g., retinoids, benzoyl peroxide), oral antibiotics, hormonal treatments, and, in severe cases, oral isotretinoin. However, these therapies often require trial and error to identify the most effective approach for individual patients, and treatment outcomes can be highly variable. Acne's potential to leave lasting scars—both physical and emotional—makes timely and effective treatment essential [5].

Acne vulgaris is a skin condition characterized by various types of lesions, and the number of these lesions depends on their specific subtypes. Given this complexity, it makes sense to explore how artificial intelligence (AI) and convolutional neural networks (CNNs) can assist in its evaluation. Recent advancements in artificial intelligence (AI) are creating new ways to combat acne. The intersection of acne treatment and AI is both intriguing and promising as it opens new doors to more personalized and effective solutions.

This chapter explores the role of artificial intelligence in acne care, focusing on its applications in the diagnosis, treatment personalization, monitoring, scar prevention, and even drug discovery. The intersection of acne treatment and AI is both intriguing and promising as it opens new doors to more personalized and effective solutions.

However, despite the promising potential of AI in acne care, there are also several ethical and practical considerations that must be addressed. While AI shows great promise in acne care, ethical concerns such as data privacy, the potential for misdiagnosis, over-reliance on technology, and unequal access to these technologies need to be carefully considered and addressed.

11.2 Acne Diagnosis by AI

Before the development of CNNs, most traditional skin detection models rely on specific color spaces like RGB (red, green, blue, which are the most common color space used in digital images), HSV (hue, saturation, value, which separate color from brightness, helping make skin detection more robust under different lighting), and YCbCr [Y: lumar component, brightness; Cb, blue-difference chroma; and Cr, red-difference chroma, which clearly separates brightness from color, helping in color-based segmentation (like detecting skin or acne)]. However, RGB is not ideal for skin detection because it mixes color and brightness information. While YCbCr separates these components, it still tends to produce inconsistent results and can be easily affected by environmental conditions. Earlier acne diagnosis systems required accurate localization of acne-prone areas [6].

For instance, Chantharaphaichit et al. introduced a facial acne detection approach using grayscale images and the HSV color space. However, this method is highly sensitive to variations in acne color, shape, and lighting, which affects its accuracy [7]. Kittigul and Uyyanonvara suggested another method based on heat mapping and adaptive thresholding, but their results still suffered from noise, often misidentifying regions like the mouth and normal skin as acne [8]. Overall, these methods depend heavily on specific color spaces and predefined thresholds, making them prone to errors and lacking strong generalization across different conditions.

For AI-based acne vulgaris diagnosis, large datasets of skin images, which are categorized by severity and lesion type, are used. These datasets are vital for dermatologists to identify the key characteristics of each acne type. Recent studies have also explored the use of deep learning techniques for better image analysis. Deep learning models, particularly CNNs, can be used to accurately classify acne and other dermatological conditions, sometimes even outperforming dermatologists in terms of accuracy. CNNs are designed to mimic the human visual processing system and excel at image classification tasks, making them ideal for detecting and diagnosing acne [9]. AI models can be trained on large datasets of labeled skin images to detect various forms of acne, including comedonal, inflammatory, and cystic acne. Once trained, AI systems can quickly and accurately identify acne lesions, categorize them, and even assess their severity. The latest AI systems are becoming more sophisticated by focusing on finer details, such as differentiating between acne and other skin conditions like rosacea or folliculitis. AI is also getting better at handling edge cases—unusual forms of acne or instances where acne is combined with other conditions (e.g., eczema or psoriasis), which were challenging to diagnose. AI's ability to consistently classify acne types and predict severity can help dermatologists make more informed treatment decisions, ultimately improving patient outcomes. In studies comparing AI systems to dermatologists, AI has demonstrated comparable or even superior accuracy in diagnosing acne lesions. Additionally, AI models can assist in monitoring the progression of acne by analyzing time-series images uploaded by patients. These systems can track changes in acne lesions over time, providing valuable insights into the effectiveness of treatments and helping clinicians adjust therapies as needed. By reducing human error and enhancing diagnostic accuracy, AI has the potential to streamline acne care and enable earlier intervention. Additionally, the use of AI in acne diagnosis can help dermatologists who may not specialize in acne management to make better-informed decisions [10].

In a study conducted by Junayed et al. (2019), the AcneNet deep learning model was utilized for classifying acne types through image analysis, significantly improving diagnostic accuracy compared to traditional manual methods, such as visual inspection and manual lesion counting, which is often time consuming and heavily influenced by clinician judgment. The new CNN model, "AcneNet," was founded on a deep residual neural network. The researchers used TensorFlow (a powerful open-source library developed by Google for numerical computation and machine learning) and Kensas (an application programming interface in Python, able to operate with TensorFlow). This model classified acne types based on image analysis into five distinct types: closed comedo, cystic, keloidalis, open comedo, and pustular forms, achieving an impressive approximate accuracy of 99.44% for the class of acne keloidalis, while the others also exceeded 94%, with fairly high precision and recall scores. Furthermore, this model demonstrated robustness in real-world applications. However, the lack of comparison with dermatologists and experts remains a limitation of the study [11].

Similarly, Shen et al. (2018) proposed an automatic diagnosis method for facial acne vulgaris using CNNs, showing that AI could classify acne severity with high precision from smartphone images [12]. A binary classifier for skin and nonskin (such as hair areas) was utilized to detect skin areas, and a seven classifiers [lesions: papule (C0), cyst (C1), blackhead (C2), normal skin (C3), pustule (C4), whitehead (C5), nodule (c6)] were employed to perform the classification task of facial acne vulgaris and healthy skin. In their experiments, Shen et al. compared the effectiveness of their CNN with the VGG16 neural network. VGG16 is a convolutional neural network architecture developed by K. Simonyan and A. Zisserman at the University of Oxford. It achieved a top 5 test accuracy of 92.7% on the ImageNet dataset, which contains over 14 million images across 1000 different categories.

The authors first compared the performance of their own binary classification CNN model with the pretrained VGG16 model. The authors found that their model's performance was slightly weaker, particularly when measuring the area under the curve (AUC) in the binary classification task, and the results were a bit poorer when applied in practical scenarios. They also realized that their model struggled with the seven-class classification task due to limitations like a small dataset and high similarity among augmented data. To overcome this, they decided to use transfer learning with the pretrained VGG16 model, which is already based on a larger dataset. By using VGG16, they were able to extract useful features from their small dataset and pass these features to a seven-class classifier to complete the multiclass classification task. Such AI-driven solutions not only support diagnosis but also provide the potential for real-time monitoring, aiding dermatologists in adjusting treatment plans based on visual data collected over time [13].

In terms of acne vulgaris mimickers, three studies on CNNs were conducted to compare rosacea and acne vulgaris, namely Aggarwal et al. [14], Goceri et al. [15], and Thomsen et al. [16], using InceptionV3, DenseNet201, and VGG16, respectively (Table 11.1). Aggarwal and colleagues made use of publicly accessible dermatological image datasets. After preprocessing and classifying the images, a specific number was selected for model training, validation, and testing using a neural network. For each skin condition, 30 images were set aside exclusively for testing. The deep learning framework adopted for this study was TensorFlow™, an open-source platform developed by Google. They retrained the InceptionV3 model—a deep convolutional neural network—specifically for this task. InceptionV3 consists of multiple computational layers designed to extract hierarchical features from input images [14]. The study's findings showed that this deep learning approach, leveraging TensorFlow™ [17] and the InceptionV3 model, effectively

Table 11.1 Studies on AI models and differential diagnosis of acne

Author	Method	Dermatoses
Aggarwal	InceptionV3	Rosacea, acne vulgaris, atopic dermatitis, psoriasis, and impetigo
Goceri	U-Net, VGGNet, InceptionV3, InceptionResNet-v2, and ResNet	Rosacea, acne vulgaris, hemangioma, psoriasis, and seborrheic dermatitis
Goceri	DenseNet201	Rosacea, acne vulgaris, hemangioma, psoriasis, and seborrheic dermatitis
Thomsen et al.	VGG16	Rosacea, acne vulgaris, psoriasis, eczema, and cutaneous T-cell lymphoma

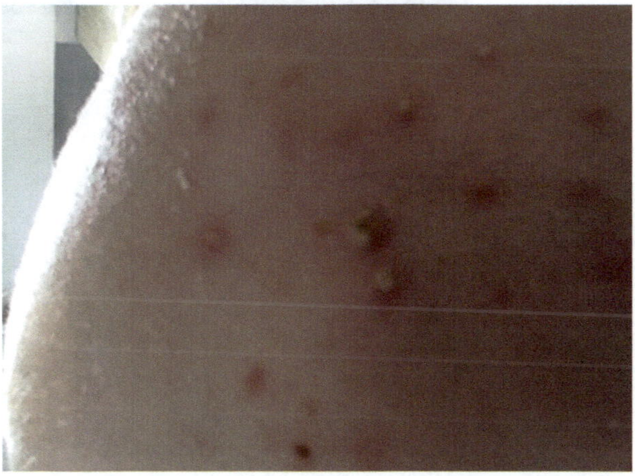

Fig. 11.1 Image showing a close-up of skin with multiple small, red to pink papules, some of which appear to have yellowish crusting or pustular tops. The distribution appears scattered. The diagnosed proposed was folliculitis or Jak-stat inhibitor-induced acneiform eruption based on the medical history of the patient [18]. The diagnosis of folliculitis was on the list of the proposed differential structures by the AI app, on which that image was uploaded. However, the second hypothesis was not, indicating the weakness of an AI model to handle tough cases only based on image analysis and the importance of medical history

distinguished between dermatological conditions such as rosacea, acne, atopic dermatitis, psoriasis, and impetigo. The model achieved strong performance across various evaluation metrics, including the Matthews correlation coefficient (MCC), F1 score, and area under the curve (AUC) [14].

It is both logical and valuable to explore how various AI models perform when applied to specific types or cases of acne. Different forms of acne—such as cystic, nodular, comedonal, or inflammatory—as well as different sites of the lesions can present unique visual characteristics and complexities that may influence how effectively a model can detect, classify, or assess severity (Figs. 11.1, 11.2, and 11.3). The first case included acneiform rash presented in a 50-year-old female patient under JAK inhibitor (tb baricitinib 4 mg S:1x2) for the treatment of alopecia areata universalis (Fig. 11.1). The second one corresponds to a young, 29-year-old female patient, who came to our office with a rash on the forehead the past 2 months. The

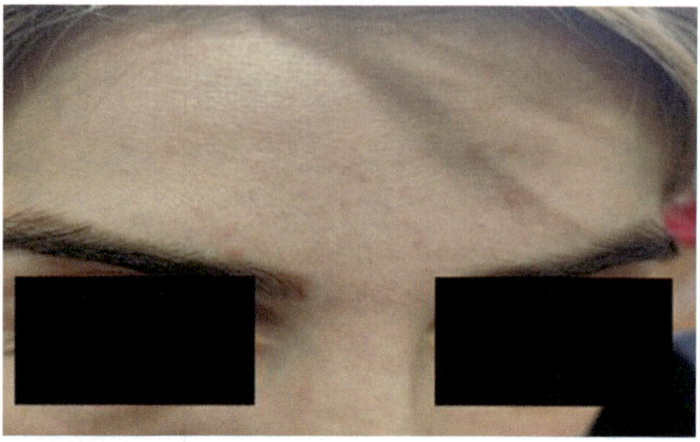

Fig. 11.2 Image showing small papules on the forehead of a young woman. When uploading such an image in the AI app, acne vulgaris is proposed as the most plausible diagnosis

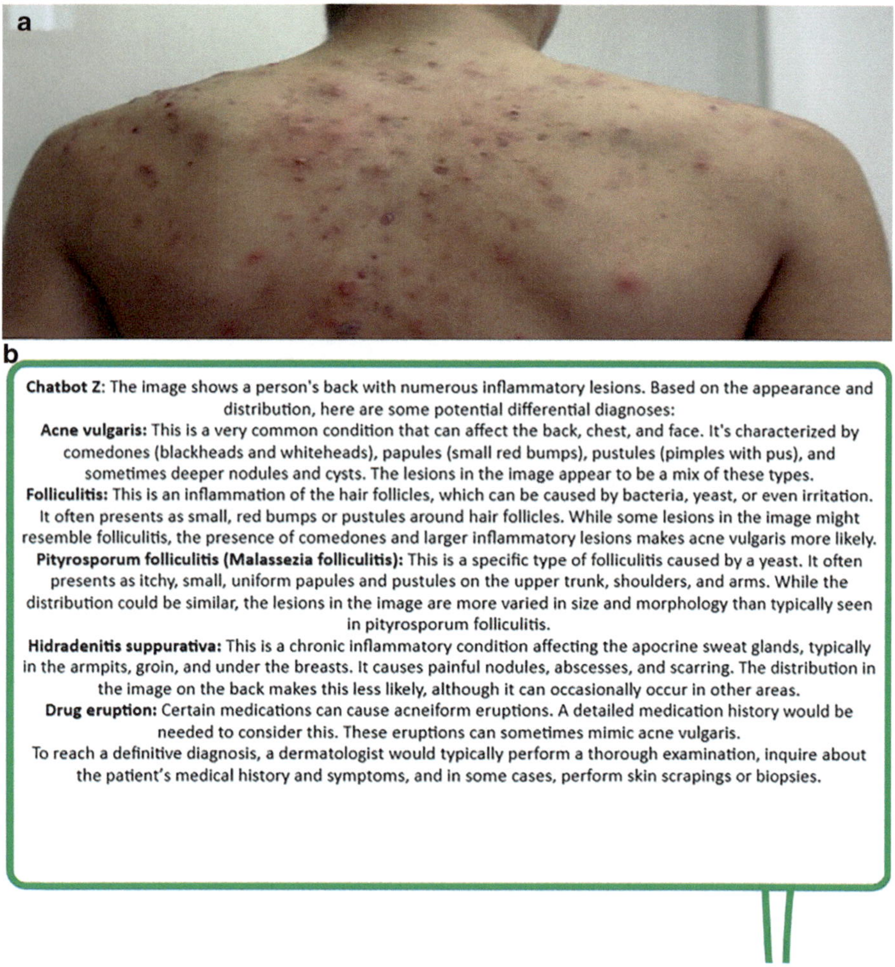

Fig. 11.3 (**a** and **b**) The differential diagnosis of a back acne generated by Chatbot Z. The model demonstrates strong capability in distinguishing acne from other similar-looking skin conditions—often referred to as acne mimickers—by analyzing factors such as lesion distribution, the degree of inflammation, and relevant medical history

two images were uploaded to an AI skin symptom checker app. This app is trained on a large database of 120,000 medical images, covering 200 skin conditions across all Fitzpatrick skin tones. The image showing a back acne was uploaded to a chatbot, asking for differential diagnosis (Fig. 11.3).

11.3 Acne Assessment Aided by AI Models

The use of CNNs in the approach to acne vulgaris was not limited to the disease diagnosis but was mainly focused on the disease severity classification. Clinicians typically rely on scoring systems in routine practice to evaluate the severity of acne, taking into account factors such as the presence of inflammatory lesions and cysts, which tend to indicate a more severe form of the condition. The Investigator's Global Assessment (IGA) scale is a widely used tool in clinical and research settings to grade acne severity, with slight variations in wording across studies or trials. It typically ranges from 0 to 4. A score of 0 (clear) indicates the absence of active acne, with no lesions or only minimal postinflammatory hyperpigmentation, while 4 (severe) denotes widespread inflammatory acne, including nodules and pustules, often with significant scarring or extensive comedonal involvement [5]. There are also more sophisticated grading systems such as the Global Acne Grading System (GAGS). GAGS offers a quantitative method for evaluating acne severity by tallying the number and type of lesions—such as comedones, papules, pustules, and nodules—across specific anatomical regions. These regions include the face (forehead, cheeks, nose, and chin), chest, back, shoulders, and upper arms. Each area is scored based on lesion count and type, contributing to a total score that reflects the overall severity of the condition. Based on the cumulative score, acne severity is categorized as follows: 0–18 indicates mild acne, 19–30 corresponds to moderate acne, 31–38 reflects severe acne, and a score of 39 or higher is classified as very severe acne [19]. Given the structure and simplicity of existing acne scoring systems, AI models—particularly those integrated into smartphone applications—tend to favor the use of the IGA scale. This preference is based on the IGA's straightforward, clinician-friendly format, which categorizes acne severity using a limited number of clearly defined stages, unlike the more complex grading systems that require counting specific lesion types across multiple body regions. This score makes it especially suitable for automated evaluations on mobile platforms, where rapid, user-accessible, and interpretable results are crucial for enhancing user engagement and supporting remote dermatological assessments.

The acne classification and assessment have been evaluated using different techniques. Chang and Liao applied a support vector machine (SVM) classifier, along with feature extraction techniques, to categorize acne vulgaris into different types, such as comedones, papules, and pustules. Before the SVM classification of skin defects, relevant features such as texture, color, and shape are extracted from the facial region of interest. The system is then trained on a labeled dataset, where each region is annotated as "comedones," etc., allowing the SVM to learn distinguishing patterns among these categories. Once trained, the SVM model uses the extracted features from a new facial image to predict the label for each region, identifying whether it is a comedone or papule or pustule, etc. [20]. Malik et al. used a similar method using an SMV classification to divide acne vulgaris into comedones, papules, etc., and then further grade acne into mild, mild to moderate, moderate to severe, and severe according to the mGAGS system (Fig. 11.4) [21]. SVM was used in the study by Chang C et al. [22] for the extraction of acne away from other skin pigmentation. A similar approach was used by Patwardhan et al. to extract features from VISIA-CR images. In all those techniques, the quality of the image played a significant role [23].

Regarding CNNs and deep learning tools, as indicated in the abovementioned section, Shen et al. employed the VGG16 model using transfer learning to classify acne patients into seven distinct categories, including normal skin, whiteheads, blackheads, pimples, pustules, cysts, and nodules, with the possibility of assigning a single patient to multiple categories [13]. Other examples of CNNs used were those of Zhao and Spoelstra. In this study, the researchers applied the 152-layer residual neural network (ResNet-152) to grade acne severity on a five-level scale—(1) clear; (2) almost clear; (3) mild; (4) moderate; and (5) severe—and compared the model's performance against the assessments made by 11 dermatologists for the same patients [24]. The characteristic of that study is that the researchers used the image rolling data augmentation approach to improve model performance by increasing the diversity of the training data. It involves extracting small patches from skin images and slightly shifting or sliding these patches across the surface, creating multiple variations of the same region. This process helps the model learn subtle differences in skin texture and appearance, improving its ability to detect and classify defects like acne or spots [25, 26]. By generating more training samples from existing data, skin patch rolling reduces the risk of overfitting. Based on the need for a more objective assessment of acne severity, frontal face images labeled with IGA scorings and more precise to three IGA categorizations were used for training. The authors evaluated neural network models inspired by three high-performing architectures: DenseNet,15 Inception v4,16, and ResNet1817. The best classification accuracy was 67% from the Inception v4 model. The authors found that the results from the abovementioned models compared favorably to the Microsoft-Nestle method, particularly in the severe (IGA 3–4) group [27].

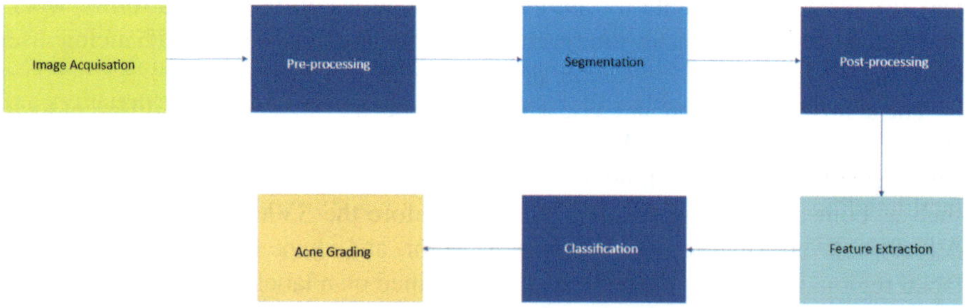

Fig. 11.4 Imaging showing the process of acne assessment using image processing techniques

Another study that focused on acne grading based on deep learning was that of Alzahrani S et al. The researchers introduced a method that combines two advanced techniques for acne analysis using 2D facial images: an attention mechanism, guided by bounding boxes from Faster R-CNN to highlight acne lesion locations, and a dilated UNet regressor for accurate lesion counting and severity grading [12]. An ensemble technique, meaning machine learning technique where multiple models or weak learners are used, is combined to create a stronger, more accurate predictive model—the AcneGrader system was used as well. This AI model achieved a prediction accuracy of 85.82% on the acne dataset [28].

Another interesting study worth mentioning is that of X. Wu et al. The authors integrated label distribution learning (LDL) with conventional classification, creating a multitask framework and a hybrid model that could simultaneously predict both the acne lesion counts and their corresponding severity levels. Unlike traditional methods that assign just one label to an instance, LDL assigns a range of neighboring labels, each reflecting varying degrees of relevance or intensity. The core of the model architecture is ResNet-50, which uses parameters that were pretrained on the ImageNet dataset to enhance performance [29]. Using high-quality images of the same database (the dataset ACNE04) as the study mentioned, another research team, Hao Wen et al., highlighted the importance of object detection for facial acne analysis, The researchers concluded that modern object detection models, specifically You Only Look Once (YOLO) and the R-CNN family (like Faster R-CNN or Mask R-CNN), are well suited for detecting exact acne lesions on facial images. While YOLO and R-CNNs are efficient models for localizing acne lesions, they have limitations related to small lesion detection, missing medical relevance, overfitting or generalization biases, and the need for high-quality images [30].

Lesion detection and aided acne grading were also performed by Kim et al., who utilized a CNN to classify acne lesions into five distinct types or perform binary classification distinguishing between inflammatory and noninflammatory lesions. The algorithm used was an enhanced version of the YOLOv3 model implemented with PaddlePaddle (PP-YOLO, which was trained on both the initial and final datasets to perform either five-class acne lesion classification or binary classification distinguishing inflammatory from noninflammatory lesions, respectively, while the images were used for training frontal and lateral view images of Korean patients. The authors validated that the proposed algorithm can assist dermatologists in detecting facial acne lesions reliably as the metric reflecting reader performance showed improvement when aided by AI compared to when readers evaluated the data on their own [31]. Another study on object detection was performed by Trivendi [32]. This research established a foundation for acne detection using deep neural networks. Several models were explored, including region-based fully convolutional network (R-FCN), Faster R-CNN, single-shot detector (SDD), and YOLO. Among these, YOLO demonstrated the highest overall performance, achieving an accuracy of 97.3%. It also outperformed others in precision (97.21%) and sensitivity (97.189%), indicating its strong ability to accurately detect acne lesions while minimizing missed cases. In contrast, Faster R-CNN and SDD showed comparatively lower performance across all evaluation metrics.

In response to AI-aided acne detection techniques, Bernhard et al. proposed a deep learning approach for predicting IGA acne severity grades that are well suited to challenging conditions, including low-resolution facial images taken with an iPhone 11 with a ring light, limited training samples, highly imbalanced acne class distributions, and the absence of detailed lesion annotations. The method enables model training using only severity grade labels, without requiring localization of acne lesions [33]. The model architecture that was used was that of the ResNet architecture, more precisely the ResNet110 with 1.7 M tunable parameters.

Regarding other CNN applications on acne classification with further implications on treatment, in the study by Yin Yang, the researchers collected 5871 digital clinical photographs from 1957 patients who visited the Hospital of Skin Diseases at the Chinese Academy of Medical Sciences between 2004 and 2016. The authors aimed to create an objective assessment model based on deep learning and according to the Chinese guidelines, which include four levels of acne classification. As part of preprocessing, the images were standardized by aligning faces horizontally and applying uniform zoom, facilitating consistent input for analysis. The classification model was built using the InceptionV3 deep learning architecture [34]. The model was initially pretrained on the ImageNet dataset, which contains 1.28 million images across 1000 categories, allowing it to retain basic visual features essential for accurate classification [35]. Then, transfer learning was applied using the acne dataset training set to enable the model to learn high-level semantic features relevant to acne diagnosis. In this study, each level of severity was linked to a recognized treatment protocol, according to which the doctors could develop clinical treatment plans and deliver standardized, targeted, and personalized care to patients according to the abovementioned Chinese guidelines. A limitation of the study is that it used images exclusively from an Asian population, which may affect how well the results can be applied to other populations. The results showed that the AI model's assessments were very similar to those of experienced dermatologists, suggesting that it performs at a professional level. Its decisions were less aligned with those of dermatology residents [34].

Regarding smartphone applications, Seité also developed a smartphone-based artificial intelligence algorithm based on performing image classification and segmentation techniques based on deep learning provided by Perfect Mobile Corp (New Taipei City, Taiwan). This AI model evaluates facial acne severity using the Global Acne Severity Scale specific to Europe [36]. Based also on smartphone images, an AI system named AcneDet was developed to automatically detect acne lesions and assess severity. The system comprises two components: a Faster R-CNN-based deep learning model for identifying four types of acne lesions—blackheads/whiteheads, papules/pustules, nodules/cysts, and acne scars—and a LightGBM machine learning model for grading acne severity based on the Investigator's Global Assessment (IGA) scale. LightGBM is an open-source framework developed by Microsoft that is widely used for classification, regression, and ranking tasks, particularly used for large datasets. The lesion counts produced by the detection model serve as input for the severity grading model. The Faster R-CNN model achieved a mean average precision (mAP) of 0.54 for lesion detection, while the LightGBM model reached a mean accuracy of 0.85 for severity assessment [37].

The highest accuracy regarding mobile applications and acne images was achieved by the Acne-RegNet system (Fig. 11.5). The app first identifies and crops out small regions or patches where acne lesions appear in the image. These patches are then classified into five different types of acne lesions using lightweight CNN models that are fast and efficient, ideal for smartphones. To improve accuracy and performance, the authors built a custom model called Acne-RegNet, which includes image enhancement techniques to clean up and brighten images, a channel attention module to help the model focus on the most important features, a region-based focal loss, which helps the model learn better from imbalanced data (since some types of acne are rarer than others), as well as model pruning and knowledge distillation, to make the model smaller and faster without losing accuracy. Combining the meta-data of patients, a personalized diagnosis was achieved, and mobile phone app was designed and implemented with the proposed acne grading method (Table 11.2) [38].

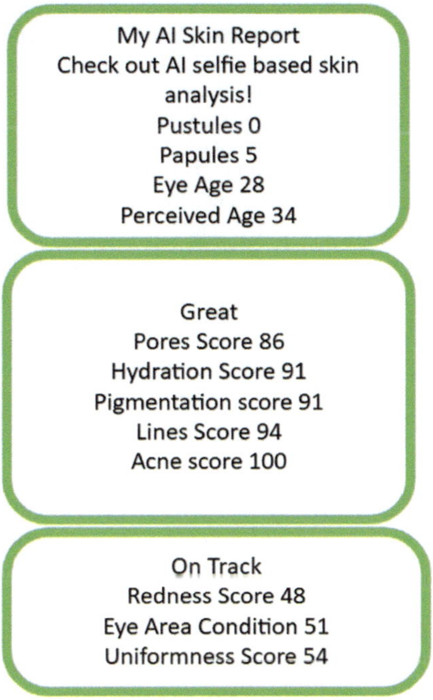

Fig. 11.5 Image showing an example of a comprehensive AI-powered skin analysis report generated by using a selfie. It evaluates key skin parameters such as pores (score: 86), hydration (91), pigmentation (91), and fine lines (94), all of which indicate excellent skin health. The acne score is perfect at 100, with no pustules and only five papules detected, suggesting minimal acne activity. However, moderate scores in redness (48), uniformness (54), and eye area condition (51) point to slight unevenness and potential sensitivity. Additionally, the app estimates an eye age of 28 and a perceived age of 34. The accompanying radar chart visualizes these results, highlighting strong areas and identifying those that could benefit from targeted skincare improvements. Examples of those apps can be found online

Table 11.2 AI models used in acne assessment

Study	System used	Scope of the study
Chang and Liao et al.,	Support vector machine	Acne classification—lesion detection
Malik et al.	Support vector machine	Acne classification—lesion detection and four severity scale classification
Shen et al.	VGG16 model	Acne classification—lesion detection
Zhao and Spoelstra et al.	ResNet-152	Acne classification (five-level scale)
Yin Yang et al.	InceptionV3 model	Acne classification (Chinese guidelines) and treatment approach
Seité et al.	Perfect Mobile Corp (New Taipei City, Taiwan) model	Acne classification—Global Acne Severity Scale
X. Wu et al.	ResNet-50 with label distribution learning	Acne classification and lesion counting
Hao Wen et al.	Object detection methods such as You Only Look Once (YOLO) and the R-CNN family (like Faster R-CNN or Mask R-CNN)	Acne lesions' exact detection
Lim et al.	Compact model based on DenseNet,15 Inception v4,16, and ResNet1817	Acne classification (IGA scores)
Kim et al.	You Only Look Once (YOLO)v3 model implemented with PaddlePaddle (PP-YOLO)	Acne lesions' exact detection
Trivedi et al.	R-FCN, Faster R-CNN, SDD, and YOLO	Object detection methods comparison in detecting acne lesions
Huynh QT et al.	Faster R-CNN and a light GBM	Acne lesions detections and acne classification (IGA scores)
Alzahrani S et al.	Faster R-CNN and a dilated UNet regressor	Acne lesions detections
Bernhard et al.	tResNet110 with 1.7 M tunable parameters	Acne classification based on low-quality images (IGA scores)
Wang et al.	Acne-RegNet	Acne classification (GAGS system)
Liu et al.	AcneGrader	Acne classification

Apps leverage CNNs to analyze images of skin conditions and provide instant feedback on acne severity, helping users better understand their skin. Aysa is an AI-powered app that analyzes images of the skin to detect a variety of conditions, including acne. It provides users with immediate feedback on potential skin conditions and helps them determine the severity of their acne. The app uses a vast database of images to compare and diagnose skin issues. LaRochePosay SpotsScanAI app—the functionality of this AI app is based on the AI algorithm created, trained, and validated on selfie images obtained from three cohorts of differently aged Asians, Africans, and Caucasians [39].As indicated by the image, it can detect the presence of pustules, discolorations, and/or skin imperfections using en face and side images and a following IGA score is produced. Numerous other applications provide insights into skin analysis, including the detection of acne vulgaris lesions (Fig. 11.5).

Vision Transformer (ViT) is a deep learning model for image recognition tasks that applies the transformer architecture, which was originally designed for natural language processing, to computer vision and was used in acne grading in a recent work [40]. This study introduces AcneDGNet, a deep learning-based model designed to perform both acne lesion detection and severity grading simultaneously. The approach begins by utilizing a vision transformer to extract robust global features from acne images captured through various sources. It then employs convolutional neural networks to identify four distinct types of acne lesions based on the Acne Grading System. Finally, it determines acne severity by integrating both global image features and localized lesion-specific information [41]. When the model is fed with a facial image, the input image first goes through the feature extraction module, which is made up of a Swin Transformer, a type of vision transformer that captures global features (big-picture understanding) from the image and then a feature pyramid network (FPN), which helps capture features at multiple scales, meaning it can detect both small and large acne lesions. Then, the multiscale feature maps created are passed into the lesion detection module, which uses a region proposal network (RPN) to focus on specific areas of the face that might contain acne and predicts the locations (bounding boxes) and types of acne lesions [42]. This fusion of global (whole-face) and regional (lesion-level) information is used to predict the overall acne severity grade (e.g., mild, moderate, severe) (Fig. 11.6).

The model was evaluated across diverse healthcare settings, including online consultations using smartphone images and offline clinical assessments using high-resolution images from digital cameras and VISIA systems. The results demonstrated that AcneDGNet significantly outperforms junior dermatologists in accuracy and achieves performance levels comparable to experienced senior dermatologists.

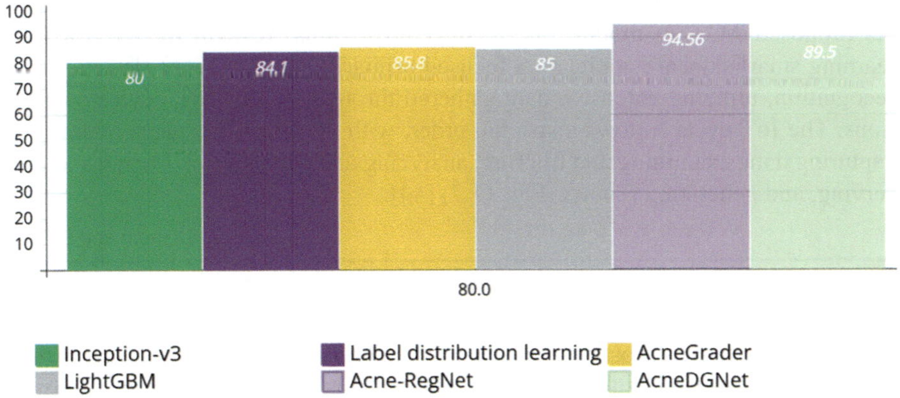

Fig. 11.6 Image showing the difference between accuracies based on the different model used each time

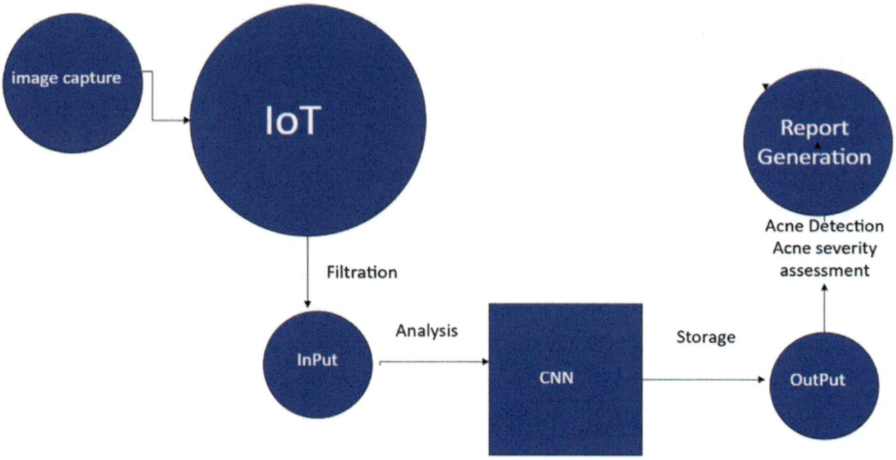

Fig. 11.7 Image showing the IoT-based AC-skin model architecture

This is the first study to test an AI-powered acne detection model in terms of healthcare facilities and real-world practice. Also, its methodology comes in contrast with the study by Bernhard et al. [33], who used only low-quality images and the object detection models that are based mainly on high-quality images as the proposed model can be based on any scenario [41].

The Internet of Things (IoT) encompasses interconnected devices that can be employed for acne grading and ongoing follow-up monitoring. In a recent study, researchers proposed a novel model, called AIC-IoT. This model is based on AI, IoT, and CC (cloud computing), technologies that play key roles in modern smart systems. More precisely, AI could be used for smart decision-making or predictive analysis; IoT refers to interconnected devices (such as sensors, wearables, or cameras) that collect and transmit data; and CC refers to the use of cloud services for data storage, processing, and analysis [43]. Toward this IoT approach, the researchers proposed AC-skin model. The architecture of this AC-skin model is a self-learning smart skincare application focused primarily on facial acne detection and recognition, utilizing extensive data gathered through various IoT device connections. The IoT cycle follows a specific order, with the lifecycle stages outlined as capturing data, examining and filtering, analyzing and aggregating, storing and preserving, and generating reports (Fig. 11.7) [44].

11.4 Acne Treatment and Follow-Up Using AI Technology

As mentioned earlier, most research on acne and AI models is based on classification, with limited studies focusing on acne diagnosis mainly comparing with rosacea [14]. The assessments provided by the AI models introduced above can be excellent tools for follow-ups of acne patients after a specific prescription is given to a patient after acne severity evaluation by a clinician. For example, AI-powered tools have significantly enhanced teledermatology by enabling accurate acne assessment through photos captured on smartphones or consumer-grade cameras, as shown in studies like those by Seité et al. [36], Huynh et al. [37], and Kim et al. [31]. This advancement allows dermatologists to remotely monitor patients, making it especially valuable for follow-ups in rural or underserved areas and in contexts where in-person visits are limited, such as during pandemic-style remote care. Additionally, automated systems like AcneGrader and Wu et al.'s model streamline clinical workflows by handling repetitive tasks such as lesion counting, severity grading, and progress tracking, freeing up clinicians to focus on treatment planning [28, 29]. Over time, consistent AI-based severity grading supports objective monitoring, allowing for data-driven treatment adjustments and early detection of worsening conditions through regular patient-submitted images. The IoT technology previously mentioned is anticipated to aid significantly in this direction. Moreover, models like Yin Yang et al.'s InceptionV3 not only classify acne but also suggest treatments aligned with clinical guidelines, moving toward precision dermatology where care can be personalized [34].

AI combined with virtual reality application can be a useful tool for acne follow-up. Virtual "before-and-after" simulations of treatment outcomes help build trust and encourage adherence, particularly among adolescents. Interactive VR tools can also lead users through skincare routines and recommend lifestyle adjustments, such as improving diet. By presenting educational content in an engaging and relatable way, these technologies boost patient motivation and promote long-term commitment to prescribed skincare regimens [45]. According to Goldust, Platforms like Viveport Human Skin VR allow users to explore detailed 3D models of skin layers and conditions such as acne, supporting both patient education and professional dermatology training. Meanwhile, EgoTouch VR/AR integrates AI with immersive AR/VR experiences for personalized acne visualization and treatment planning. Similarly, DermaAI utilizes advanced AI-based imaging to grade acne severity and predict treatment responses, further enhancing diagnostic accuracy and patient care [46]. However, validation of effectiveness is still limited in those practices that seem to be utilized soon.

In contrast to virtual reality technologies, which are less accessible, chatbots and large language models have become the traditional AI helpers. ChatGPT has sparked global interest by creating realistic and intelligent-sounding text, often indistinguishable from human-written content. In a study entitled "An Interesting Conversation with ChatGPT about Acne Vulgaris," ChatGPT generated a detailed write-up with largely correct information in an easy-to-understand language [47]. The accuracy and thoroughness of ChatGPT's responses to commonly asked questions about acne were evaluated. Using ChatGPT version 4.0, 85 responses were rated, with 74 receiving positive feedback for correctness and completeness (87.1%). The results indicate that while ChatGPT can offer basic information on acne, it still needs expert oversight to guarantee its accuracy and comprehensiveness. The identified errors highlight the necessity of verifying AI-generated content before relying on it as a reference [48] (Fig. 11.8).

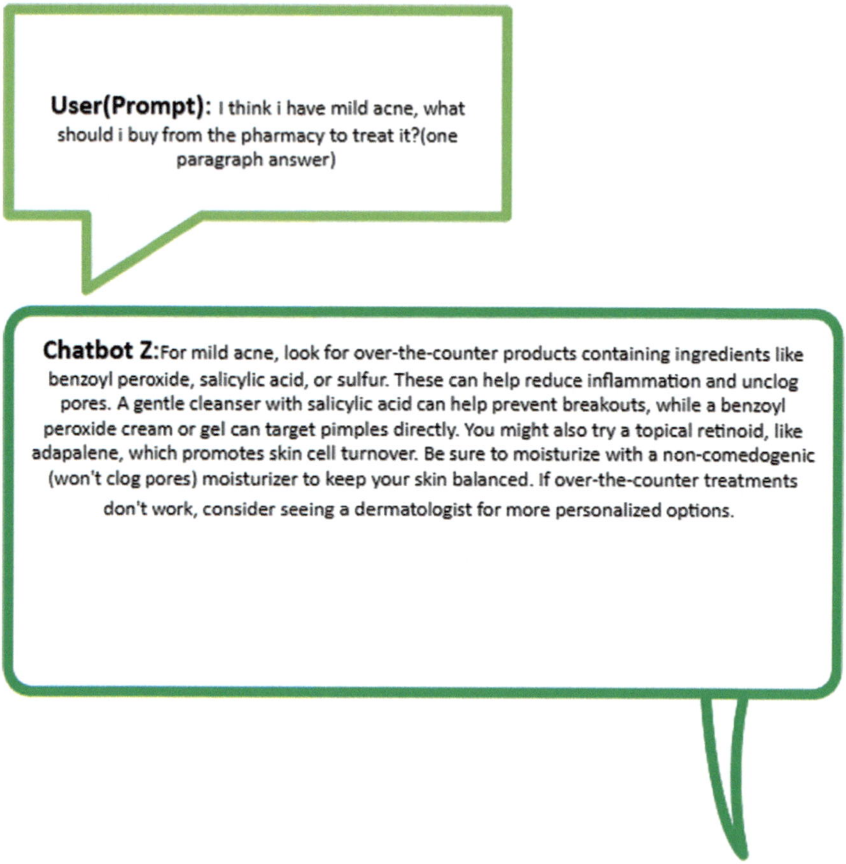

Fig. 11.8 Image showing a query requesting treatment advice for over-the-counter topical use. The phrase "I think" should prompt the chatbot to conduct further research. The chatbot's lack of presentation of contraindications for these topical treatments, along with its limited access to the patient's full medical history, may lead to inaccurate or mixed responses

References

1. Vasam M, Korutla S, Bohara RA. Acne vulgaris: a review of the pathophysiology, treatment, and recent nanotechnology based advances. Biochem Biophys Rep. 2023;36:101578. https://doi.org/10.1016/j.bbrep.2023.101578.
2. Carter KF, Dufour LT, Ballard CN. Identifying primary skin lesions. Nursing (Brux). 2003;33:68–9. https://doi.org/10.1097/00152193-200312000-00048.
3. Cardili RN, Roselino AM. Elementary lesions in dermatological semiology: literature review. An Bras Dermatol. 2016;91:629–33. https://doi.org/10.1590/abd1806-4841.20164931.
4. Geng R, Sibbald RG. Acne vulgaris: clinical aspects and treatments. Adv Skin Wound Care. 2024;37:67–75. https://doi.org/10.1097/ASW.0000000000000089.
5. Bae IH, Kwak JH, Na CH, Kim MS, Shin BS, Choi H. A comprehensive review of the acne grading scale in 2023. Ann Dermatol. 2024;36:65. https://doi.org/10.5021/ad.23.094.

6. Moncho-Santonja M, Aparisi-Navarro S, Defez B, Peris-Fajarnés G. Segmentation of acne vulgaris images techniques: a comparative and technical study. Appl Sci. 2023;13:6157. https://doi.org/10.3390/app13106157.
7. Chantharaphaichi T, Uyyanonvara B, Sinthanayothin C, Nishihara A. Automatic acne detection for medical treatment. In: 2015 6th International Conference of Information and Communication Technology for Embedded Systems (IC-ICTES). IEEE; 2015. p. 1–6. https://doi.org/10.1109/ICTEmSys.2015.7110813.
8. Kittigul N, Uyyanonvara B. Automatic acne detection system for medical treatment progress report. In: 2016 7th International Conference of Information and Communication Technology for Embedded Systems (IC-ICTES). IEEE; 2016. p. 41–4. https://doi.org/10.1109/ICTEmSys.2016.7467119.
9. Vaz JM, Balaji S. Convolutional neural networks (CNNs): concepts and applications in pharmacogenomics. Mol Divers. 2021;25:1569–84. https://doi.org/10.1007/s11030-021-10225-3.
10. Omiye JA, Gui H, Daneshjou R, Cai ZR, Muralidharan V. Principles, applications, and future of artificial intelligence in dermatology. Front Med (Lausanne). 2023;10 https://doi.org/10.3389/fmed.2023.1278232.
11. Junayed MS, Jeny AA, Atik ST, Neehal N, Karim A, Azam S, et al. AcneNet - a deep CNN based classification approach for acne classes. In: 2019 12th International Conference on Information & Communication Technology and System (ICTS). IEEE; 2019. p. 203–8. https://doi.org/10.1109/ICTS.2019.8850935.
12. Alzahrani S, Al-Bander B, Al-Nuaimy W. Attention mechanism guided deep regression model for acne severity grading. Computers. 2022;11:31. https://doi.org/10.3390/computers11030031.
13. Shen X, Zhang J, Yan C, Zhou H. An automatic diagnosis method of facial acne vulgaris based on convolutional neural network. Sci Rep. 2018;8:5839. https://doi.org/10.1038/s41598-018-24204-6.
14. Aggarwal SLP. Data augmentation in dermatology image recognition using machine learning. Skin Res Technol. 2019;25:815–20. https://doi.org/10.1111/srt.12726.
15. Goceri E. Diagnosis of skin diseases in the era of deep learning and mobile technology. Comput Biol Med. 2021;134:104458. https://doi.org/10.1016/j.compbiomed.2021.104458.
16. Thomsen K, Christensen AL, Iversen L, Lomholt HB, Winther O. Deep learning for diagnostic binary classification of multiple-lesion skin diseases. Front Med (Lausanne). 2020;7 https://doi.org/10.3389/fmed.2020.574329.
17. Novac O-C, Chirodea MC, Novac CM, Bizon N, Oproescu M, Stan OP, et al. Analysis of the application efficiency of TensorFlow and PyTorch in convolutional neural network. Sensors. 2022;22:8872. https://doi.org/10.3390/s22228872.
18. Ballanger F, Auffret N, Leccia M-T, Claudel JP, Dréno B. Acneiform lesions but not acne after treatment with Janus kinase inhibitors: diagnosis and management of Janus Kinase-acne. Acta Derm Venereol. 2023;103:adv11657. https://doi.org/10.2340/actadv.v103.11657.
19. Alsulaimani H, Kokandi A, Khawandanh S, Hamad R. Severity of acne vulgaris: comparison of two assessment methods. Clin Cosmet Investig Dermatol. 2020;13:711–6. https://doi.org/10.2147/CCID.S266320.
20. Chang C-Y, Liao H-Y. Automatic facial skin defects detection and recognition system. In: 2011 Fifth International Conference on Genetic and Evolutionary Computing. IEEE; 2011. p. 260–3. https://doi.org/10.1109/ICGEC.2011.67.
21. Malik AS, Humayun J, Kamel N, Yap FB-B. Novel techniques for enhancement and segmentation of acne vulgaris lesions. Skin Res Technol. 2014;20:322–31. https://doi.org/10.1111/srt.12122.
22. Chang C-Y, Liao H-Y. Automatic facial spots and acnes detection system. J Cosmet Dermatol Sci Appl. 2013;03:28–35. https://doi.org/10.4236/jcdsa.2013.31A006.
23. Patwardhan SV, Kaczvinsky JR, Joa JF, Canfield D. Auto-classification of acne lesions using multimodal imaging. J Drugs Dermatol. 2013;12:746–56.
24. Zhao THZ, Zhang H, Spoelstra J. A computer vision application for assessing facial acne severity from selfie images arXiv:1907.07901. 2019. n.d.

25. Mumuni A, Mumuni F. Data augmentation: a comprehensive survey of modern approaches. Array. 2022;16:100258. https://doi.org/10.1016/j.array.2022.100258.
26. Hao R, Namdar K, Liu L, Haider MA, Khalvati F. A comprehensive study of data augmentation strategies for prostate cancer detection in diffusion-weighted MRI using convolutional neural networks. J Digit Imaging. 2021;34:862–76. https://doi.org/10.1007/s10278-021-00478-7.
27. Lim ZV, Akram F, Ngo CP, Winarto AA, Lee WQ, Liang K, et al. Automated grading of acne vulgaris by deep learning with convolutional neural networks. Skin Res Technol. 2020;26:187–92. https://doi.org/10.1111/srt.12794.
28. Liu S, Fan Y, Duan M, Wang Y, Su G, Ren Y, et al. AcneGrader: an ensemble pruning of the deep learning base models to grade acne. Skin Res Technol. 2022;28:677–88. https://doi.org/10.1111/srt.13166.
29. Wu X, Wen N, Liang J, Lai Y-K, She D, Cheng M-M, et al. Joint acne image grading and counting via label distribution learning. In: 2019 IEEE/CVF International Conference on Computer Vision (ICCV). IEEE; 2019. p. 10641–50. https://doi.org/10.1109/ICCV.2019.01074.
30. Wen H, Yu W, Wu Y, Zhao J, Liu X, Kuang Z, et al. Acne detection and severity evaluation with interpretable convolutional neural network models. Technol Health Care. 2022;30:143–53. https://doi.org/10.3233/THC-228014.
31. Kim DH, Sun S, Cho SI, Kong H-J, Lee JW, Lee JH, et al. Automated facial acne lesion detecting and counting algorithm for acne severity evaluation and its utility in assisting dermatologists. Am J Clin Dermatol. 2023;24:649–59. https://doi.org/10.1007/s40257-023-00777-5.
32. Trivedi NK, Maheshwari H, Tiwari RG, Gautam V, Agarwal AK, Sharma M. Deep acne: advancing automated acne identification through deep neural networks. In: 2024 1st International Conference on Advanced Computing and Emerging Technologies (ACET). IEEE; 2024. p. 1–5. https://doi.org/10.1109/ACET61898.2024.10730442.
33. Bernhard R, Bletterer A, Le Caro M, García Álvarez E, Kostov B, Herrera ED. Automatic acne severity grading with a small and imbalanced data set of low-resolution images. Dermatol Ther (Heidelb). 2024;14:2953–69. https://doi.org/10.1007/s13555-024-01283-0.
34. Yang Y, Guo L, Wu Q, Zhang M, Zeng R, Ding H, et al. Construction and evaluation of a deep learning model for assessing acne vulgaris using clinical images. Dermatol Ther (Heidelb). 2021;11:1239–48. https://doi.org/10.1007/s13555-021-00541-9.
35. Chawla S, Nakov P, Ali A, Hall W, Khalil I, Ma X, et al. Ten years after ImageNet: a 360° perspective on artificial intelligence. R Soc Open Sci. 2023;10 https://doi.org/10.1098/rsos.221414.
36. Seité S, Khammari A, Benzaquen M, Moyal D, Dréno B. Development and accuracy of an artificial intelligence algorithm for acne grading from smartphone photographs. Exp Dermatol. 2019;28:1252–7. https://doi.org/10.1111/exd.14022.
37. Huynh QT, Nguyen PH, Le HX, Ngo LT, Trinh N-T, Tran MT-T, et al. Automatic acne object detection and acne severity grading using smartphone images and artificial intelligence. Diagnostics. 2022;12:1879. https://doi.org/10.3390/diagnostics12081879.
38. Wang J, Luo Y, Wang Z, Hounye AH, Cao C, Hou M, et al. A cell phone app for facial acne severity assessment. Appl Intell. 2023;53:7614–33. https://doi.org/10.1007/s10489-022-03774-z.
39. Zhang Y, Jiang R, Kezele I, Flament F, Elmozino E, Zhang J, et al. A new procedure, free from human assessment, that automatically grades some facial skin signs in men from selfie pictures. Application to changes induced by a severe aerial chronic urban pollution. Int J Cosmet Sci. 2020;42:185–97. https://doi.org/10.1111/ics.12602.
40. Al-hammuri K, Gebali F, Kanan A, Chelvan IT. Vision transformer architecture and applications in digital health: a tutorial and survey. Vis Comput Ind Biomed Art. 2023;6:14. https://doi.org/10.1186/s42492-023-00140-9.
41. Gao N, Wang J, Zhao Z, Chu X, Lv B, Han G, et al. Evaluation of an acne lesion detection and severity grading model for Chinese population in online and offline healthcare scenarios. Sci Rep. 2025;15:1119. https://doi.org/10.1038/s41598-024-84670-z.
42. Liao Z, Fan N, Xu K. Swin transformer assisted prior attention network for medical image segmentation. Appl Sci. 2022;12:4735. https://doi.org/10.3390/app12094735.

43. Khalid U, Chen L, Khan AA, Chen B, Mehmood F, Yasir M. A smart facial acne disease monitoring for automate severity assessment using AI-enabled cloud-based internet of things. Discov Comput. 2025;28:12. https://doi.org/10.1007/s10791-025-09503-7.
44. Khalid U, Li C, Ayub Khan A, Mehmood F. AC-skin: facial acne detection-based on intelligent learning and large data collection of internet of things (IoT) for smart skincare. IEEE Sensors J. 2024;24:30769–77. https://doi.org/10.1109/JSEN.2024.3414148.
45. Rong Q, Lian Q, Tang T. Research on the influence of AI and VR Technology for Students' concentration and creativity. Front Psychol. 2022;13 https://doi.org/10.3389/fpsyg.2022.767689.
46. Goldust M. AI-powered virtual reality in acne vulgaris. J Cosmet Dermatol. 2025:24. https://doi.org/10.1111/jocd.70104.
47. Deoghare S. An interesting conversation with ChatGPT about acne vulgaris. Indian Dermatol Online J. 2024;15:137–40. https://doi.org/10.4103/idoj.idoj_77_23.
48. Bettoli V, Naldi L, Santoro E, Valetto MR, Bolzon A, Cassalia F, et al. ChatGPT and acne: accuracy and reliability of the information provided—The AI - check study. J Eur Acad Dermatol Venereol. 2025:39. https://doi.org/10.1111/jdv.20324.

AI-Powered Approach to Rosacea

12

Eirini Kyrmanidou and Elizabeth Lazaridou

12.1 Key Elements of Rosacea

Rosacea is a chronic inflammatory skin disease that predominantly affects women aged 20–50 years. The prevalence of this skin disease is estimated to range from 0.2% to 22% of the population of North America and Europe. In America, around 16 million people are affected by rosacea [1]. This skin disease is often characterized by various symptoms, including subjective symptoms such as facial flushing, burning sensation, and objective symptoms such as persistent redness (erythema), the appearance of small red bumps known as papules, as well as pustules that can resemble acne. Additionally, individuals with rosacea may develop visible blood vessels or telangiectasia, and in some cases, even granulomas on their face, which can further contribute to the condition's aesthetic impact and patient's quality of life [2].

Rosacea is categorized into four distinct phenotypes: erythematotelangiectatic, papulopustular, granulomatous, and ocular (Fig. 12.1). Each type displays unique features, but distinguishing between them can often be a challenging task for both patients and healthcare professionals. Erythematotelangiectatic rosacea is marked by persistent erythema and visible blood vessels, while papulopustular rosacea features inflamed papules and/or pustules. Granulomatous rosacea is characterized by thickened skin, and ocular rosacea affects the eyes, leading to irritation and redness. Rosacea shares clinical similarities to other skin conditions, and misdiagnosis as acne, lupus, and dermatitis are not uncommon [3, 4].

Elevated vascular permeability as a consequence of increased vasomotor function, combined with an increased release of angiogenic substances from the mast cells, contributes to the development of the disease and the resulting

E. Kyrmanidou · E. Lazaridou (✉)
Second Dermatology Department, School of Health Sciences, Aristotle University of Thessaloniki, Thessaloniki, Greece
e-mail: bethlaz@auth.gr

E. Karampinis et al. (eds.), *Artificial Intelligence Applications in Dermatology*,
https://doi.org/10.1007/978-3-032-15614-3_12

facial erythema. Inflammatory responses involving hair follicle mites (*Demodex folliculorum*) may also be involved in the development of the disease [5].

Furthermore, the absence of specific biological markers for rosacea complicates the diagnostic process, often leading to delayed treatment. However, advancements in technology, particularly dermoscopy, have provided clinicians with valuable tools. This diagnostic tool enables healthcare providers to observe vascular changes in the skin more clearly, thereby enhancing diagnostic accuracy. The most common rosacea dermoscopic findings were linear vessels and *Demodex* tails, presenting as white mass protruding out of the hair follicle [6] (Fig. 12.1). Overall, understanding the nuances of rosacea is crucial for effective management and treatment as early recognition and appropriate intervention can significantly improve the quality of life for those affected by this often-misdiagnosed skin condition [7].

In the past decade, significant advancements in AI-driven computer-aided diagnosis have revolutionized the detection of a wide array of skin diseases, ensuring high accuracy and efficiency. These technological innovations have made it easier for healthcare professionals to identify conditions at earlier stages, improving patient outcomes. Meanwhile, the COVID-19 pandemic has further accelerated the growth of telemedicine, allowing patients to access medical consultations remotely, thus enhancing the delivery of healthcare services in new ways. However, the aim of most studies was the evaluation and diagnosis of skin malignancies [8]. Recently, artificial intelligence is increasingly being employed to accurately classify a range of noncancerous skin diseases, including inflammatory skin diseases, enhancing diagnostic precision and enabling healthcare professionals to provide better patient care and treatment options.

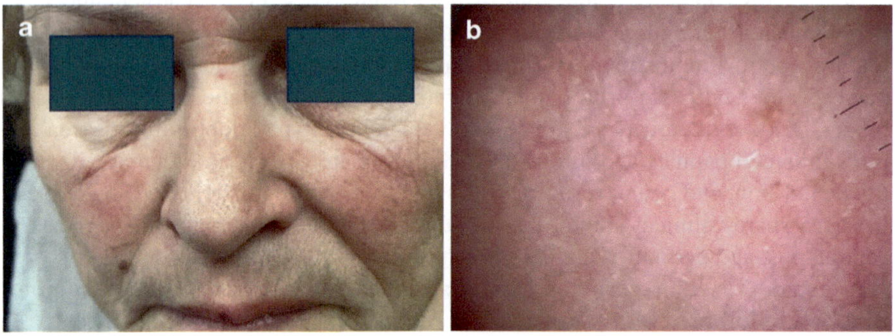

Fig. 12.1 Erythematotelangiectatic rosacea: (**a**) clinical picture; (**b**) dermoscopic picture: thin telangiectasias are visible (white circle), as well as *Demodex* tails (black arrows) (Dermlite DL200 Hybrid)

12.2 AI Models in Rosacea Diagnosis

Artificial intelligence has the potential to deliver impartial clinical evaluations and accurate outcome forecasts by systematically analyzing dermatological images. This capability aids healthcare professionals in making subjective decisions, ultimately enhancing patient care and treatment effectiveness in dermatology. Convolutional neural networks (CNNs) have seen remarkable advancements in recent years, establishing themselves as a cornerstone in the field of medical image analysis. These sophisticated algorithms function by emulating the activity of neurons in the human brain, enabling them to recognize intricate patterns within complex datasets. This capability is particularly valuable in dermatology, where accurate image interpretation can lead to improved diagnosis and treatment. Innovations such as GoogleNet have further propelled the efficiency of CNNs by introducing parallel convolution layers that utilize varying kernel sizes [9]. This design allows the network to capture a more comprehensive array of features from the images, optimizing performance and accuracy. As a result, CNNs are transforming the landscape of medical imaging, paving the way for enhanced patient care [10] (Table 12.1).

First, Binol et al. developed a hybrid AI method used to efficiently detect rosacea lesions from facial images with a combination of classical multidimensional scaling (MDS)—a technique that selects the most representative data information and a deep CNN, specifically the Inception-ResNet-v2 model, which was used to classify image patches as either rosacea or nonrosacea. This was an efficient AI model that maintained high diagnostic accuracy while using only a small, carefully selected subset of the training data [11].

Table 12.1 Studies on different methods of AI-approached diagnosis of rosacea

Author	Method	Dermatoses
Aggarwal	InceptionV3	Rosacea, acne vulgaris, atopic dermatitis, psoriasis, and impetigo
Binol et al.	Inception-ResNet-v2	Rosacea
Binol et al.	Ros-Net	Rosacea
Goceri	U-Net, VGGNet, InceptionV3, InceptionResNet-v2, and ResNet	Rosacea, acne vulgaris, hemangioma, psoriasis, and seborrheic dermatitis
Goceri	DenseNet201	Rosacea, acne vulgaris, hemangioma, psoriasis, and seborrheic dermatitis
Thomsen et al.	VGG-16	Rosacea, acne vulgaris, psoriasis, eczema, and cutaneous T-cell lymphoma
Park et al	ResNet-101, DarkNet-19, DarkNet-53, ResNet-50, and GoogleNet	Rosacea
Ge et al.	Gradient Boosting Machine (GBM) algorithm	Rosacea

Ros-Net was the first framework to be introduced in automatic identification of rosacea lesions from photographic images. Binol et al. presented an identification system designed to enhance accuracy and efficiency. By utilizing transfer learning techniques on a pretrained deep learning model, Ros-Net can adapt to various applications, making it a powerful tool for recognizing patterns and improving performance across diverse domains [12].

Transfer learning is a powerful technique that allows leveraging the knowledge gained from one domain and applying it to a different task [13]. In Ros-Net, this transfer is achieved by utilizing the Inception-ResNet-v2 and ResNet neural networks. By transferring the features learned from these models, performance is enhanced in new tasks, leading to more efficient and effective machine learning solutions. Furthermore, Binol et al. developed an innovative anatomically directed region of interest (ROI) specifically focused on facial areas that are particularly susceptible to rosacea. This method is distinguished by its incorporation of 12 carefully selected anthropometric landmarks that correspond to key facial features. By utilizing this targeted approach, they were able to enhance the precision of lesion identification significantly. One of the most notable outcomes of this advancement was a marked reduction in the false-positive rate, which is crucial for accurate diagnosis and treatment planning in rosacea patients. The effectiveness of the novel ROI was rigorously validated through a leave-one-patient-out cross-validation technique, ensuring that the findings are both reliable and applicable in clinical settings. The proposed framework evaluated the probability of a skin lesion being located within an impacted region by analyzing various environmental factors and distribution patterns to enhance accuracy and effectiveness. The proposed framework by Binol et al. demonstrates a strong capability in identifying facial skin affected by rosacea, showcasing its potential in dermatological assessments. However, it currently falls short in providing precise demarcation of lesions, which is crucial for accurate diagnosis and treatment planning [12].

Following, Park et al. introduced an innovative methodology known as the "Five Accurate CNNs-based Evaluation System" (FACES). This system is designed to enhance the detection of rosacea from clinical images by leveraging the strengths of the top five CNN models in deep learning, namely ResNet-101, DarkNet-19, DarkNet-53, ResNet-50, and GoogleNet. By assigning weights based on the accuracy of each model, FACES effectively synthesizes their outputs. The classification process employs a majority rule, ensuring that the final diagnosis reflects the consensus of the most reliable models. According to this majority rule, if the number of models indicating rosacea is equal to or greater than 3, the decision by the majority rule denotes rosacea. This integrated approach not only improves the precision of rosacea detection but also sets a new standard for utilizing multiple CNNs in medical image analysis, paving the way for better patient outcomes [14].

Clinical images were gathered from a cohort of 40 rosacea patients alongside 59 control subjects at the Johns Hopkins University Hospital. This comprehensive collection aimed to enhance the understanding of rosacea's clinical manifestations, employing advanced imaging techniques to analyze and compare the dermatological characteristics between the two groups. A total of 600 images for each group were collected and inserted for training purposes through the 19 pretrained CNNs. Finally, depending on accuracy outcomes, the top 5 CNN-based models were selected to be applied into FACES. The classification of rosacea was established through a consensus approach involving the five CNN models. When three or more of these models agreed on a diagnosis, it was deemed sufficient to confirm the presence of rosacea, ensuring a robust and reliable classification process grounded in collaborative model evaluation. The proposed FACES system showed a higher accuracy in diagnosing rosacea lesions, reaching 92.7%, compared to the Ros-Net (90.2%) [12] (Fig. 12.2). However, this system's effectiveness could have been better assessed through a comparison with evaluations made by experienced dermatologists. Additionally, important demographic factors such as race, age, and gender have to be included, which may significantly influence the performance and accuracy of this tool. Future studies should address these limitations to enhance the reliability and applicability of the findings [14].

Ge et al. analyzed physiological monitoring data and results from dermoscopic examination to uncover critical markers that are indicative of rosacea [15]. Researchers opted for the Gradient Boosting Machine (GBM) algorithm due to its ability to enhance the accuracy of predictive models. GBM works by refining a series of base learners or decision trees, thereby minimizing overall prediction loss and improving diagnostic precision. The integration of machine learning techniques, such as GBM, not only promises to follow the diagnostic process but also enhances the potential for personalized treatment plans. GBM improves diagnostic precision by combining many learners into a strong predictive model. Each learner improves upon the last by learning from its mistakes, which leads to highly accurate and reliable predictions—crucial for diagnosing conditions like rosacea [16]. Dermoscopic images combined with skin physiological evaluations, including

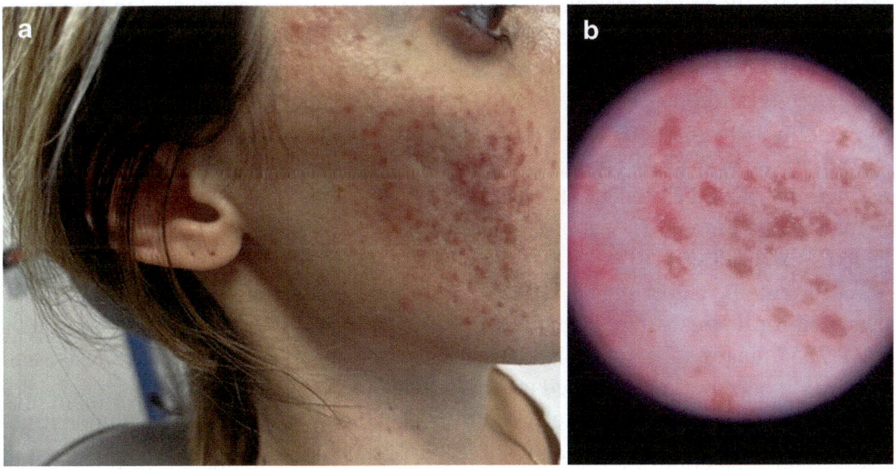

Fig. 12.2 Papulopustular rosacea mimicking acne: (**a**) clinical picture; (**b**) dermoscopy picture with the absence of comedones and polygonal perifollicular vessels, perifollicular scaling, and follicular pustules

percutaneous water loss, cuticle moisture content, pH, lipid, and erythema value in the central forehead, left cheek, right cheek, and jaw of the 495 participants, were measured. The study population consisted of 350 patients with facial skin diseases, among them 150 with rosacea, 100 with acne, and 100 with facial dermatitis, and 100 controls. From the statistical analysis, the melanin index from the physiological skin detection, and the vascular polygons, yellow halos around hair follicles and pustules from the dermoscopic analysis showed valuable prognostic indications in the differential diagnosis of rosacea. Interestingly, the dermoscopic features mentioned achieved a 100% positive prediction rate within the rosacea group, highlighting the strong diagnostic value of dermoscopy for this condition. In contrast, these features were far less common in other groups, appearing in only 8% of acne cases, 4% of dermatitis cases, and 1% of healthy controls, underscoring their specificity to rosacea. Furthermore, a man–machine comparison of GBM model prediction versus three resident doctors was carried out, supporting the predominance of the deep learning model developed in the diagnosis of inflammatory facial diseases. In the validation set of 45 cases, the research highlights that the GBM accurately carries out the differential diagnosis of rosacea in both dichotomous (rosacea and nonrosacea) and four classifications (rosacea, acne, seborrheic dermatitis, and normal). The total accuracy rate of GBM model prediction was 84.4% [15].

Thus, researchers indicate that integrating traditional skin physiological detection techniques and dermatoscopy with advanced machine learning algorithms significantly elevates clinicians' diagnostic efficiency for rosacea. This innovative approach allows for more accurate assessments, leading to timely treatment decisions and improved patient outcomes in dermatological care.

Thomsen et al. used the VGG-16 model, developed by the Oxfords Geometry Group (VGG), to improve the diagnostic accuracy of GPs in identifying five multiple-lesion skin diseases, rosacea included. A total of 19,641 images were inserted into the model for analysis. Since the research was conducted in Denmark, the images involved mainly patients with Fitzpatrick skin types II and III. The VGG-16 model, a convolutional neural network renowned for its effectiveness in image recognition tasks, demonstrated remarkable performance, especially in distinguishing between acne and rosacea lesions, reaching a sensitivity of 85.42 and specificity of 89.53%. Researchers admit that although the VGG-16 did not reach the heights of other pioneer studies, like that conducted by Esteva et al. in melanoma identification [17], it shows great potential, especially in classifying multiple-lesion skin diseases [18].

Furthermore, Goceri et al. introduced a tailored MobileNet model specifically designed for the real-time diagnosis of five prevalent skin diseases. The researchers used 725 images of seborrheic dermatitis, rosacea, hemangioma, psoriasis, and acne. By incorporating advanced techniques such as dilated convolutions and Leaky Rectified Linear Unit (LeakyReLU) activations, the model enhances feature extraction capabilities, improving diagnostic accuracy. Generally, LeakyReLU is used in neural networks, especially deep learning models, to introduce nonlinearity, which is essential for the model to learn complex patterns [19]. Additionally, the integration of a novel mobile app further optimizes performance, making it a valuable tool for dermatologists and healthcare professionals aiming to provide timely and effective patient care in skin disease management. Goceri et al. have also tested multiple models like ResNet and Inception-ResNet-v2, which incorporate advanced architectures and residual connections, and tend to outperform simpler models like U-Net in rosacea classification tasks. Those models enabled automated diagnosis from digital photographs. However, as indicated by the authors, the identification of advantages of those models and the creation of a new one that combines them are necessary [20].

Lastly, Aggarwal et al. utilized publicly available dermatological image datasets. After preprocessing and categorizing the images, the following numbers were selected for model development, testing, and evaluation using a neural network. For each dermatological condition, 30 images were reserved exclusively for the testing phase. The deep learning framework employed was TensorFlow™, an open-source library developed by Google. The InceptionV3 model, a deep convolutional neural network, was retrained for this task. InceptionV3 comprises a series of computational layers, each with specific input and output, facilitating the extraction of hierarchical features from the images. The results demonstrated that employing a deep learning-based approach using TensorFlow™ [21] and InceptionV3 enables the differentiation of dermatological images to rosacea, acne, atopic dermatitis, psoriasis, and impetigo categories with notable performance metrics [22] (Table 12.1).

A FACES study achieved the greatest accuracy [14]. However, there are many limitations to those studies. In certain studies, the performance of the AI model was not compared with that of experienced dermatologists to validate the tested method. Therefore, further comparative testing is needed to confirm the suitability of our detection tool for clinical use. Additionally, factors such as race, age, or gender are strongly linked to the development of rosacea and may influence AI model classification accuracy. Also, in certain studies such as that of Ge et al., it was based mainly on female rosacea patients [15]. Overfitting bias was acknowledged in the study of Thomson et al. [18]. In many studies, clinical photos were captured using a digital camera to cover the entire face. However, a single photo may not capture the full extent of the skin lesion, potentially misrepresenting or distorting the features of rosacea [14].

12.3 AI Assessment of Facial Erythema

Although these methods effectively detect rosacea, the studies outlined in Table 12.1 mainly emphasize general diagnosis rather than specific subtypes. The boundary between these subtypes is quite obscure, and these subtypes may overlap or transform from one subtype to another, especially erythematotelangiectatic and papulopustular (Fig. 12.2). In the study by Zhao et al., the researchers used a CNN model, namely ResNet-50, to differentiate between three subtypes of rosacea, achieving classification accuracies of 83.9%, 74.3%, and 80.0%, respectively. Notably, 28.1% (54 out of 192) of the papulopustular cases were incorrectly identified as erythematotelangiectatic. This performance discrepancy may be attributed to the clinical overlap in symptoms between the two subtypes, which often makes them difficult to distinguish. This example highlights that the diagnostic challenges faced in clinical practice are similarly difficult for AI models to address. In this study, the comparison dataset included conditions such as acne, facial eczema, seborrheic dermatitis, lupus erythematosus, chronic solar dermatitis, corticosteroid-induced dermatitis, and lupus miliaris disseminatus faciei [2]. However, specific comparison metrics—for instance, the classification accuracy between rosacea and lupus erythematosus—were not detailed. It is strongly recommended that CNNs be trained to recognize specific rosacea subtypes using differential diagnosis images commonly seen in clinical settings [23]. This approach would enhance the clinical applicability and usefulness of AI models in real-world practice (Table 12.2).

Interestingly, despite the varying lesion types associated with different rosacea subtypes, the CNNs developed appear capable of accurately identifying features such as redness, telangiectasia, pustules, papules, and even phymatous changes—all aligning with a rosacea diagnosis. In comparative analyses, conditions like acne vulgaris (distinguished by the presence of comedones) and seborrheic dermatitis (often identified by lesion location) were commonly used. This suggests that the high performance of these CNN models may partly stem from their ability to distinguish rosacea based on contrasting features found in the comparative diseases (Table 12.2). Therefore, the comparison with dermatologists' performance is always essential as head-to-head testing against dermatologists provides a clear metric of the AI model performance.

Regarding rosacea subtype diagnosis, a recently published study showed that integrating advanced deep learning architectures—specifically Swin transformers (Swin-Tiny, Swin-Small, and Swin-Base)—with pretrained convolutional neural networks (VGG19, ResNet-50, and DenseNet201) enhances the accuracy of rosacea type classification. Among all models evaluated, Swin-Base achieved the best results, with a test accuracy of 99%, while the researchers added explainable AI techniques to build further trust in the use of AI for diagnosis [24].

Regarding rosacea mimickers, studies focusing on AI models that are used to detect diseases such as lupus erythematosus and photodermatitis seem to be missing, highlighting an important gap in the literature [2]. They are used for developing and training CNN classifiers for differentiating photodermatitis subtypes, such as polymorphic light eruption, photoallergic and phototoxic reactions, porphyrias, and photo-exacerbated dermatoses like lupus and rosacea. The use of AI for analyzing

Table 12.2 Rosacea subtypes and differential diagnoses

Rosacea subtype	Differential diagnoses
Erythematotelangiectatic	Seborrheic dermatitis, lupus erythematosus, photodermatitis, contact dermatitis, carcinoid syndrome
Papulopustular	Acne vulgaris, perioral dermatitis, folliculitis, seborrheic dermatitis
Phymatous	Acne keloidalis nuchae, sebaceous hyperplasia, cutaneous lymphoma
Granulomatous	Cutaneous sarcoidosis, lupus miliaris disseminatus faciei, tuberculosis, leprosy

facial redness is still in its early stages and has been primarily limited to rosacea-related research.

The type of imaging modality employed—such as reflectance confocal microscopy (RCM), dermoscopy, or VISIA—plays a significant role in rosacea diagnosis as each provides distinct imaging features valuable for assessment. A study by Huang et al. (2022) demonstrated that integrating data from these three noninvasive imaging tools using a multilayer perceptron (MLP) model enhanced diagnostic accuracy for rosacea. Specifically, the MLP model achieved an area under the receiver operating characteristic curve (AUROC) of 0.8385 when combining RCM, dermoscopy, and VISIA data, surpassing the performance of any single modality [25].

Apart from AI models based on the macroscopic clinical image, the diagnosis can be based on microscopy—for example, in the presence of *Demodex* mites in the skin of the patients. A similar approach was followed in the study of *Demodex blepharitis* and the meibography images. AI algorithms can rapidly process meibography images to detect and quantify gland atrophy patterns, providing a consistent and reproducible assessment. This automation facilitates the identification of patients with *Demodex blepharitis* and the evaluation of the extent to which *Demodex* infestation affects meibomian gland morphology. In a dry eye unit, such AI-driven tools can streamline diagnostic workflows, enabling timely and accurate assessments that inform treatment decisions [26]. A similar approach can be used in case of facial skin and demodicosis, but further studies need to be done in this direction by recognizing specific structures on skin, measuring its morphology and making AI correlations of the presence or absence of *Demodex* mites.

12.4 Rosacea Severity Assessment Using AI

Apart from diagnosis, AI algorithms have been used to assess the severity of many dermatoses providing subjective scores in faster ways that a clinician, no matter how expert one is, can achieve. The currently used Investigator's Global Assessment (IGA) lacks specificity as it does not take into account the subtypes or phenotypes of rosacea, nor does it consider the extent of area involvement. To address these limitations, the Rosacea Area and Severity Index (RASI) was developed to provide a more detailed evaluation of rosacea features across four facial regions—cheeks, forehead, nose, and chin—with adjustments based on each area's relative importance to derive an overall severity score (RASI) that evaluates primary rosacea symptoms such as papules, pustules, erythema, telangiectasias, and phyma, along with the extent of lesion spread. While RASI offers a more comprehensive approach, it still relies on visual assessment, which introduces subjectivity and often fails to detect subtle differences in erythema, especially in mild cases [27].

To improve objectivity, computer-aided analysis using technologies like the VISIA® system is often employed. Various devices—such as chromameters, high-frequency ultrasound, and laser speckle contrast imaging—are also used to detect and quantify erythema. The VISIA® system specifically helps in objectively evaluating rosacea-related erythema by providing

(i) Feature count: total number of erythema spots, regardless of size or intensity.
(ii) Absolute score: a combined measure reflecting number, size, area, and intensity.
(iii) Percentile scores: comparisons against a larger database.

However, the system has limitations. It struggles to fully segment or identify diffuse or gradient-pattern erythema, which leads to inaccurate or imprecise results, making it less reliable in representing the real clinical picture for many rosacea patients. Another study found that the absolute score and percentile of the red area showed significant correlations with the IGA and clinical erythema assessment (CEA) [28]. However, the red area did not show a significant correlation with the numerical score or telangiectasia. Specifically, in patients with erythematotelangiectatic rosacea, the red area had the strongest correlation with both IGA and CEA, particularly in individuals aged 51–60 [29].

Currently, there is no work published on AI assessment of rosacea patients. AI models trained on VISIA images can be the future of rosacea assessment as VISIA generates high-quality, detailed facial images that can serve as a rich dataset for AI algorithms. Currently, there is no study based on an AI algorithm that assesses the severity of rosacea.

12.5 AI Approaches Involved in Rosacea Treatment and Follow-Up

In parallel with assessment, there are no currently published studies regarding AI technology aiding in clinician decisions tailoring treatment planning in patients with rosacea. While included in the follow-up and treatment, patient education is an important tool that has been proved to be a rather efficient chatbot.

More specifically, researchers evaluated the reliability and clinical applicability assessment for four categories of questions posed by patients with rosacea. Those questions were related to potential triggers, medication practices, special manifestations, and skin care routine. Notably, high scores were achieved especially in case of clinical applicability and more specifically in case of potential triggers, with questions on food and other practices that may exacerbate or cause rosacea flare. This can be extremely useful in terms of patient education as the chatbots can be really useful in quickly answering patients' questions and aiding patients' follow-up. The question "What dietary considerations should be taken into account for rosacea?" received a perfect score—100%—for both clinical applicability and accuracy, based on expert evaluations using a five-point scale for reliability and a three-point scale for clinical relevance [30]. It is worth mentioning that this study is based on ChatGPT 3.5's generative ability. Therefore, the development and release of more advanced AI chatbots would be expected to provide even more sophisticated answers to the same questions (Fig. 12.3).

Indeed, recent progress in natural language processing has significantly improved the ability of these tools to deliver more context-aware and detailed answers across

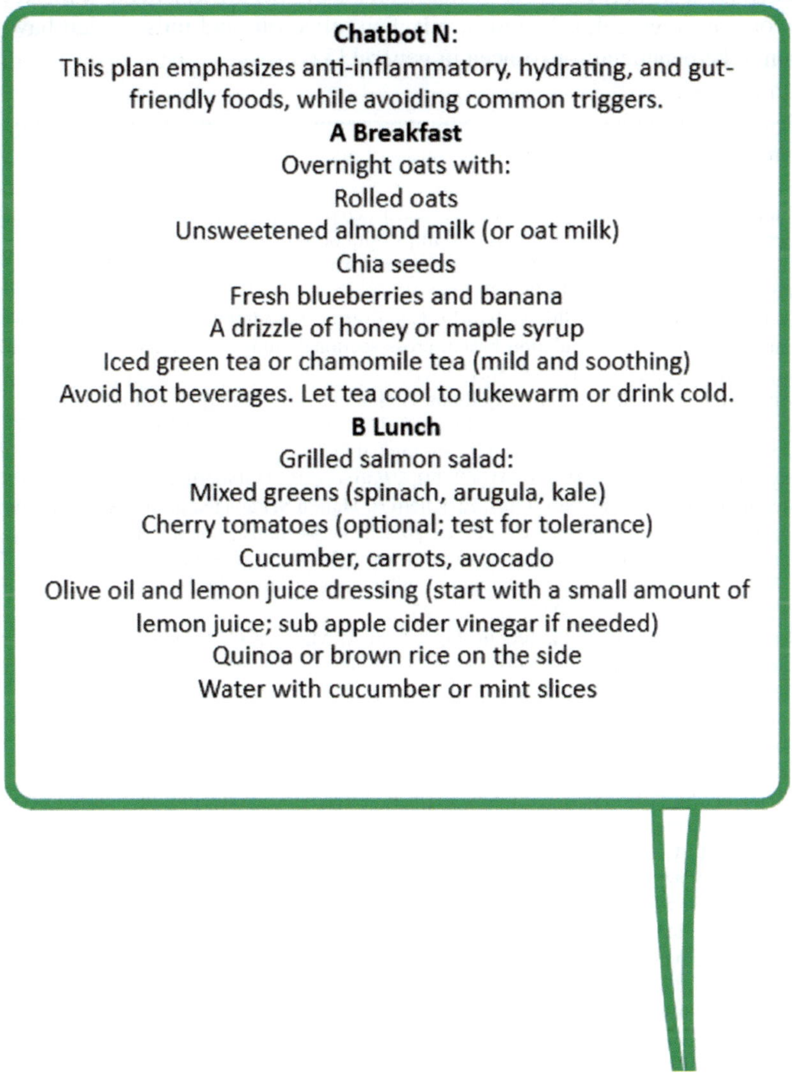

Fig. 12.3 Image showing meal examples for patients with rosacea. The input to the chatbot N is "Design a sample rosacea-friendly meal plan," while the chatbot's output is, except for breakfast and lunch, it presents snacks, dinner, and desserts, suitable for rosacea patients

various types of questions compared to the previous versions. As large language models, they are trained on extensive datasets, allowing them to understand queries and generate accurate, timely responses. As a result, ChatGPT 4.5 offers improved performance compared to ChatGPT 3.5 [31]. According to Fig. 12.3, chatbots can provide very useful suggestions. The response is in line with diet recommendations, meaning avoidance of alcohol and spicy foods and cinnamaldehyde-containing foods, such as tomatoes, citrus fruits, chocolate, cheese, and meat while the plan also contains vegetables, legumes, oily fish, olive oil, and nuts, which have been proven to be beneficial for rosacea in general [32].

References

1. Rainer BM, Kang S, Chien AL. Rosacea: epidemiology, pathogenesis, and treatment. Dermatoendocrinol. 2017;9:e1361574. https://doi.org/10.1080/19381980.2017.1361574.
2. Two AM, Wu W, Gallo RL, Hata TR. Rosacea. J Am Acad Dermatol. 2015;72:749–58. https://doi.org/10.1016/j.jaad.2014.08.028.
3. Li J, Wang B, Deng Y, Shi W, Jian D, Liu F, et al. Epidemiological features of rosacea in Changsha, China: A population-based, cross-sectional study. J Dermatol. 2020;47:497–502. https://doi.org/10.1111/1346-8138.15301.
4. Mikkelsen CS, Holmgren HR, Kjellman P, Heidenheim M, Karppinnen A, Bjerring P, et al. Rosacea: a clinical review. Dermatol Rep. 2016;8 https://doi.org/10.4081/dr.2016.6387.
5. Maden S. Rosacea: an overview of its etiological factors, pathogenesis, classification and therapy options. Dermato. 2023;3:241–62. https://doi.org/10.3390/dermato3040019.
6. Stefanou E, Gkentsidi T, Spyridis I, Errichetti E, Manoli S, Papageorgiou C, et al. Dermoscopic spectrum of rosacea. JEADV Clin Pract. 2022;1:38–44. https://doi.org/10.1002/jvc2.6.
7. van Zuuren EJ, Arents BWM, van der Linden MMD, Vermeulen S, Fedorowicz Z, Tan J. Rosacea: new concepts in classification and treatment. Am J Clin Dermatol. 2021;22:457–65. https://doi.org/10.1007/s40257-021-00595-7.
8. Ruggiero A, Martora F, Fabbrocini G, Villani A, Marasca C, Megna M, et al. The role of teledermatology during the COVID-19 pandemic: a narrative review. Clin Cosmet Investig Dermatol. 2022;15:2785–93. https://doi.org/10.2147/CCID.S377029.
9. Yamashita R, Nishio M, Do RKG, Togashi K. Convolutional neural networks: an overview and application in radiology. Insights Imaging. 2018;9:611–29. https://doi.org/10.1007/s13244-018-0639-9.
10. Shi X, De-Silva V, Aslan Y, Ekmekcioglu E, Kondoz A. Evaluating the learning procedure of CNNs through a sequence of prognostic tests utilising information theoretical measures. Entropy. 2021;24:67. https://doi.org/10.3390/e24010067.
11. Binol H, Niazi MKK, Plotner A, Sopkovich J, Kaffenberger B, Gurcan MN. A multidimensional scaling and sample clustering to obtain a representative subset of training data for transfer learning-based rosacea lesion identification. In: Hahn HK, Mazurowski MA, editors. Medical imaging 2020: computer-aided diagnosis. SPIE; 2020. p. 38. https://doi.org/10.1117/12.2549392.
12. Binol H, Plotner A, Sopkovich J, Kaffenberger B, Niazi MKK, Gurcan MN. Ros-NET: a deep convolutional neural network for automatic identification of rosacea lesions. Skin Res Technol. 2020;26:413–21. https://doi.org/10.1111/srt.12817.
13. Chato L, Regentova E. Survey of transfer learning approaches in the machine learning of digital health sensing data. J Pers Med. 2023;13:1703. https://doi.org/10.3390/jpm13121703.
14. Park S, Chien AL, Lin B, Li K. FACES: A deep-learning-based parametric model to improve rosacea diagnoses. Appl Sci. 2023;13:970. https://doi.org/10.3390/app13020970.
15. Ge L, Li Y, Wu Y, Fan Z, Song Z. Differential diagnosis of rosacea using machine learning and dermoscopy. Clin Cosmet Investig Dermatol. 2022;15:1465–73. https://doi.org/10.2147/CCID.S373534.
16. Natekin A, Knoll A. Gradient boosting machines, a tutorial. Front Neurorobot. 2013;7 https://doi.org/10.3389/fnbot.2013.00021.
17. Esteva A, Kuprel B, Novoa RA, Ko J, Swetter SM, Blau HM, et al. Dermatologist-level classification of skin cancer with deep neural networks. Nature. 2017;542:115–8. https://doi.org/10.1038/nature21056.

18. Thomsen K, Christensen AL, Iversen L, Lomholt HB, Winther O. Deep learning for diagnostic binary classification of multiple-lesion skin diseases. Front Med (Lausanne). 2020;7 https://doi.org/10.3389/fmed.2020.574329.
19. Montesinos López OA, Montesinos López A, Crossa J. Fundamentals of artificial neural networks and deep learning. In: Multivariate statistical machine learning methods for genomic prediction. Cham: Springer; 2022. p. 379–425. https://doi.org/10.1007/978-3-030-89010-0_10.
20. Goceri E. Diagnosis of skin diseases in the era of deep learning and mobile technology. Comput Biol Med. 2021;134:104458. https://doi.org/10.1016/j.compbiomed.2021.104458.
21. Novac O-C, Chirodea MC, Novac CM, Bizon N, Oproescu M, Stan OP, et al. Analysis of the application efficiency of TensorFlow and PyTorch in convolutional neural network. Sensors. 2022;22:8872. https://doi.org/10.3390/s22228872.
22. Aggarwal SLP. Data augmentation in dermatology image recognition using machine learning. Skin Res Technol. 2019;25:815–20. https://doi.org/10.1111/srt.12726.
23. Zhao Z, Wu C-M, Zhang S, He F, Liu F, Wang B, et al. A novel convolutional neural network for the diagnosis and classification of rosacea: usability study. JMIR Med Inform. 2021;9:e23415. https://doi.org/10.2196/23415.
24. Anjali T, Abhishek S, Remya S. A novel framework for rosacea detection using Swin Transformers and explainable artificial intelligence. Alex Eng J. 2025;118:36–58. https://doi.org/10.1016/j.aej.2024.12.080.
25. Huang Y, He J, Zhang S, Tang Y, Wang B, Jian D, et al. A novel multi-layer perceptron model for assessing the diagnostic value of non-invasive imaging instruments for rosacea. PeerJ. 2022;10:e13917. https://doi.org/10.7717/peerj.13917.
26. Liu X, Fu Y, Wang D, Huang S, He C, Yu X, et al. Uneven index: a digital biomarker to prompt demodex blepharitis based on deep learning. Front Physiol. 2022;13 https://doi.org/10.3389/fphys.2022.934821.
27. Wienholtz NKF, Thyssen JP, Christensen CE, Thomsen SF, Karmisholt KE, Jemec GBE, et al. Validity and reliability of the Rosacea Area and Severity Index: A novel scoring system for clinical assessment of rosacea severity. J Eur Acad Dermatol Venereol. 2023;37:573–80. https://doi.org/10.1111/jdv.18721.
28. Tan J, Liu H, Leyden JJ, Leoni MJ. Reliability of Clinician Erythema Assessment grading scale. J Am Acad Dermatol. 2014;71:760–3. https://doi.org/10.1016/j.jaad.2014.05.044.
29. Pan Y, Jia K, Yan S, Jiang X. Effectiveness of VISIA system in evaluating the severity of rosacea. Skin Res Technol. 2022;28:740–8. https://doi.org/10.1111/srt.13194.
30. Yan S, Du D, Liu X, Dai Y, Kim M-K, Zhou X, et al. Assessment of the reliability and clinical applicability of ChatGPT's responses to patients' common queries about rosacea. Patient Prefer Adherence. 2024;18:249–53. https://doi.org/10.2147/PPA.S444928.
31. Tsai C-Y, Cheng P-Y, Deng J-H, Jaw F-S, Yii S-C. ChatGPT v4 outperforming v3.5 on cancer treatment recommendations in quality, clinical guideline, and expert opinion concordance. Digit Health. 2024;10 https://doi.org/10.1177/20552076241269538.
32. Searle T, Ali FR, Carolides S, Al-Niaimi F. Rosacea and diet: what is new in 2021? J Clin Aesthet Dermatol. 2021;14:49–54.

Artificial Intelligence and Bullous Dermatoses

13

Emmanouil Karampinis and Efterpi Zafiriou

13.1 Bullous Dermatoses

The diagnosis of a blistering eruption traditionally involves a combination of clinical, histological, and immunological parameters that need to be assessed. In daily practice, thorough clinical evaluation helps rule out transient blistering caused by bacterial, viral, or parasitic infections, as well as those blisters associated with eczema, guiding the diagnosis toward a potential autoimmune blistering disease [1]. Key laboratory techniques for diagnosing include histological examination of a biopsy from an early intact blister to distinguish between intraepidermal and subepidermal blister formation, along with direct immunofluorescence (DIF) microscopy to identify the composition and site of immune reactants in the patient's skin or mucosa. Bullous pemphigoid is the most prevalent autoimmune blistering disorder affecting the subepidermal layer, while its mimicker being pemphigus vulgaris is an uncommon autoimmune disorder characterized by the formation of painful blisters and erosions on the skin and mucous membranes, with the oral cavity being the most frequently affected area. The exact etiopathogenesis of bullous pemphigoid remains largely unclear [2]. However, in some cases, the onset or worsening of the disease has been linked to specific trigger factors, including drugs, physical factors, vaccines, and infections that interact with various predisposing factors, such as comorbidities, HLA genetics, and aging, which contribute to the development of the

E. Karampinis (✉)
Second Dermatology Department, School of Health Sciences, Aristotle University of Thessaloniki, Thessaloniki, Greece

Department of Dermatology, Faculty of Medicine, School of Health Sciences, University General Hospital of Larissa, University of Thessaly, Larissa, Greece

E. Zafiriou
Department of Dermatology, Faculty of Medicine, School of Health Sciences, University General Hospital of Larissa, University of Thessaly, Larissa, Greece
e-mail: zafevi@o365.uth.gr

E. Karampinis et al. (eds.), *Artificial Intelligence Applications in Dermatology*,
https://doi.org/10.1007/978-3-032-15614-3_13

pathogenic cascade of the disease and the resulting formation of the bulla. Bullous pemphigoid usually resolves on its own within a few months, though it can persist for up to 5 years. Treatment aims to alleviate symptoms such as pain and itching associated with the bullous lesions. The primary treatment for bullous pemphigoid is systemic corticosteroids, although the specific approach depends on the patient's comorbidities and the severity of the disease [3]. How can AI integrate into the approach to such a complex disease?

13.2 AI and Bullous Diseases Diagnoses

The AI solitary image-based approach for bullous dermatoses can be challenging, mainly due to the different stages bullous lesions can undergo, as in the early stages, the blisters may be intact and more difficult to differentiate, creating a clinical image based on the patient's skin texture with variable shape or size. Once the blisters rupture, the skin may present with erosions or ulcers, which are more common in later stages of bullous diseases [1]. These changes can mimic skin conditions such as eczema or infected wounds, which may confuse AI models if they cannot "consider" medical history and if they have not been specifically trained to identify post-rupture changes (Fig. 13.1).

Many studies have proved that the construction of a convolutional neural network (CNN) architecture had achieved higher diagnosis accuracy than dermatologists. One of the first attempts was performed based on the Chinese population. To address the variability in the presence of different dermatoses in Chinese

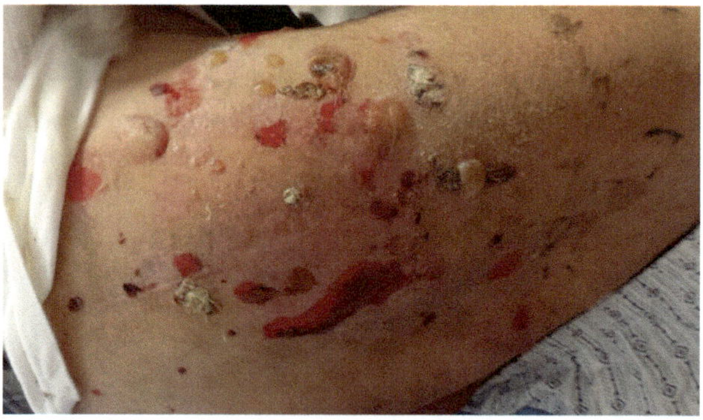

Fig. 13.1 Image showing multiple skin lesions on the upper arm and shoulder characterized by fluid-filled blisters (bullae), some intact and others ruptured, with serous or yellowish content. Also, extensive erosions and ulcerations where blisters have ruptured, leaving raw, erythematous, and oozing skin, can be noted. Crusted areas and scabs, likely from dried serum, blood, or secondary infection, overlay some lesions. The surrounding skin appears inflamed and reddened, with excoriations. As indicated by the image, the lesions in cases of bullous dermatoses can be at different stages of development, making AI-based diagnosis challenging. AI systems rely on patterns within images to make diagnoses, and the diversity of lesion stages (ranging from early blisters to healed or crusted lesions) can make it difficult for AI to interpret them accurately

individuals, a large image database called the Xiangya-Derm database was created. Using a CNN, six common subtypes of dermatoses were selected for analysis, including psoriasis, basal cell carcinoma, seborrheic keratosis, pemphigus, eczema, and lupus erythematosus. The database consisted of 5660 clinical images. To evaluate the performance of Xy-SkinNet, an artificial neural network that was trained to be a six-category model for these six common types of diseases and confirm its clinical effectiveness, a comparison was conducted with 31 dermatologists. Xy-SkinNet's top differential diagnosis was pemphigus, achieving a top 1 accuracy rate of 80.0%. This high performance may be because pemphigus has fewer variations in its clinical manifestations compared to other conditions like eczema or lupus erythematosus, which can be more complex and have a wider range of presentations [4]. High performances were also noted in studies that focused on the performance of CNNs in the case of diagnosis of common dermatologic conditions in real-life experience or based on mobile phone applications [5]. Also, there was a study focusing on AI-diagnosed pemphigus in the early stage of the disease [6]. However, in all the above-mentioned studies, bullous diseases were not compared with each other [4–6].

Evaluations of an AI system that differentiates bullous dermatoses and therefore can have promising results in clinical practice are

- *Deep learning-aided diagnosis of autoimmune blistering diseases:* According to this study, autoimmune blistering diseases were categorized into three primary groups: pemphigus, pemphigoid, and common differential diagnoses such as bullous lupus and urticaria, forming the first level of the taxonomy. Within these groups, there are eight distinct disease manifestations, making up the second layer (bulla, blisters, erosions, etc.). The distinction between pemphigus and pemphigoid is determined by the skin layer affected, with pemphigus occurring due to impairment of the upper layers of the skin and pemphigoid due to deeper layers of damage. Differentiation, on the other hand, within the second layer is based on the specific structural proteins targeted. The dataset consisted of 1670 clinically validated open-source images obtained from online repositories, showcasing a variety of disease manifestations from oral mucosal lesions to active cutaneous blisters. To optimize algorithm training, the data was randomly split into training (80%), validation (10%), and test (10%) sets, ensuring a well-balanced distribution for model learning and evaluation. A prototype for blister classification is developed using a CNN, specifically implementing the GoogleNet Inception v3 architecture, which has been pretrained on approximately 1.28 million images to achieve 80% accuracy. The system included three loops. The first loop included trains on the ISIC dataset (a dataset used as a global initiative aimed at improving skin cancer detection to recognize skin cancers and is usually used for training machine learning algorithms to assist in diagnosing skin cancer, particularly melanoma). This loop helped the model behave as an integrated feature extractor and learn useful features before working on blister images. The second loop included training on an augmented dataset to balance underrepresented disease classes, improving sensitivity rather than just accuracy, and the third loop included fine-tuning on the authors' original main dataset (blistering eruptions), as the GoogleNet Inception v3 architecture has been trained on a large dataset (ISIC). Most classes showed high sensitivity (above 65%), except for the pemphigus classes, which have a sensitivity of around 50%. In the first-layer partition, both pemphigus and pemphigoid maintain high sensitivity, similar to dermatologists, demonstrating the algorithm's ability to effectively distinguish between major disease classes [7].

- *AI-provided instant differential diagnosis of pemphigus vulgaris and bullous pemphigoid: qualitative study*. This study availed a dermatological dataset of 17,735 clinical images and 346 patient metadata for bullous dermatoses. A two-stage diagnostic framework was employed—first stage as a clinical image classification model to distinguish bullous dermatoses from five common skin diseases and normal skin, and second stage a multimodal classification model that integrated clinical images and patient metadata to further differentiate pemphigus vulgaris from bullous pemphigus. The classification model and multimodal classification model achieved areas under the receiver operating characteristic curve scores of 0.998 and 0.942, respectively, outperforming the average performance of 27 junior dermatologists (sensitivity: 0.68; specificity: 0.78) and competing with 69 senior dermatologists' performance (sensitivity: 0.80; specificity: 0.87). The AI-based diagnostic framework, utilizing clinical images and patient metadata, achieved expert-level accuracy in identifying pemphigoid and pemphigus [8].

As mentioned, the diagnostics needs that AI is called to cover are mainly focused on the differential between blistering and bullous disorders. However, as indicated by the limited number of studies that exist in this area, as well as the fact that the two existing studies are in the form of preprint, the research on this topic is still limited [7, 8]. Large datasets, including blistering disorder images such as pemphigus vulgaris, bullous pemphigoid, herpes gestationis, and linear IgA dermatosis, do not exist to the extent of other skin entities as in the case of skin cancer. Also, the complexity of these disorders, along with the variations in clinical presentation and progression, makes it challenging for AI models to reliably classify and differentiate them, especially when the models are trained on limited and unverified data. Also, the integration of patient's metadata is crucial to guide diagnosis. Interestingly, there are studies in the authors' use AI models to assess not the clinical image for diagnosis but other exams, including histopathology evaluation, immunofluorescent staining, and Tzanck smear used to confirm or exclude the presence of pemphigus vulgaris. More specifically:

- *TzanckNet: a convolutional neural network to identify cells in the cytology of erosive-vesiculobullous diseases*: The Tzanck smear test is used in bullous dermatoses to help differentiate blistering conditions on the skin by identifying acantholytic cells, which indicate loss of adhesion between skin cells in case of pemphigus or/and multinucleated giant cells, especially in viral infections that can mimic bullous diseases as herpes infections. Hyphae indicating fungal infections can also be identified by this test. Tzanck smear test cannot be used to differentiate pemphigus from pemphigoid. The authors of this study presented TzanckNet, an AI model that was trained on a retrospective dataset of 2260 Tzanck smear images collected between December 2006 and December 2019. It is a CNN (ResNet50), pretrained on ImageNet (a large visual database designed for use in visual object recognition software research), with the final classification layer being replaced with six output nodes corresponding to the six cell types commonly encountered in the test (correspond to the six cell types). It was then evaluated using a prospective validation dataset of 359 images collected from 15 patients in January 2020. The model is designed to identify six cell types: acantholytic cells, eosinophils, hyphae, multinucleated giant cells, normal keratinocytes, and tadpole cells. Across 359 images, TzanckNet made 2154 predictions, achieving an accuracy of 94.3% and a sensitivity of 83.7%, as well as specificity of 97.3%. Therefore, an application using this CNN can be a useful tool for a clinician to assess a Tzanck smear segment quickly (Fig. 13.2) [9].

Immunofluorescence staining is the gold standard for diagnosing autoimmune blistering diseases by differentiating between pemphigus and pemphigoid based on antibody deposition.

- AI analyzers of immunofluorescence staining images:
  A deep learning approach to direct immunofluorescence pattern recognition in autoimmune bullous diseases: This study analyzed direct immunofluorescence (DIF) images from skin biopsies of patients suspected of having autoimmune blistering diseases, collected between January 2022 and January 2024. 5-mm punch biopsies were taken, prepared, and classified by experienced dermatologists into intercellular, linear staining patterns, or negative cases. To enhance diagnostic accuracy, a transfer learning framework for image classification was applied to pretrain deep neural networks with five-fold cross-validation. The researchers evaluated six CNN architectures: (1)

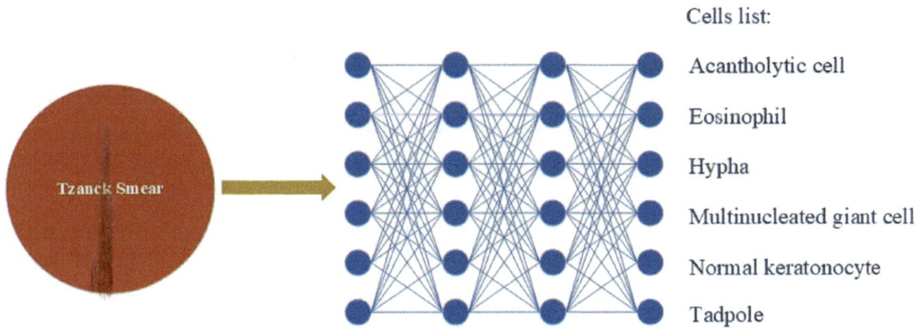

Fig. 13.2 A diagram illustrating the functioning of the proposed TzanckNet. TzanckNet takes a Tzanck smear image as input and determines which of the six cell types are present or absent in the image. Depending on this cell-type finding, a diagnosis can be predicted

EfficientNetB0 and EfficientNetB4, which optimize depth, resolution, and width; (2) ResNet18 and ResNet50, incorporating residual connections for improved gradient flow and stability; (3) DenseNet121 and DenseNet201, utilizing densely connected layers for efficient feature reuse; and (4) a vision transformer, leveraging attention-based deep learning. The dataset was divided into 436 training images and 93 test images. The Swin Transformer achieved the highest validation accuracy (98.5%), while the best-performing model reached 94.6% accuracy on the test set, with 95.3% sensitivity and 97.5% specificity in classifying blistering diseases. The study confirmed that CNNs effectively identify DIF patterns, supporting automated analysis and reporting. This approach improves diagnostic consistency, speed, data processing, and cost-efficiency, highlighting the potential of deep learning integration to refine DIF-based autoimmune blistering disease diagnostics and streamline dermatological workflows [10].

Use of convolutional neural networks for the detection of u-serrated patterns in direct immunofluorescence images to facilitate the diagnosis of epidermolysis bullosa acquisita: Also, the recognition of certain serrated patterns of immunodepositions observed between epidermolysis bullosa acquisita and bullous pemphigoid is a significant feature. The U-shaped pattern is observed on epidermolysis bullosa acquisita and represents the deposition of immune complexes of IgG and C3 along the dermal–epidermal junction. On the contrary, the N-shaped deposition in bullous pemphigoid and other anti-BP180-associated pemphigoid diseases represents a more superficial deposition of immune complexes at the roof of the blister. This study explores the potential of convolutional neural networks (CNNs) for identifying u-serrated patterns, which aid in diagnosing epidermolysis bullosa acquisita (EBA). Researchers trained and validated nine widely used CNN models using 220,800 manually annotated direct immunofluorescence (DIF) image patches derived from 106 images of 46 patients. The dataset was divided into 10 subsets, with 9 subsets used for training and the remaining subsets serving as the validation set. This process was repeated 10 times, each time using a different validation subset. The top-performing CNN model achieved 89.3% specificity and 89.3% sensitivity in classifying u-serrated DIF image patches, demonstrating expert-level diagnostic accuracy. The results demonstrate the high accuracy of CNN-based techniques in recognizing u-serrated patterns. This method could be a valuable tool for clinicians and pathologists, aiding in the detection of u-serrated patterns in DIF images and enhancing the diagnostic accuracy of EBA [11].

No study assessing AI models and dermoscopy of bullous was found, presenting an additional gap in the integration of AI technology in the assessment of bullous dermatoses. In most cases, the dermoscopy presentation of bullous pemphigoid presents with yellowish-pink translucent areas, prominent follicular and eccrine openings, and an erythematous background, often accompanied by a distorted pigment network and perifollicular pigmentation. The dermoscopy of other mimickers, such as bullous fixed drug eruptions, exhibits a dark brown pigment network with clusters of black, brown, and blue dots and globules. Dermoscopy also reveals prominent eccrine openings and an irregularly shaped margin [12]. In this case, the medical history of recent drug exposure guides the diagnosis rather than the dermoscopy. However, a study with a CNN trained on different dermoscopy images of bullous dermatoses does not currently exist, and by analyzing distinct dermoscopic patterns, such a model could help the clinician distinguish bullous pemphigoid, bullous fixed drug eruptions, herpes labialis, pompholyx, and other mimickers with greater accuracy [13]. Such platforms providing real-time diagnostic assistance, presenting probabilistic percentages for each possible condition in case of bullous dermatoses, similar to how AI is currently used to differentiate skin cancer mimickers, could contribute to a more effective workflow in case of bullous and vesiculobullous disorders (Fig. 13.3).

As observed in Fig. 13.3, we uploaded this image to two open AI chatbots asking for differential diagnosis percentages. The first chatbot attempt presented the best first alternative, the severe contact dermatitis (allergic or irritant) at a rate of 30% and reported irritants or allergens such as poison ivy/oak and chemicals as potential triggers. Following there was the diagnosis of bullous impetigo (~25%), bullous pemphigoid (~20%), bullous drug eruption (~10%), erythema multiforme/Stevens–Johnson syndrome spectrum (~5%), pemphigus vulgaris (~5%), and other possibilities such as herpes zoster, insect bites, thermal, or chemical burns (~5%). As indicated, the chatbot provided a complete list of vesiculobullous diseases, suggesting certain medical history points for the clinicians to focus as exposure to chemicals, older aging, and recent medications (Fig. 13.3). The second chatbot's (Perplexity, AI) attempt in the same question regarding the same image provided a similar list with slight differences and position replacements while it placed the right diagnosis in the first place of its differential. More specifically, the chatbot presented as possible diagnosis bullous pemphigoid (40–50%), dermatitis herpetiformis (15–20%), Stevens–Johnson syndrome/toxic epidermal necrolysis (10–15%), severe drug reaction causing widespread blistering and mucosal involvement,

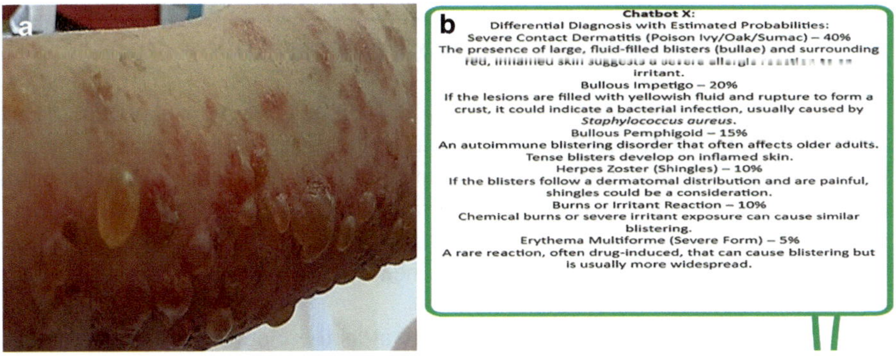

Fig. 13.3 An image of a patient's arm featuring several fluid-filled blisters (bullae) on reddened, inflamed skin (**a**), alongside the chatbot's response when asked about the differential diagnosis of the lesions shown in the image (**b**)

staphylococcal scalded skin syndrome (5–10%), bullous impetigo (5–10%), linear IgA dermatosis (5%), contact dermatitis (5%), and erythema multiforme (1–5%). The difference between the first and second is based on the different patterns and information from the data they were trained on. As indicated above, those percentages and information can be helpful as AI-differential diagnoses can serve as a supplementary tool that highlights potential conditions and guides clinicians on the additional tests that they need to follow to confirm or exclude diseases from the generated list [14]. However, given the unknown source of the training data and the model used, although this information may appear informative, it should be approached with caution and not accepted blindly.

13.3 AI and Bullous Disease Grading

Apart from bullous disease differential diagnoses, disease grading is also an important aspect of clinical assessment. There are many scores developed to evaluate the severity of the disease. The Pemphigus Disease Area Index (PDAI) is a scoring system designed to measure disease activity and damage by assigning scores to the skin, scalp, and mucous membranes by evaluating erosions, blisters, or erythema across 12 areas. Studies have examined PDAI severity thresholds, classifying patients into mild, moderate, and severe categories. Additionally, there is also the Autoimmune Bullous Skin Disorder Intensity Score (ABSIS), which was initially developed for pemphigus assessment but later widely used for all autoimmune bullous diseases. The Bullous Pemphigoid Disease Area Index (BPDAI), created by the International Bullous Diseases Group (IBDG) in 2007, specifically evaluates bullous pemphigoid. It uses a 0–360-point scale based on four key factors: affected body surface area percentage, peak pruritus numerical rating scale score, disease extent index, and area index. Contrary to the AI-calculated PASI score, there is no established AI-driven grading system that can complement existing clinical assessments in bullous pemphigoid or other bullous disorders [15].

13.4 AI and Bullous Disease Treatment and Follow-Up

To our knowledge, no study exists focusing on AI-aided treatment approach in case of bullous autoimmune dermatoses. It is anticipated that AI-driven predictive models would have the ability to analyze complex datasets, including clinical records and specific molecular signatures, to tailor treatment strategies for bullous dermatoses, giving the AI-aided personalized approach. A question emerges about the quality of the answer of the available chatbots when asked about the treatment approach to challenging bullous cases (Fig. 13.4).

A treatment challenge occurs in this patient as there are antipsoriatic medications (e.g., TNF-α inhibitors such as adalimumab or infliximab) that have been reported to exacerbate bullous pemphigoid and vice versa (rituximab and dupilumab treating bullous pemphigoid may exacerbate psoriasis [16]). In case you ask

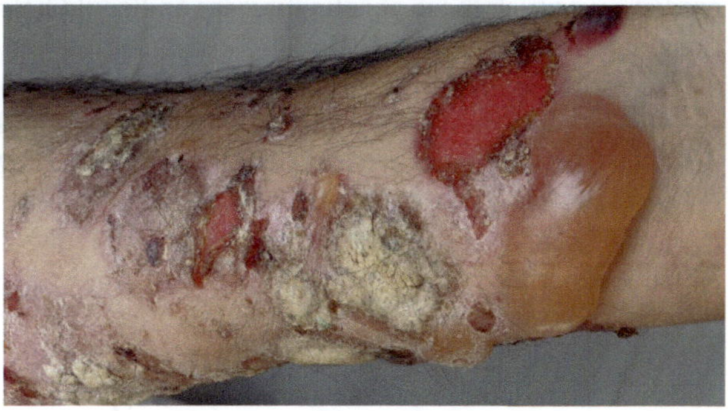

Fig. 13.4 A 36-year-old patient with chronic psoriasis presenting with intense bullae as presented in the image. The immunofluorescence staining of the blistering lesions guides the diagnosis of bullous pemphigoid

a chatbot (ChatGPT, OpenAI) what would be the best treatment option in this dilemma, at the beginning, it would analyze treatment characteristics in each case and would conclude with a table as a summary of the best approach. In the two columns of preferred treatment, the medication for both diseases, methotrexate, exists. According to a recent systematic review on coexisting psoriasis and BP, including topical treatments, immunosuppressants, antibiotics, biologics, and vitamins, the authors concluded that systemic immunosuppressants like corticosteroids and methotrexate remain the preferred treatment options, followed by azathioprine and cyclosporine, and they advise a gradual dosage tapering to minimize the risk of psoriasis or bullous pemphigoid flare-ups [16]. Comparing the chatbot answer and the review report, they present some overlap in treatment recommendations. However, a review written by specialists considers individual patient differences and long-term safety concerns that the clinicians must take into account when encountering such difficult cases, limiting the AI chatbot recommendations to a tool for initial guidance.

AI offers promising advancements in follow-up practices for bullous dermatoses. A follow-up system with AI, as the Genetic Progression Score (GPS), which is an advanced AI-driven model designed to predict the transition from preclinical to clinical stages in autoimmune bullous diseases such as bullous pemphigoid and pemphigus vulgaris, represents a promising future technology [17]. This score, by leveraging genome-wide association studies to analyze genetic differences between affected individuals and healthy controls, would help to identify genetic variants linked to disease susceptibility and progression. By detecting genetic markers, GPS can assess the likelihood of developing bullous diseases, considering interactions between genetic predisposition, environmental triggers, and immune responses. This predictive approach enhances long-term disease monitoring, contributing to improved patient outcomes in autoimmune bullous disorders [18]. The most relevant study whose approach aligns with personalized medicine principles considering genetic parameters in bullous dermatoses is SpliceAI prediction model for junctional epidermolysis bullosa (JEB). Regarding this study, SpliceAI predicts splice site mutation consequences in patients with JEB and mutations LAMB3 (Laminin Subunit Beta 3) identified premature termination complexes, which generally result in nonfunctional protein. The authors report that such AI tools may predict severity in those genetic diseases and could help in choosing cases for additional laboratory analysis [19].

13.5 Limitations and Attention Points Regarding the Use of AI Models in Bullous Dermatoses

When studies are conducted on AI algorithms, there should be additional features taken into consideration by the bioengineers or AI experts.

1. Blisters and bulla can take skin of color appearance; therefore, diagnostic challenges may occur in the case of dark-skinned individuals [20].
2. Autoimmune blistering disorders, apart from cutaneous symptoms, can have systemic involvement, and that data should be taken into consideration as well to construct a more accurate AI model [3].
3. The lighting in which images of bullous lesions are captured plays a crucial role in the accuracy of AI models. The reflected light can alter the appearance of blisters (bullae) and erosions, leading to misinterpretations. Bullae have a smooth, fluid-filled surface that can create reflections. These reflections can be tricky for AI models to interpret because they might alter the real structure of the lesion.
4. Currently, there is no study on bullous disorders grading or bullous dermoscopy and AI or treatment planning powered by AI tools, while databases with images of different types of bullous dermatoses are not extensive and, therefore, AI models cannot train adequately.

References

1. Holtsche MM, Boch K, Schmidt E. Autoimmune bullous dermatoses. J Dtsch Dermatol Ges. 2023;21:405–12. https://doi.org/10.1111/ddg.15046.
2. Patrício P, Ferreira C, Gomes MM, Filipe P. Autoimmune bullous dermatoses: a review. Ann N Y Acad Sci. 2009;1173:203–10. https://doi.org/10.1111/j.1749-6632.2009.04737.x.
3. van Beek N, Zillikens D, Schmidt E. Bullous autoimmune dermatoses. Dtsch Arztebl Int. 2021; https://doi.org/10.3238/arztebl.m2021.0136.
4. Huang K, Jiang Z, Li Y, Wu Z, Wu X, Zhu W, et al. The classification of six common skin diseases based on Xiangya-Derm: development of a Chinese database for artificial intelligence. J Med Internet Res. 2021;23:e26025. https://doi.org/10.2196/26025.
5. Pangti R, Mathur J, Chouhan V, Kumar S, Rajput L, Shah S, et al. A machine learning-based, decision support, mobile phone application for diagnosis of common dermatological diseases. J Eur Acad Dermatol Venereol. 2021;35:536–45. https://doi.org/10.1111/jdv.16967.
6. Vagh M, Kasat D. Detection of pemphigus vulgaris in development stage of skin erosion. In: Smart computing techniques and applications; 2021. p. 175–83. https://doi.org/10.1007/978-981-16-0878-0_18.
7. Cai D, Ardakany AR, Ay F. Deep learning-aided diagnosis of autoimmune blistering diseases 2021. https://doi.org/10.1101/2021.11.27.21266845.

8. He X, Su J, Wang G, Zhang K, Alexander N, Christophe HSU, et al. AI-provided instant differential diagnosis of pemphigus vulgaris and bullous pemphigoid: qualitative study (Preprint). 2020. https://doi.org/10.2196/preprints.24845.
9. Noyan MA, Durdu M, Eskiocak AH. TzanckNet: a convolutional neural network to identify cells in the cytology of erosive-vesiculobullous diseases. Sci Rep. 2020;10:18314. https://doi.org/10.1038/s41598-020-75546-z.
10. Capurro N, Pastore VP, Touijer L, Odone F, Cozzani E, Gasparini G, et al. A deep learning approach to direct immunofluorescence pattern recognition in autoimmune bullous diseases. Br J Dermatol. 2024;191:261–6. https://doi.org/10.1093/bjd/ljae142.
11. Shi C, Meijer JM, Azzopardi G, Diercks GFH, Guo J, Petkov N. Use of convolutional neural networks for the detection of u-serrated patterns in direct immunofluorescence images to facilitate the diagnosis of epidermolysis bullosa acquisita. Am J Pathol. 2021;191:1520–5. https://doi.org/10.1016/j.ajpath.2021.05.024.
12. Gharib K, Nassar A, Youssef A, Bessar H. Dermoscopic approach for differential diagnosing of autoimmune bullous disease: pemphigus vulgaris, pemphigus foliaceus, and IgA pemphigus. Int J Dermatol. 2023;62:770–5. https://doi.org/10.1111/ijd.16623.
13. Manuelyan K, Dragolov M, Drenovska K, Shahid M, Vassileva S. Artificial intelligence in autoimmune bullous dermatoses. Clin Dermatol. 2024;42:426–33. https://doi.org/10.1016/j.clindermatol.2024.06.008.
14. Karampinis E, Toli O, Georgopoulou K-E, Kampra E, Spyridonidou C, Roussaki Schulze A-V, et al. Can artificial intelligence "hold" a dermoscope?—the evaluation of an artificial intelligence chatbot to translate the dermoscopic language. Diagnostics. 2024;14:1165. https://doi.org/10.3390/diagnostics14111165.
15. Boulard C, Duvert Lehembre S, Picard-Dahan C, Kern JS, Zambruno G, Feliciani C, et al. Calculation of cut-off values based on the autoimmune bullous skin disorder intensity score (ABSIS) and pemphigus disease area index (PDAI) pemphigus scoring systems for defining moderate, significant and extensive types of pemphigus. Br J Dermatol. 2016;175:142–9. https://doi.org/10.1111/bjd.14405.
16. Hsieh C-Y, Tsai T-F. Management of coexisting bullous pemphigoid and psoriasis: a review. Am J Clin Dermatol. 2022;23:869–79. https://doi.org/10.1007/s40257-022-00719-7.
17. Xue Y, Wang D, Peng D. Bioinformatics technologies in autophagy research. Adv Exp Med Biol. 2021;1208:387–453. https://doi.org/10.1007/978-981-16-2830-6_18.
18. Moingeon P. Artificial intelligence-driven drug development against autoimmune diseases. Trends Pharmacol Sci. 2023;44:411–24. https://doi.org/10.1016/j.tips.2023.04.005.
19. Wen D, Balacco D, Hunjan M, Bardhan A, Harper N, Ogboli M, et al. BG05 Artificial intelligence prediction of splice site mutation consequences in junctional epidermolysis bullosa: signposts to severity. Br J Dermatol. 2023;188 https://doi.org/10.1093/bjd/ljad113.145.
20. Sanfilippo E, Gonzalez Lopez A, Saardi KM. Erythrodermic bullous pemphigoid in skin of color treated with dupilumab. J Drugs Dermatol. 2023;22:685–6. https://doi.org/10.36849/JDD.7196.

Part IV

Artificial Intelligence in Cosmetic Dermatology

Skin Care Guided by AI

14

Vasiliki-Sofia Grech and Efstathios Rallis

14.1 Introduction

The incorporation of artificial intelligence (AI) into dermatology has fundamentally transformed the field of skincare, enabling data-driven, personalized approaches that enhance diagnostic precision, therapeutic efficacy, and the development of dermatological and cosmetic formulations. This chapter explores the evolution of AI applications in skincare, beginning with its foundational role in natural language processing (NLP)-based ingredient analysis and AI-driven chatbots for dermatological guidance. As computational methodologies have advanced, AI has increasingly been integrated into more sophisticated domains, including deep learning-based real-time skin analysis, predictive modeling for individualized skincare regimens, and intelligent home-based skincare systems.

Recent advancements have facilitated the deployment of AI in high-precision dermatological applications, including bioprinted skin models for ethical and scalable cosmetic safety assessments, genetic profiling for personalized skincare interventions, and AI-enhanced formulation strategies for dermatological and cosmetic products. These innovations allow AI-driven systems to dynamically evaluate skin health, forecast dermatological changes over time, and optimize skincare recommendations based on genetic predispositions, environmental exposures, and real-time physiological parameters.

Despite the transformative potential of AI in dermatology, its integration poses significant challenges. These include algorithmic bias in the representation of diverse skin phenotypes, data security and privacy concerns surrounding biometric information, and ethical considerations in AI-driven clinical and cosmetic decision-making. This chapter provides a comprehensive review of both foundational and

V.-S. Grech (✉) · E. Rallis
Department of Biomedical Sciences, School of Health and Care Sciences, University of West Attica, Athens, Greece

E. Karampinis et al. (eds.), *Artificial Intelligence Applications in Dermatology*,
https://doi.org/10.1007/978-3-032-15614-3_14

cutting-edge AI applications in skincare, critically assessing their scientific underpinnings, technological implications, and clinical relevance while addressing key limitations and future directions in AI-driven dermatological research and practice.

14.2 AI in Skincare Recommendation Systems

14.2.1 Natural Language Processing in Skincare Recommendation

As the range of available skincare formulations continues to expand, the manual assessment of both naturally derived and synthetic ingredients for various skin types and dermatological concerns has become increasingly impractical [1, 2]. In response to this challenge, AI has been integrated into cosmetic dermatology to streamline skincare recommendation processes. Among the simplest methods through which AI aids in this field are natural language processing (NLP) and machine learning (ML). NLP facilitates the extraction of relevant insights from unstructured text sources, such as patient reviews and dermatological literature, by converting natural language into structured, machine-readable data. This structured data is then processed through ML algorithms, which identify patterns in ingredient efficacy and consumer preferences, ultimately enabling more personalized and effective skincare recommendations [3].

To further enhance the accuracy of AI-generated skincare recommendations, advanced filtering techniques that leverage the extraction of relevant insights from textual data are employed. Content-based filtering and neural collaborative filtering analyze historical consumer interactions, ingredient performance, and user satisfaction trends to optimize recommendations. These methodologies enable AI to detect product tolerability and efficacy patterns, ensuring more precise and individualized skincare solutions [4, 5].

Additionally, the ingredient frequency-inverse product frequency (IF-IPF) method identifies key skincare ingredients by evaluating how often this ingredient appears in highly effective products (ingredient frequency) while reducing the influence of other commonly used ingredients found in many formulations (inverse product frequency). This approach highlights distinctive and impactful ingredients, enhancing AI-driven skincare recommendations by prioritizing those most strongly associated with positive dermatological outcomes [6]. By incorporating these AI-driven methodologies, skincare recommendation systems enhance the precision of product selection, facilitating a more seamless alignment between consumer needs and evidence-based dermatological insights, ultimately contributing to advancements in both clinical and cosmetic dermatology.

14.2.2 AI-Driven Skin Analysis for Precision Skincare Recommendations

While ingredient-based skincare recommendations primarily rely on preexisting product information and user feedback, advancements in AI have introduced image-based AI-driven skin analysis, which evaluates individual skin characteristics to enhance personalization. This evolution from text-based analysis to image-based deep learning models marks a significant breakthrough in dermatological AI.

Deep learning algorithms, such as YOLOv4, refine facial recognition and skin feature extraction by reducing image noise and enhancing texture classification, allowing for more accurate skin assessments [7]. Similarly, the U-Net model, originally developed for biomedical image segmentation, has been adapted for dermatological applications, enabling the precise evaluation of skin morphology, wrinkles, pores, and other structural features beyond traditional color-based image processing [8, 9].

A major advancement in 2024 saw the development of an AI system that integrates both ingredient-based and skin condition-based analysis, surpassing earlier models by utilizing deep neural networks (DNNs) to analyze sequential ingredient data rather than relying solely on product descriptions. Building upon established dermatological classification systems, such as the Baumann skin typing system, AI models categorize skin into 12 distinct types, incorporating factors such as oiliness, dryness, pigmentation, wrinkles, and sensitivity. This classification enables product recommendations that are not only tailored to individual skin characteristics but also optimized for cosmetic formulation efficacy. The recommendation system further employs a similarity-based matching strategy, systematically comparing a user's skin profile with product efficacy predictions. By analyzing sequential ingredient data rather than relying solely on product descriptions, AI skincare systems provide highly personalized and objective product recommendations, marking a significant shift toward precision skincare solutions (Figs. 14.1 and 14.2) [1].

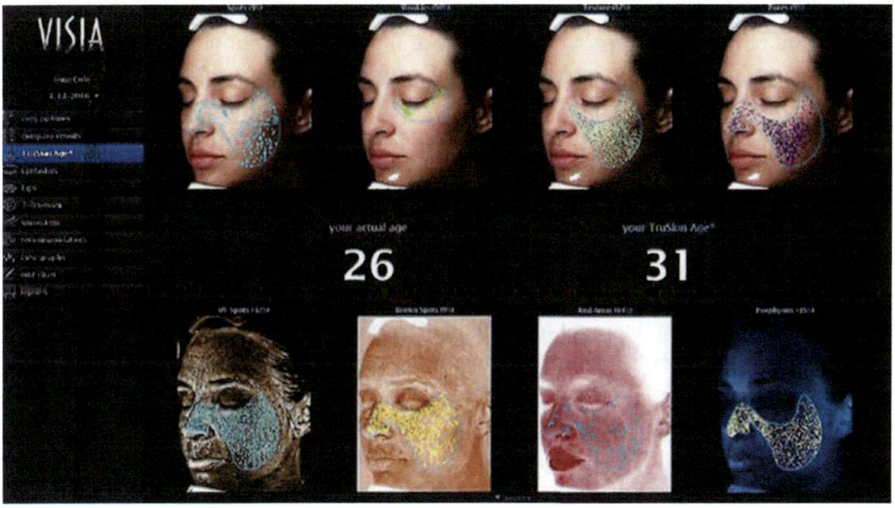

Fig. 14.1 Canfield's VISIA captures high-quality, standardized facial images that are then analyzed with AI and computer vision algorithms to produce objective analysis of spots, wrinkles, texture, pores, UV spots, brown spots, red areas, porphyrins, lip lines, and eyelashes. VISIA uses Canfield's RBX technology for visualization and measurement of red and brown skin components. Age simulation models incorporating AI are integrated into VISIA to predict future facial appearance in shape, color, and texture based on multiethnic aging data. Algorithmic VISIA measures have been shown to be precise, providing objective information on skin surface characteristics, and effective in the measurement of conditions such as rosacea

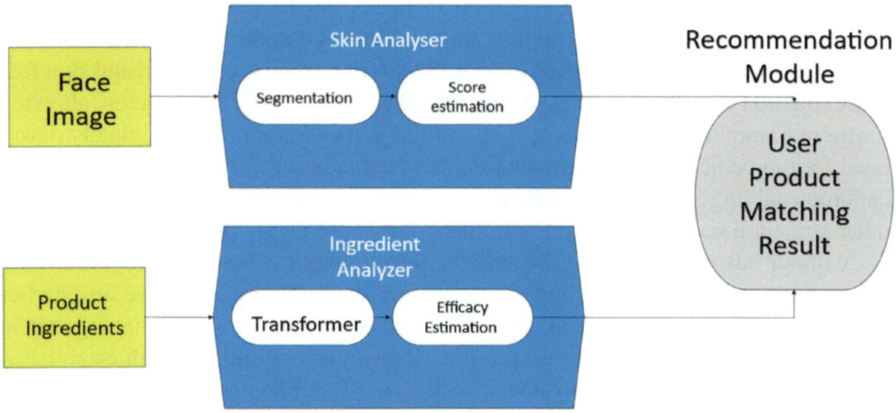

Fig. 14.2 Image showing a skincare recommendation system powered by AI that uses image segmentation and heat maps to detect six common skin issues—pores, redness, acne, wrinkles, pigmentation, and dark circles—while also analyzing product ingredients to provide personalized skincare advice

14.2.3 Virtual Try-On Technology and AI-Driven Makeup Applications

Cosmetic makeup has long been utilized to enhance facial aesthetics and serve as a form of self-expression. Over time, the practice of cosmetic application has evolved in response to cultural and societal influences, incorporating technological advancements to improve precision and personalization. While traditional makeup application has required a multidisciplinary approach, the integration of AI and computational methods has significantly expanded the capabilities of virtual cosmetic simulations, offering enhanced accuracy and individualized recommendations.

One of the earliest AI-driven approaches to virtual makeup application was cosmetic transfer, a computational technique introduced in 2007. This method employed mathematical modeling to compare pre- and post-makeup images, enabling the digital replication of cosmetic effects onto a target face. The algorithm processed these modifications at the pixel level, using three aligned images with identical two-dimensional geometry to achieve realistic virtual applications [10]. Although this approach successfully simulated makeup placement, limitations in accuracy and realism were noted, necessitating further refinements in digital cosmetic modeling.

Subsequent advancements in AI have facilitated the development of more sophisticated algorithms capable of assessing facial morphology, skin tone, and eye color to optimize virtual makeup application. These models analyze multiple facial characteristics to generate objective, personalized cosmetic recommendations. A notable AI-driven system was developed to evaluate 23 distinct facial traits, including hair attributes, based on user-generated images. By utilizing deep learning, the system provides tailored makeup suggestions in alignment with established cosmetic principles. The reliability of this system has been validated through expert assessments, with professional makeup artists confirming its accuracy across diverse demographic groups [11].

Further refinements in virtual try-on technology have introduced a multilayered evaluation framework, integrating style adherence, feature similarity, and facial aesthetics to improve recommendation precision. The style component ensures that suggested cosmetic applications align with professional makeup techniques, while the similarity metric refines recommendations based on facial feature recognition. The final stage incorporates human perception of facial aesthetics, optimizing the accuracy of selected cosmetic effects. Additionally, AI-based frameworks now incorporate feature extraction and prior data modeling, improving makeup transfer accuracy even in low-resolution images or cases where facial pose and expression vary [12].

The integration of AI into virtual makeup applications represents a significant advancement in both dermatology and cosmetic science. These models enhance the precision, reproducibility, and personalization of makeup recommendations, facilitating objective, data-driven cosmetic assessments that can be tailored to individual facial characteristics. As AI technology continues to evolve, virtual try-on systems are expected to play an increasingly pivotal role in dermatological and aesthetic consultations, supporting both consumer applications and professional practice.

14.2.4 AI-Powered Chatbots for Skincare Consultations

AI-driven chatbots have become valuable tools in dermatology, providing instant and accessible support for a wide range of skincare concerns. These systems have evolved from basic question-answering models to sophisticated AI-driven consultation platforms capable of offering more personalized and evidence-based guidance. Early chatbot applications relied on pretrained language models to assist users with general skincare inquiries, whereas more advanced systems now integrate predictive modeling to assess long-term skin health outcomes, emotional satisfaction, and behavior-driven interventions [13].

One of the most effective applications of AI chatbots in dermatology and skincare has been their role in managing common dermatological conditions, such as rosacea. Performance evaluations of AI chatbots in dermatological consultations have demonstrated accuracy levels ranging from 92.22% to 97.78%, closely aligning with expert dermatological assessments. These chatbots have also provided comprehensive coverage of essential topics, including treatment options, skincare regimens, and dietary triggers, with clinical applicability scores between 98.61% and 100%, confirming their effectiveness as a supplementary dermatological support system [13].

Despite their strengths, AI-driven chatbots have inherent limitations, particularly in managing adverse reactions and complex dermatological conditions that require direct clinical evaluation. Future advancements in AI chatbot technology will incorporate real-time dermatological imaging and advanced patient-specific analysis, moving beyond static text-based responses to provide more dynamic, personalized, and clinically relevant skincare guidance. As these technologies continue to develop, AI-powered chatbots are expected to play an increasingly integral role in dermatological consultations, patient education, and remote skincare management [13].

14.2.5 AI-Driven Prediction of Long-Term Skincare Effects

Advancements in AI have facilitated the development of predictive modeling systems capable of assessing the long-term impact of skincare routines. By analyzing product formulations and their effects on various skin types, AI can forecast how continued use of specific products may influence skin health over time. Models such as SkincareMirror utilize predictive algorithms to evaluate the potential evolution of an individual's skin based on their chosen skincare products. These systems integrate multiple data sources, including product function labels to identify key ingredients and their dermatological effects, user images to monitor real-time skin conditions and changes over time, and efficacy ratings to assess how different formulations contribute to long-term skin health [14].

By incorporating large datasets and ongoing skin assessments, AI-driven models generate personalized predictions that allow users to visualize potential skincare outcomes before committing to a regimen. The ability to anticipate the effects of specific ingredients facilitates more informed decision-making, reducing the reliance on trial and error when selecting products. This approach also provides visual forecasts of skincare results, enabling users to better understand the potential dermatological effects of different formulations. Studies suggest that male consumers, who traditionally engage less in skincare routines, benefit significantly from AI-assisted decision-making. The integration of image-based deep learning into skincare prediction models represents a shift toward more personalized, data-driven dermatological analysis, improving the accuracy and effectiveness of long-term skincare planning [14].

14.2.6 AI-Driven Emotional Satisfaction Analysis in Skincare

The integration of artificial intelligence in skincare now extends beyond assessing dermatological efficacy to evaluating consumer emotional responses during product use. By utilizing electroencephalography (EEG) and galvanic skin response (GSR) data, AI-driven models analyze user reactions to different skincare textures and formulations, providing valuable insights into overall satisfaction. These advancements allow both dermatologists and skincare brands to refine product recommendations based not only on clinical effectiveness but also on sensory appeal. Since consumer satisfaction is influenced by both measurable skin improvements and emotional experiences, AI-driven emotional analysis enables a more personalized approach, ensuring that skincare products align with both dermatological needs and user preferences [15].

One of the earliest AI applications in this field involved convolutional neural network (CNN)-based deep learning models analyzing EEG data to predict user satisfaction with skincare products. In controlled studies, EEG data was collected as participants applied creams with different textures, and brain activity was analyzed across four frequency bands—alpha, beta, low gamma, and high gamma—to assess user preferences. The AI model demonstrated 75.4% accuracy in predicting product satisfaction [16]. Further research incorporating EEG and GSR data has expanded AI's capability to evaluate consumer experiences with emollients, lip balms, and fragrances, enhancing user satisfaction [15]. This advancement represents a shift from AI-driven skincare recommendations focused solely on efficacy to AI-driven consumer preference modeling, ultimately improving both dermatological outcomes and patient satisfaction.

14.2.7 AI in Preventive Skincare and Behavioral Interventions

AI is emerging as a pivotal tool in preventive dermatology by predicting long-term skin damage and encouraging protective behaviors. AI-driven face-aging applications have demonstrated effectiveness in motivating younger individuals to adopt healthier skincare habits by visually illustrating the cumulative effects of UV exposure over time. Studies have shown that AI-based interventions significantly influence behavior, particularly among adolescents, who respond more strongly to appearance-based education than conventional health messaging. For instance, mobile applications that simulate the impact of sun damage have been associated with a noticeable increase in daily sunscreen use among young individuals. Additionally, AI-powered educational tools have improved awareness of skin health, leading to a significant rise in the number of students engaging in regular self-examinations. By providing personalized, visual representations of potential skin damage, AI serves as a persuasive motivator for behavioral change in skincare routines [17].

Beyond reinforcing sunscreen use and self-examinations, AI has contributed to the reduction of harmful skincare behaviors, such as indoor tanning. Research indicates that students exposed to AI-driven interventions were less likely to engage in tanning bed use, highlighting AI's potential in discouraging practices that accelerate skin aging and increase the risk of skin cancers, including melanoma [17]. These findings emphasize the role of AI based strategies in promoting long-term skincare awareness and disease prevention, particularly when introduced at an early age. As AI technology continues to evolve, further refinement of these interventions will enhance their effectiveness, making them adaptable for broader applications in personalized skincare education and preventive dermatology.

14.3 State-of-the-Art Skincare Using AI and Genetic Insights

Advancements in genetics and AI have transformed personalized dermatology, leading to the development of DNA-based expert systems that analyze genetic markers to provide individualized skin-health recommendations. These systems utilize machine learning algorithms to categorize skincare products based on their ingredient composition and relevance to genetic traits associated with specific skin phenotypes. Techniques such as random forests, support vector machines, and logistic regression refine product recommendations by aligning formulations with an individual's genetic predispositions, ensuring optimal skincare choices based on scientifically validated data. Additionally, genetic algorithms further enhance this process by selecting products containing ingredients tailored to the user's unique dermatological profile. Research suggests that this approach improves ingredient relevance by incorporating up to 71% more components aligned with a person's genetic characteristics. However, the integration of genetic data into skincare also presents ethical and privacy considerations, particularly regarding data security and potential disparities in product accessibility. As precision medicine continues to advance, the combination of genetic insights and AI in dermatology represents a promising frontier, offering a more targeted and scientifically informed approach to skin health management [18].

Beyond genetic predispositions, epigenetic research has introduced new dimensions to dermatological care, particularly through the study of DNA methylation—an epigenetic modification that regulates gene expression and responds to external environmental factors such as UV exposure, pollution, and diet. The ability to analyze DNA methylation in dermatology has been enhanced by noninvasive sampling techniques, reducing the need for traditional biopsies. Methods such as tape stripping facilitate the collection of epidermal cells while preserving their methylation profiles, making large-scale studies on skin aging and UV-induced damage more feasible. This innovation allows for the identification of molecular biomarkers associated with skin deterioration, enabling scientifically optimized and personalized skincare interventions [19].

AI-driven genetic analysis is also redefining skincare by leveraging insights from single-nucleotide polymorphisms (SNPs), the most common form of genetic variation, which influence key skin characteristics such as collagen production, pigmentation, and inflammation. Variations in the MMP1 gene, for example, are associated with collagen degradation, while SNPs in the SOD2 gene indicate susceptibility to oxidative stress. AI-powered tools process vast genetic datasets, identifying patterns and correlations that traditional methods may overlook. This enables dermatologists to predict individual skin responses to treatments and customize therapies accordingly—for instance, recommending collagen-boosting regimens for individuals with MMP1 variations or antioxidant-rich skincare for those predisposed to oxidative damage [20].

AI continues to refine personalized skincare protocols by integrating new genetic insights and identifying complex interactions between multiple SNPs. For example, variations in the TYR gene influence pigmentation, while IL-6 SNPs are linked to inflammatory responses. ML algorithms can detect these interactions, allowing dermatologists to develop highly personalized treatment plans, such as anti-inflammatory skincare regimens for individuals prone to excessive inflammation or tailored laser therapy settings to minimize pigmentation risks in patients with specific TYR variations. As more SNP-related data becomes available, AI-powered diagnostic tools will further refine skincare strategies, ushering in an era of unprecedented precision in dermatological treatments [20].

Table 14.1 Skincare recommendation systems, a comparative overview of AI-driven skincare applications, including ingredient analysis, virtual try-ons, predictive models, and genetic insights

Application type	AI techniques used	Advantages
Ingredient analysis	NLP, content-based filtering, neural collaborative filtering	Provides accurate ingredient-based recommendations
Image analysis	Deep learning (YOLOv4, U-Net), facial recognition	Enhances personalization by analyzing individual skin features
Virtual try-on	GANs, super-resolution AI	Enables real-time, personalized makeup simulations
Chatbots	Pretrained NLP models, machine learning	Offers instant support and guidance
Predictive models	Deep neural networks, reinforcement learning	Predicts long-term skincare outcomes based on patterns
Emotion recognition	EEG analysis, deep learning on brain activity, GSR sensors	Enhances user experience by recommending skincare based on emotional responses
Behavioral interventions	Face-aging simulations, reinforcement learning, predictive modeling	Encourages healthier skincare habits through visual simulations and personalized recommendations
Genetic insights	Random forests, support vector machines, logistic regression, ML on SNPs	Allows highly personalized skincare based on genetic phenotype; identifies SNPs linked to collagen production, pigmentation, and inflammation

By combining AI with genetic and epigenetic analysis, dermatology is advancing toward a future in which skincare is not only personalized but also predictive and highly targeted. These innovations ensure optimal skin health through scientifically validated, data-driven approaches, paving the way for more effective and individualized dermatological care. Table 14.1 provides a comprehensive summary of AI-driven skincare recommendation systems.

14.4 AI-Driven Devices in Skincare

14.4.1 AI-Powered At-Home Skincare Devices

AI-driven at-home skincare technologies have significantly advanced personalized dermatological care by integrating high-resolution imaging, real-time data analysis, and smart dispensing systems. These innovations surpass traditional product recommendations by enabling precise assessment of individual skin conditions through multispectral imaging, LED sensors, and AI-powered evaluations. Handheld skin scanners, for example, utilize advanced imaging techniques to detect dermatological concerns such as hyperpigmentation, fine lines, dryness, and uneven skin texture at a microscopic level. These systems facilitate targeted interventions by dispensing customized serums or corrective formulations exclusively to affected areas, thereby enhancing treatment efficacy and minimizing unnecessary product use [21, 22].

The integration of the Internet of Things (IoT) has further expanded the capabilities of home-based skincare technology. IoT, as a network of interconnected devices with embedded sensors, software, and data-processing capabilities, enables seamless communication between smart skincare devices, mobile applications, and cloud-based analytical platforms [23]. This connectivity allows for real-time data exchange, facilitating dynamic and highly personalized skincare solutions. AI algorithms process cloud-based data to analyze skin profiles, assess lifestyle factors, and evaluate environmental conditions, such as humidity, pollution, and UV exposure, to generate adaptive skincare recommendations. One example of this innovation is the development of smart skincare mixers, which formulate and dispense single-use applications of moisturizers, serums, or sunscreens based on real-time skin assessments, ensuring formulations are tailored to specific dermatological needs. This approach not only optimizes ingredient efficacy but also reduces reliance on multiple skincare products [21, 22].

Furthermore, AI-powered mobile applications have enhanced home-based dermatological care by transforming smartphones into advanced diagnostic tools. Facial analysis technology assesses skin texture, pigmentation, under-eye circles, wrinkles, and hydration levels, continuously refining skincare regimens based on sequential scans. Some applications integrate lifestyle tracking, accounting for variables such as sleep patterns, dietary habits, and stress levels, to provide a more comprehensive and individualized approach to skincare management. By leveraging AI insights in conjunction with IoT-based connectivity, these innovations bring clinical-grade skin analysis into everyday routines, making personalized skincare more accessible and precise [21, 22].

As AI-driven skincare technology evolves, the cost of high-precision skin analysis continues to decline, increasing accessibility to advanced dermatological diagnostics. A key development in this area is the low-cost miniature skin spectrum measurement system (LMSSMS), which integrates a compact spectral device, DNN, and a mobile application to deliver highly accurate (94.7%) skin assessments at a fraction of traditional costs. By analyzing erythema index and melanin index, LMSSMS enables precise cosmetic shade matching and personalized skincare recommendations. The increasing affordability of AI-driven diagnostics democratizes access to data-driven skincare solutions, allowing a broader population to benefit from reliable tools for tailored product selection, sun protection, and dermatological care [24]. This transformation shifts professional-grade skin analysis from an exclusive luxury to a widely available resource, with profound implications for both clinical and consumer skincare applications.

14.4.2 IoT-Enabled Wearables and Smart Mirrors for Skincare

The integration of AI into wearable skincare technology has led to significant advancements in real-time, noninvasive skin health monitoring. One of the most notable innovations is electronic skin (E-skin), which incorporates multifunctional sensors capable of detecting subtle changes in hydration, temperature, and UV exposure. By continuously tracking these parameters, E-skin provides valuable dermatological insights that support proactive skincare management. For instance, hydration sensors monitor moisture levels to prevent transepidermal water loss and skin dryness, while UV sensors track cumulative sun exposure and generate personalized alerts to reduce the risk of photodamage. These wearables are further enhanced by their connectivity to the IoT, enabling seamless synchronization with mobile applications that provide real-time feedback and tailored skincare recommendations [25].

Beyond passive monitoring, AI enhances E-skin functionality by analyzing large datasets to predict and prevent potential dermatological concerns. By identifying patterns in hydration fluctuations, excessive UV exposure, or temperature-related changes in skin physiology, AI-driven models can recommend personalized skincare interventions. For example, a decline in hydration levels may prompt recommendations for moisture-retaining formulations, while frequent UV exposure can trigger reminders for sunscreen application and photoprotection measures. The combination of IoT and AI in E-skin technology enhances precision and personalization, transforming skincare management into a dynamic, responsive system that adapts to individual skin health needs [25].

Another major AI-driven advancement in skincare is the development of smart mirrors, which are redefining dermatological assessment and cosmetic product selection. These AI-enabled devices incorporate facial recognition, augmented reality, and algorithmic analysis to evaluate facial morphology, detect cutaneous changes, and provide personalized skincare insights. Equipped with high-resolution imaging systems and adjustable LED lighting, smart mirrors improve the visualization of dermatological features such as texture irregularities, pigmentation, fine lines, and hydration levels, enabling users to make more informed decisions about skincare and cosmetic applications. Through IoT connectivity, these devices can integrate with mobile applications, allowing users to track skin changes longitudinally and receive continuously updated recommendations based on evolving dermatological needs [23, 26].

In retail and consumer skincare settings, smart mirrors enhance the user experience by offering virtual try-on technology and AI-driven product recommendations. Systems such as HiMirror assess skin health metrics to suggest optimal skincare products, while platforms like Modiface specialize in augmented reality simulations for real-time visualization of cosmetic effects. Despite their growing role in consumer skincare, the current adoption of smart mirrors remains limited in dermatological practice. Future advancements should focus on integrating interactive touchscreens, voice recognition, and improved AI algorithms to enhance diagnostic accuracy and facilitate more clinically relevant skin health assessments. As AI-driven skincare technology continues to evolve, these innovations have the potential to bridge the gap between cosmetic dermatology and evidence-based dermatological care, offering more precise, personalized, and accessible skincare solutions [23, 26].

14.4.3 AI-Powered Office-Based Skincare Systems

The integration of AI into office-based skincare devices has significantly enhanced dermatological diagnostics and aesthetic treatments. These systems employ high-resolution imaging, cross-polarized and ultraviolet lighting, and AI-driven software to conduct comprehensive skin evaluations. By analyzing multiple parameters, including wrinkles, texture, UV damage, pores, pigmentation, general spots, brown spots, red areas, porphyrins, and vascular conditions, AI-powered devices generate precise assessments and personalized treatment plans. Through comparisons with extensive dermatological databases, these systems improve diagnostic accuracy and provide tailored skincare recommendations [21, 22].

A key advantage of AI-driven office-based devices is their ability to visualize both surface and subsurface skin conditions, enabling early detection of skin damage and facilitating preventive care strategies. Some models incorporate age prediction algorithms, assisting dermatologists in identifying early signs of premature aging and recommending targeted interventions to maintain skin health. These predictive tools help optimize treatment protocols by assessing the effectiveness of specific therapies and guiding individualized skincare regimens [21, 22].

One of the most impactful innovations in this field is the development of three-dimensional imaging systems, which create detailed models of the skin's surface, allowing high-precision evaluation of fine lines, enlarged pores, and pigmentation irregularities. These systems utilize multidirectional LED illumination to capture subtle textural changes and early signs of aging, making them particularly effective for tracking treatment progress. Additionally, specialized models focus on the analysis of atrophic acne scars, aiding in the evaluation of resurfacing treatments, while others provide close-up imaging to assess the efficacy of antiaging procedures [21, 22].

The introduction of portable, handheld imaging devices has further improved the accessibility of AI-powered dermatological analysis. These compact tools provide a flexible and efficient alternative to traditional large-scale imaging equipment, enabling real-time, in-depth skin assessments. Their ability to deliver immediate diagnostic insights enhances patient consultations, allowing dermatologists to recommend customized treatments during clinical visits [21, 22].

Beyond improving diagnostic precision, AI-powered office-based systems contribute to patient engagement by providing visual representations of skin conditions. Patients can compare images before and after treatments, track improvements over time, and gain a clearer understanding of the effects of prescribed skincare regimens. Additionally, some systems incorporate treatment outcome simulations, allowing patients to make more informed decisions regarding their therapeutic options [21, 22].

As AI technology continues to advance, office-based imaging systems will further refine personalized skincare assessments, optimizing both dermatological care and aesthetic treatments. By integrating advanced scientific methodologies with real-time data analysis, these AI-powered systems facilitate a more data-driven approach to skin health, improving both diagnostic accuracy and treatment efficacy in professional dermatology settings.

In Table 14.2, an overview of AI-driven skincare devices is presented, highlighting their key technologies, main functions, and applications in both clinical dermatology and consumer skincare.

Table 14.2 AI-driven skincare devices: technologies, functions, and applications

AI-driven device type	Key technologies used	Main functions	Clinical and consumer applications
At-home skincare devices	High-resolution imaging, multispectral imaging, LED sensors, AI-driven evaluations, IoT integration	Real-time skin analysis, targeted treatment dispensing, adaptive skincare recommendations	Personalized skincare regimens, ingredient optimization, cost-effective dermatological diagnostics
IoT-enabled wearables	E-skin with hydration, temperature, and UV sensors, AI data analysis, IoT connectivity	Noninvasive skin health monitoring, hydration tracking, UV exposure detection, predictive skincare interventions	Proactive skin health management, prevention of photodamage and dehydration, personalized skincare adjustments
Smart mirrors	Facial recognition, augmented reality, algorithmic analysis, high-resolution imaging, LED lighting, IoT integration	Personalized skincare insights, virtual try-ons, dermatological assessment, real-time skincare tracking	Consumer skincare product selection, aesthetic consultations, integration into retail environments
AI-powered office-based skincare systems	High-resolution imaging, cross-polarized and ultraviolet lighting, AI-driven software, three-dimensional imaging	Advanced dermatological diagnostics with detailed surface and subsurface skin visualization, individualized treatment planning, and AI-driven comparison of extensive dermatological databases to enhance diagnostic accuracy and generate personalized skincare recommendations	Early detection of skin damage, monitoring treatment efficacy, patient engagement in dermatological care

14.5 AI-Driven Optimization of Cosmetic Ingredients in Skincare

The integration of AI and ML into cosmetic ingredient development has significantly improved the selection, functionality, and formulation of skincare products. These technologies enable a precise, data-driven approach to ingredient optimization, enhancing product efficacy, stability, and safety [27].

A primary application of AI in skincare formulation is the selection and optimization of surfactants, which play a crucial role in cleansing and emulsification. ML models analyze extensive datasets to predict critical micelle concentration and phase behavior, allowing for the identification of surfactant combinations that improve product stability and cleansing performance while minimizing irritation. This predictive capability optimizes formulation processes, ensuring enhanced compatibility and reduced dermatological sensitivity [27].

AI also plays a critical role in the development of polymers, which influence the viscosity, texture, and film-forming properties of skincare products. By modeling molecular interactions, ML algorithms predict polymer behavior within formulations, ensuring that creams, gels, and serums achieve the desired consistency, spreadability, and performance without compromising stability. These predictive models assist in selecting polymers that enhance skin feel and product longevity [27].

In fragrance formulation, AI models analyze molecular structures to predict odor profiles, stability, and ingredient compatibility. This enables the precise selection of fragrance compounds that enhance sensory appeal while maintaining formulation integrity. Additionally, AI supports the optimization of preservative systems by identifying antimicrobial agents that ensure microbial stability while minimizing the risk of irritation or allergic reactions [27].

The application of AI in hydrogel development has led to advancements in hydration and active ingredient delivery in dermatology. ML models predict hydrogel swelling behavior, rheological properties, and controlled release mechanisms, leading to formulations that provide superior moisture retention and prolonged release of active ingredients. These AI-driven optimizations contribute to improved therapeutic outcomes in dermatological applications [27].

Beyond formulation advancements, AI enhances product safety by detecting potentially hazardous ingredients. ML algorithms screen extensive ingredient databases to identify sensitizing agents, allergens, and unsafe preservatives, ensuring that skincare formulations comply with safety regulations while maintaining efficacy. By predicting ingredient interactions and potential adverse effects, AI minimizes the likelihood of irritation and facilitates the replacement of harmful substances with safer alternatives [27].

As AI continues to evolve, its integration into ingredient selection and formulation processes will further advance the development of safer, more effective, and consumer-tailored skincare products. These innovations contribute to dermatological science by refining product formulations with data-driven precision, ensuring both safety and performance in skincare applications.

Ensuring the safety of skincare products is a critical aspect of dermatology, as cosmetics are a common cause of allergic contact dermatitis (ACD), a type IV hypersensitivity reaction. Symptoms typically manifest 48–72 h after exposure and may include erythema, vesiculation, and edema, often affecting delicate areas such as the eyelids due to their thin stratum corneum. In some cases, allergens transferred from the hands can lead to secondary eyelid dermatitis, highlighting the complexity of cosmetic-induced reactions. While many formulations exclude common allergens, nonspecific irritation remains a challenge, with conditions such as status cosmeticus causing persistent burning or stinging sensations with nearly all cosmetic applications [28].

The ability to predict the skin sensitization potential of cosmetic ingredients is essential for minimizing ACD and other adverse reactions. Historically, animal-based methods such as the guinea pig maximization test (GPMT), the Bühler test, and the local lymph node assay (LLNA) were standard in safety evaluations.

However, ethical concerns and regulatory restrictions have led to the development of alternative approaches. The European Union's 2013 ban on animal testing for cosmetics has driven a transition toward new approach methodologies (NAMs), including in vitro assays such as the human cell line activation test (h-CLAT), direct peptide reactivity assay (DPRA), LuSens, myeloid U937 skin sensitization test (MUSST), and KeratinoSens [29, 30]. While these in vitro models provide valuable insights, they primarily assess specific adverse outcome pathways and do not fully replace animal or human trials, necessitating the use of in silico models for comprehensive risk evaluation [29].

14.5.1 In Silico Models for Skin Sensitization

In silico models utilize computational simulations and ML algorithms to predict skin sensitization risks based on extensive databases of chemical structures, historical epidemiological data, and experimental findings. The Cosmetic Ingredient Database (CosIng), an online resource from the European Commission, compiles structural alerts and published data to construct predictive models. However, the accuracy of these models depends on high-quality input data, requiring extensive validation. ML techniques such as K-step yard sampling, decision trees, artificial neural networks, support vector machines, AdaBoost, logistic regression, iterative least-squares linear discriminant, consensus methods, and Bayesian networks contribute to the development of predictive models. These algorithms analyze chemical reactivity, metabolism, and exposure potential, allowing dermatologists and toxicologists to evaluate bioactivity and biochemical pathways of cosmetic ingredients [31].

Beyond individual ingredient assessment, in silico models facilitate high-throughput screening of chemical libraries, reducing the need for physical experimentation. These approaches align with the principles of replacement, reduction, and refinement (3Rs) by minimizing reliance on animal testing while improving efficiency in risk evaluation [32].

14.5.2 Applications of In Silico Models in Cosmetic Formulation

In silico modeling extends beyond ingredient-level safety evaluations to whole-product assessments, incorporating factors such as exposure levels, application frequency, and formulation characteristics. Sensitization risks vary depending on the type of cosmetic product, with leave-on formulations such as creams and foundations resulting in greater exposure compared to rinse-off products like shampoos and body washes. The substantial difference in exposure levels between these categories necessitates the use of quantitative in silico models to assess dose–response relationships rather than relying solely on binary classifications [31].

Modern quantitative models predict sensitization potency, allowing for more refined risk evaluations and adherence to regulatory safety standards. These models assist in determining safe concentration levels, optimizing formulations, and ensuring consumer protection against adverse dermatological reactions. By enabling comparative analysis of different ingredients, in silico models contribute to the development of safer and more effective cosmetic formulations [31, 33].

A comparative analysis of multiple in silico models against human datasets has demonstrated predictive accuracies ranging from 70% to 80%, aligning with results from traditional LLNA studies. Variability in mispredictions among different models suggests that a multimodel approach may further enhance reliability. These findings underscore the growing potential of in silico tools as cost-effective, nonanimal alternatives for assessing cosmetic ingredient sensitization risks [34].

Although human-based skin sensitization tests, such as the human maximization test (HMT) and the human repeat insult patch test (HRIPT), provide direct results, challenges related to inconsistent data, ethical concerns, and subjective interpretations persist. While animal testing has traditionally been used as a predictive model, it presents ethical dilemmas and limitations in accuracy. Despite advancements in nonanimal testing methods, some regulatory bodies, including those in Brazil, Canada, Japan, China, and the United States, continue to mandate animal testing in certain contexts [31].

14.5.3 AI-Powered Bioprinted Skin for Cosmetic Ingredient Testing and Safety Assessment

Bioprinted skin is transforming cosmetic ingredient testing by providing a precise, ethical, and scalable alternative to traditional animal testing [35]. Advanced 3D and four-dimensional (4D) bioprinting technologies enable the replication of the epidermis, dermis, and hypodermis, along with complex skin structures such as hair follicles and sebaceous glands. These advancements allow for more accurate evaluations of skincare formulations, ensuring both efficacy and safety. The integration of artificial intelligence and ML further optimizes bioprinting by refining printing parameters, enhancing bioink composition, and improving quality control, thereby increasing the reproducibility and reliability of bioprinted models [36, 37].

The introduction of 3D laser-assisted bioprinting has enabled the incorporation of sensory neurons within these models, allowing them to mimic neuroinflammatory responses to potential irritants. For example, when capsaicin, a known neurosensitizing agent, was applied to an innervated bioprinted skin model within a basic moisturizer formulation, a significant release of neuropeptides and proinflammatory cytokines, such as substance P and calcitonin gene-related peptide (CGRP), was observed. This response closely mirrored human in vivo reactions, demonstrating the model's ability to replicate real skin responses accurately. The increased presence of CGRP in the culture medium further supports the predictive accuracy of bioprinted skin models for evaluating cosmetic and therapeutic formulations. Human skin equivalents (HSEs) like bioprinted skin provide reliable and reproducible platforms for screening potential inflammatory responses, ensuring skincare product safety before market release. Future advancements, including the integration of human-derived neurons, are expected to enhance the biological accuracy and applicability of these models in dermatology [38].

The emergence of 4D bioprinting introduces an additional dimension to bioprinted skin, allowing printed structures to adapt dynamically to external stimuli over time. Unlike traditional 3D bioprinting, where structures remain static after fabrication, 4D bioprinting incorporates time as a variable, enabling skin models to respond to environmental factors such as temperature, humidity, pH, and light exposure. These dynamic properties improve the accuracy of cosmetic formulation testing under real-world conditions and have significant potential for personalized skincare development. Additionally, 4D bioprinted skin models are promising tools for wound healing research, drug delivery system optimization, and inflammatory response studies, further advancing safety assessments in dermatology [37].

Beyond replicating healthy skin, bioprinting has facilitated the creation of disease-specific models, such as those for atopic dermatitis. These constructs enable researchers to investigate skin barrier dysfunction, immune responses, and inflammation, improving the ability to screen new formulations for individuals with sensitive or inflamed skin. By ensuring better compatibility and reducing irritation risks, these models contribute to the development of more targeted and effective dermatological treatments [39].

The integration of artificial intelligence with 4D bioprinting is further advancing personalized skincare by tailoring formulations to individual sensitivities, genetic predispositions, and environmental factors. This synergy between AI and bioprinting is shaping the future of precision dermatology, enabling safer, more effective skincare products while laying the foundation for next-generation dermatological research and therapeutic applications.

14.6 Bias and Limitations in AI-Guided Skincare

AI has become an essential component of dermatology, particularly in facial analysis and age estimation. However, research indicates that AI-driven models frequently exhibit inherent biases that compromise their accuracy and clinical applicability. Similar to human observers, AI systems tend to overestimate the age of individuals with smiling expressions and specific textural changes. Nevertheless, these biases are often more pronounced in AI algorithms, leading to greater inaccuracies, particularly among older adults, women, and individuals displaying positive facial expressions. AI-powered skincare tools frequently incorporate age estimation algorithms to personalize treatment recommendations. If these systems systematically misinterpret age due to biases related to skin texture, facial expressions, or demographic factors, they may generate inaccurate assessments of skin health and suggest inappropriate skincare regimens. Such inaccuracies not only affect treatment efficacy but also hinder inclusivity, as individuals may receive recommendations that do not align with their actual dermatological needs. These discrepancies arise from AI's reliance on predefined visual patterns rather than a comprehensive contextual understanding of skin aging, underscoring fundamental limitations in current ML models [40].

Another major limitation in AI-guided dermatology is the underrepresentation of diverse skin types and ethnic backgrounds in training datasets, which directly impacts diagnostic accuracy. A 2023 study highlighted the challenges associated with developing representative datasets, emphasizing the insufficient inclusion of minority populations in clinical research. Structural differences, such as the increased number of corneocyte layers observed in Black individuals, variations in lipid composition, and differences in transepidermal water loss, significantly influence skin permeability, barrier function, and absorption of topical agents. Despite these well-documented physiological differences, the lack of diversity in clinical studies has resulted in gaps in understanding racial and ethnic variations in dermatological conditions and treatment responses. This underrepresentation increases the likelihood of misdiagnoses, suboptimal treatment recommendations, and biased skincare formulations. Addressing these disparities requires greater inclusion of diverse populations in dermatological research and AI training datasets to enhance diagnostic accuracy and optimize skincare efficacy [41].

Additionally, one more critical limitation in AI-driven dermatology is the continued reliance on the Fitzpatrick skin phototype (FST) scale, introduced in 1975 to classify skin tones into six categories based on an individual's reaction to UV exposure. Originally developed for phototherapy risk assessment in predominantly Caucasian populations, this classification system remains widely used in AI training datasets despite its inadequacy in accurately representing skin of color. A 2024 review found that only 30% of AI dermatology programs reported data related to skin of color, highlighting a substantial gap in representation. The FST scale frequently misclassifies darker skin tones, particularly among Black individuals, leading to inaccuracies in cancer risk assessments, lesion identification, and overall dermatological evaluations. These biases in AI training data contribute to reduced diagnostic accuracy for individuals with skin of color, further exacerbating existing healthcare disparities [42].

To address these shortcomings, alternative classification systems have been proposed. The Monk Scale, introduced as a more inclusive alternative to the FST scale, categorizes skin tones into ten distinct groups based on color and ethnic background, providing a more precise and equitable classification framework. Recognizing the importance of reducing AI bias, major technology companies have begun integrating the Monk Scale into AI-driven dermatological models to improve fairness and representation. By combining the Monk Scale and FST, AI systems can better account for skin tone diversity, thereby reducing algorithmic bias and enhancing dermatological and cosmetic care for individuals of all skin types [42].

Advancing AI-driven skincare systems requires a multifaceted approach, including the development of well-distributed datasets that incorporate a broader range of skin types, the adoption of more inclusive classification tools, and the continuous refinement of ML algorithms to mitigate biases. Ensuring comprehensive representation in AI training datasets is essential for achieving accurate skin assessments, promoting fairness in AI applications, and delivering equitable dermatological and cosmetic care to individuals of all skin tones and ethnicities.

14.7 Fairness and Data Security in AI-Guided Skincare

The integration of AI in skincare has raised significant concerns regarding data security, transparency, and privacy. Many AI-driven systems function as black boxes, where the decision-making process remains opaque, making it difficult to validate their fairness and reliability [43]. This lack of transparency is particularly problematic in facial analysis technologies used for skin assessments, as inaccurate or biased evaluations can disproportionately affect certain demographic groups. Without comprehensive oversight and accountability, these systems may reinforce biases and produce unreliable results, necessitating the implementation of safeguards to ensure fairness in dermatological applications [44].

One major concern in AI-guided skincare is the unequal accuracy of facial analysis across phenotypic and demographic subgroups. Studies have demonstrated that error rates are significantly higher for individuals with darker skin tones, particularly among women, compared to lighter-skinned individuals. These disparities accentuate the need for dermatological models that are fair, accountable, and free from bias to prevent misclassification and inaccurate assessments. Beyond dermatology and cosmetology, AI influences multiple sectors, including hiring decisions, financial approvals, and judicial outcomes, highlighting the importance of algorithmic transparency and fairness in ensuring ethical decision-making across various domains [45].

In addition to concerns about fairness, data privacy remains a growing challenge in skincare applications that rely on artificial intelligence. The beauty industry frequently collects and processes sensitive biometric data, facial analysis records, and consumer behavior tracking to provide personalized skincare recommendations. These datasets often include location, demographic details such as age and gender, skin characteristics, allergy information, purchase history, and online activity. The extensive collection of such data introduces ethical and security risks, particularly concerning the potential for data breaches, unauthorized access, or misuse of personal information [46].

In this context, a 2024 survey of cosmetic medicine professionals revealed widespread concerns regarding the handling of sensitive data in AI-driven skincare technologies. Nearly half of the respondents expressed apprehension about privacy risks, underscoring the necessity of implementing strong protective measures to safeguard user information [47]. To mitigate these risks, companies must establish robust data protection strategies, including anonymization and de-identification techniques to prevent the misuse of personal information. Encryption protocols should be employed to ensure the secure storage and transmission of sensitive data, and stringent access controls must be implemented to restrict unauthorized usage [48].

Informed consent is another critical component of data security, requiring companies to communicate transparently with users about how their data is collected, stored, and utilized. Organizations must ensure that data is not repurposed without explicit authorization, reinforcing trust and ethical responsibility in dermatological applications. Establishing strict data governance frameworks, implementing quality control mechanisms, and adhering to privacy regulations are essential for maintaining ethical standards in AI-driven skincare technologies. Compliance with established data protection laws and ethical AI standards is fundamental to responsible data usage, while the incorporation of privacy-by-design principles ensures that security measures are integrated from the initial stages of system development rather than applied retroactively [48].

By prioritizing data security, transparency, and fairness, AI-driven skincare technologies can provide accurate, ethical, and privacy-conscious solutions. These measures will not only enhance the reliability of dermatological applications but also foster trust between consumers, healthcare professionals, and technology providers, ensuring the responsible use of artificial intelligence in dermatology.

14.8 Conclusion

The integration of AI into skincare and dermatology has significantly advanced research methodologies, diagnostic precision, and personalized treatment approaches. AI-driven technologies now play a pivotal role in ingredient selection, predictive modeling, virtual skin analysis, and at-home skincare management, bridging the gap between scientific innovation and individualized skincare solutions. These advancements have redefined dermatological care, enabling data-driven, adaptive, and highly personalized regimens that cater to diverse consumer needs.

Despite these breakthroughs, challenges remain, particularly in addressing algorithmic bias, ensuring data security, and enhancing AI's applicability across varied skin types and conditions. The reliance on outdated classification models, such as the Fitzpatrick scale, highlights the urgent need for more inclusive and representative frameworks like the Monk Skin Tone Scale to improve dermatological assessments. Moreover, as AI-powered skincare systems continue to evolve, safeguarding biometric data and personal information remains a paramount ethical and regulatory concern.

The future of AI in skincare, as seen in Fig. 14.3 as well, will depend on continuous advancements in transparency, data integrity, and algorithmic fairness. Refining ML models to eliminate disparities, incorporating more diverse datasets, and developing robust security protocols will be essential in optimizing AI's role in dermatology. By overcoming these challenges, AI will further enhance the precision, accessibility, and reliability of dermatological science, shaping the next generation of personalized skincare solutions while maintaining ethical and scientific rigor.

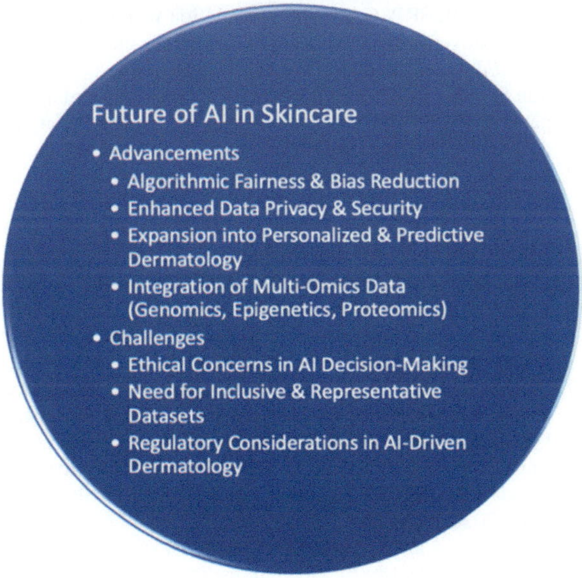

Fig. 14.3 Future of AI in skincare: key advancements and challenges

References

1. Lee J, et al. Deep learning-based skin care product recommendation: a focus on cosmetic ingredient analysis and facial skin conditions. J Cosmet Dermatol. 2024;23(6):2066–77. https://doi.org/10.1111/jocd.16218.
2. Olivia S. Post-pandemic beauty: The growing role of ingredients. 2022 [cited 2024 June]; Available from: https://www.teknoscienze.com/Contents/Riviste/Sfogliatore/HPC4_2022/46/.
3. Pai VV, Pai RB. Artificial intelligence in dermatology and healthcare: an overview. Indian J Dermatol Venereol Leprol. 2021;87(4):457–67. https://doi.org/10.25259/IJDVL_518_19.
4. Rubasri S, et al. Cosmetic product selection using machine learning. In: 2022 International Conference on Communication, Computing and Internet of Things (IC3IoT); 2022.
5. He X, et al. Neural collaborative filtering. In: Proceedings of the 26th International Conference on World Wide Web. 2017, International World Wide Web Conferences Steering Committee: Perth, Australia; 2017. p. 173–82.
6. Nakajima Y, et al. Recommender system based on user evaluations and cosmetic ingredients. In: 2019 4th International Conference on Information Technology (InCIT); 2019.
7. Li HH, et al. Based on machine learning for personalized skin care products recommendation engine. In: 2020 International Symposium on Computer, Consumer and Control (IS3C); 2020.
8. Ronneberger O, Fischer P, Brox T. U-net: convolutional networks for biomedical image segmentation. In: Medical image computing and computer-assisted intervention–MICCAI 2015: 18th international conference, Munich, Germany, October 5–9, 2015, proceedings, part III 18. Springer; 2015.
9. Yoon H, et al. Deep-learning-based morphological feature segmentation for facial skin image analysis. Diagnostics (Basel). 2023;13(11) https://doi.org/10.3390/diagnostics13111894.
10. Tong W-S, et al. Example-based cosmetic transfer. In: 15th Pacific conference on computer graphics and applications (PG'07); 2007. p. 211–8.
11. Flament F, et al. Developing an Artificial Intelligence (A.I)-based descriptor of facial appearance that fits with the assessments of makeup experts. Skin Res Technol. 2021;27(6):1081–91. https://doi.org/10.1111/srt.13061.

12. Lin K, et al. SRPSGAN: super-resolution with pose and expression robust spatial-aware generative adversarial network for makeup transfer. Multimed Tools Appl. 2024;83(4):10147–65. https://doi.org/10.1007/s11042-023-15440-8.
13. Yan S, et al. Assessment of the reliability and clinical applicability of ChatGPT's responses to patients' common queries about rosacea. Patient Prefer Adherence. 2024;18:249–53. https://doi.org/10.2147/ppa.S444928.
14. Shi C, et al. A personalized visual aid for selections of appearance building products with long-term effects. In: Proceedings of the 2022 CHI conference on human factors in computing systems. New Orleans: Association for Computing Machinery; 2022. p. Article 74.
15. Balconi M, et al. Touching to feel: brain activity during in-store consumer experience. Front Psychol. 2021;12 https://doi.org/10.3389/fpsyg.2021.653011.
16. Kim J, et al. Emotion recognition while applying cosmetic cream using deep learning from EEG data; cross-subject analysis. PLoS One. 2022;17(11):e0274203. https://doi.org/10.1371/journal.pone.0274203.
17. Brinker TJ, et al. Effect of a face-aging Mobile app-based intervention on skin cancer protection behavior in secondary schools in Brazil: a cluster-randomized clinical trial. JAMA Dermatol. 2020;156(7):737–45. https://doi.org/10.1001/jamadermatol.2020.0511.
18. Liu X, et al. A DNA-based intelligent expert system for personalised skin-health recommendations. IEEE J Biomed Health Inform. 2020;24(11):3276–84. https://doi.org/10.1109/JBHI.2020.2978667.
19. Banila C, et al. A noninvasive method for whole-genome skin methylome profiling. Br J Dermatol. 2023;189(6):750–9. https://doi.org/10.1093/bjd/ljad316.
20. Haykal D. Leveraging single nucleotide polymorphism profiling for precision skin care: how SNPs shape individual responses in cosmetic dermatology. J Cosmet Dermatol. 2025;24(1):e16750. https://doi.org/10.1111/jocd.16750.
21. Elder A, et al. The role of artificial intelligence in cosmetic dermatology-current, upcoming, and future trends. J Cosmet Dermatol. 2021;20(1):48–52. https://doi.org/10.1111/jocd.13797.
22. Elder A, et al. Artificial intelligence in cosmetic dermatology: an update on current trends. Clin Dermatol. 2024;42(3):216–20. https://doi.org/10.1016/j.clindermatol.2023.12.015.
23. Fatima H, et al. Internet-of-mirrors (IoM) for connected healthcare and beauty: a prospective vision. Internet of Things. 2024;28:101415. https://doi.org/10.1016/j.iot.2024.101415.
24. Hsu LC, et al. Developing low-cost Mobile device and apps for accurate skin Spectrum measurement via low-cost Spectrum sensors and deep neural network technology. Sensors (Basel). 2022;22(22) https://doi.org/10.3390/s22228844.
25. Frasier K, et al. The role of wearable technology in real-time skin health monitoring. JEADV Clin Pract. 2024; https://doi.org/10.1002/jvc2.587.
26. Yum, J., et al. Improving user-centered Interface for smart mirror as a product-service system design. 2022. Cham: Springer International Publishing.
27. Xin H, et al. Applications of artificial intelligence and machine learning on critical materials used in cosmetics and personal care formulation design. Curr Opin Colloid Interface Sci. 2024;73:101847. https://doi.org/10.1016/j.cocis.2024.101847.
28. Fisher AA. "Status cosmeticus": a cosmetic intolerance syndrome. Cutis. 1990;46(2):109–10.
29. Kalicinska J, et al. Artificial intelligence that predicts sensitizing potential of cosmetic ingredients with accuracy comparable to animal and in vitro tests-how does the Infotechnomics compare to other "omics" in the cosmetics safety assessment? Int J Mol Sci. 2023;24(7) https://doi.org/10.3390/ijms24076801.
30. Gilmour N, et al. Development of a next generation risk assessment framework for the evaluation of skin sensitisation of cosmetic ingredients. Regul Toxicol Pharmacol. 2020;116:104721. https://doi.org/10.1016/j.yrtph.2020.104721.
31. Ta GH, Weng CF, Leong MK. In silico prediction of skin sensitization: quo vadis? Front Pharmacol. 2021;12:655771. https://doi.org/10.3389/fphar.2021.655771.
32. Gellatly N, Sewell F. Regulatory acceptance of in silico approaches for the safety assessment of cosmetic-related substances. Comput Toxicol. 2019;11:82–9. https://doi.org/10.1016/j.comtox.2019.03.003.

33. Grech VS, Kefala V, Rallis E. Cosmetology in the era of artificial intelligence. Cosmetics. 2024;11(4):135.
34. Golden E, et al. Evaluation of the global performance of eight in silico skin sensitization models using human data. ALTEX. 2021;38(1):33–48. https://doi.org/10.14573/altex.1911261.
35. Cadau S, et al. New bioprinted skin, cosmetic in vitro model. J Cosmet Sci. 2017;68(1):85–90.
36. Castro Thomazi V, Maurmann N, Pranke P. Bioprinting for skin: current approaches, technological advancements and the role of artificial intelligence: bioprinting for skin: approaches, advancements and artificial intelligence. Int J Adv Med Biotechnol – IJAMB. 2024;6(2):114–30. https://doi.org/10.52466/ijamb.v6i2.135.
37. Damiati LA, et al. 4D printing in skin tissue engineering: a revolutionary approach to enhance wound healing and combat infections. Bioprinting. 2025;45:e00386. https://doi.org/10.1016/j.bprint.2025.e00386.
38. Freer M, et al. Development of a mammalian neurosensory full-thickness skin equivalent and its application to screen sensitizing stimuli. Bioeng Transl Med. 2023;8(3):e10484. https://doi.org/10.1002/btm2.10484.
39. Ahn M, et al. 3D biofabrication of diseased human skin models in vitro. Biomater Res. 2023;27(1):80. https://doi.org/10.1186/s40824-023-00415-5.
40. Ganel T, Sofer C, Goodale MA. Biases in human perception of facial age are present and more exaggerated in current AI technology. Sci Rep. 2022;12(1):22519. https://doi.org/10.1038/s41598-022-27009-w.
41. Salminen AT, Manga P, Camacho L. Race, pigmentation, and the human skin barrier-considerations for dermal absorption studies. Front Toxicol. 2023;5:1271833. https://doi.org/10.3389/ftox.2023.1271833.
42. Fliorent R, et al. Artificial intelligence in dermatology: advancements and challenges in skin of color. Int J Dermatol. 2024;63(4):455–61. https://doi.org/10.1111/ijd.17076.
43. Grzybowski A, Jin K, Wu H. Challenges of artificial intelligence in medicine and dermatology. Clin Dermatol. 2024;42(3):210–5. https://doi.org/10.1016/j.clindermatol.2023.12.013.
44. Khalil A, et al. Investigating bias in facial analysis systems: a systematic review. IEEE Access. 2020;8:130751–61. https://doi.org/10.1109/ACCESS.2020.3006051.
45. Buolamwini J, Gebru T. Gender shades: intersectional accuracy disparities in commercial gender classification. In: FAT; 2018.
46. Revieve. Personalization and Data Privacy Balance in the Beauty Industry. 2021; Available from: https://www.revieve.com/resources/personalization-data-privacy-balance-in-beauty.
47. Haykal D, et al. Exploring the landscape of AI adoption in cosmetic medicine and surgery: insights from the 25th IMCAS Congress (International Master Course in Aging Science). J Cosmet Dermatol. 2024; https://doi.org/10.1111/jocd.16316.
48. Authors A, Luz G, Olaoye G. Data quality and data privacy challenges in AI applications. 2024. Available online: https://www.researchgate.net/publication/378904709_Data_quality_and_data_privacy_challenges_in_AI_applications. Accessed 1 June 2024.

Applications of Toxin and Fillers and AI Use

15

Vasiliki-Sofia Grech and Efstathios Rallis

15.1 Botulinum Toxin: Mechanisms, Applications, and Clinical Considerations

Botulinum toxin is a powerful neurotoxin produced by *Clostridium botulinum*, a Gram-positive, spore-forming, obligate anaerobic bacterium. Since its clinical introduction in the late 1970s, Botox has become a critical tool in the treatment of neurological and muscular disorders, owing to its ability to regulate neuromuscular activity and induce temporary muscle relaxation. This mechanism not only serves as the basis for its extensive therapeutic applications but also drives its growing use in aesthetic medicine [1].

Botulinum toxin exerts its pharmacological effects by inhibiting neuromuscular transmission at the presynaptic level, thereby preventing muscle contraction. Once internalized by the nerve terminal, the toxin cleaves SNARE proteins, which are essential for synaptic vesicle fusion with the presynaptic membrane and the subsequent release of acetylcholine into the synaptic cleft. By disrupting this process, botulinum toxin effectively blocks cholinergic neurotransmission, leading to temporary flaccid paralysis. This mechanism forms the basis for its clinical applications in treating conditions characterized by excessive muscular activity, as well as in aesthetic medicine for reducing dynamic wrinkles caused by repetitive facial muscle movements [2]. In addition to its neuromuscular effects, botulinum toxin has been shown to modulate pain perception by inhibiting the release of proinflammatory mediators such as bradykinin, prostaglandins, histamine, and serotonin. This inhibition reduces peripheral and central sensitization, contributing to its therapeutic efficacy in the management of chronic pain disorders, including migraines and neuralgias [1].

V.-S. Grech (✉) · E. Rallis
Department of Biomedical Sciences, School of Health and Care Sciences, University of West Attica, Athens, Greece

E. Karampinis et al. (eds.), *Artificial Intelligence Applications in Dermatology*,
https://doi.org/10.1007/978-3-032-15614-3_15

The clinical effects of botulinum toxin vary depending on the therapeutic indication. In aesthetic applications, the onset of action typically occurs within 3–14 days, with maximal effects observed around 2 weeks post injection. The duration of efficacy generally ranges from 3 to 5 months. In contrast, when used for autonomic dysfunctions such as primary focal hyperhidrosis and overactive bladder, its effects can persist for 6–9 months [3, 4].

Botulinum toxin is commercially available in lyophilized powder form in four primary formulations: OnabotulinumtoxinA, AbobotulinumtoxinA, IncobotulinumtoxinA, and RimabotulinumtoxinB. Each formulation differs in potency, diffusion characteristics, and clinical applications. Proper reconstitution with sterile, preservative-free saline is essential to ensure accurate dosing and minimize the risk of unintended diffusion. Improper dilution or injection technique may lead to suboptimal therapeutic outcomes or adverse effects, such as eyelid ptosis, due to unintended spread of the toxin to adjacent muscle groups [1].

Botulinum toxin injections are generally well tolerated; however, they can be associated with mild, self-limiting adverse effects such as transient erythema, ecchymosis, edema, localized injection site pain, and flu-like symptoms. Less common complications include unintended muscle weakening, leading to conditions such as blepharoptosis or eyebrow ptosis, particularly in the periorbital region. Hypersensitivity reactions, though rare, may present as localized pruritus, urticaria, or angioedema. Severe systemic adverse effects, including anaphylaxis and generalized neuromuscular weakness, are exceedingly uncommon but have been reported [1].

In aesthetic practice, botulinum toxin is highly valued for its ability to reduce dynamic wrinkles by temporarily paralyzing targeted muscles. Achieving natural and well-balanced results necessitates an in-depth understanding of facial anatomy and skillful injection techniques [5].

A comprehensive patient assessment is crucial for achieving optimal botulinum toxin outcomes. Evaluating muscle strength, thickness, and contraction patterns before treatment allows for precise dose selection and accurate injection placement [2]. Superficial injections are ideal for fine lines, whereas deeper injections are required for hyperactive muscles, such as the corrugator supercilii and masseter [5]. Additionally, dose adjustments may be necessary, as male patients typically require higher doses due to greater muscle mass [2].

Proper injection technique is essential in minimizing complications while ensuring natural and balanced results. Strategic placement of injections helps prevent adverse effects such as brow or eyelid ptosis, while techniques such as the staggered or zigzag injection pattern in larger muscles improve toxin distribution and overall efficacy [2, 3]. Post-treatment guidelines—such as advising patients to avoid excessive facial movement and remain upright for several hours—further help reduce unintended toxin diffusion, enhancing both safety and effectiveness [2].

The selection of treatment areas and appropriate dosing is critical in optimizing outcomes. Botulinum toxin is commonly used in the upper face, including the glabellar complex (procerus and corrugator muscles) to soften frown lines, the frontalis to smooth forehead wrinkles, and the orbicularis oculi to reduce lateral canthal lines (crow's feet). In the lower face, injections into the masseter muscle are frequently performed to address hypertrophy and enhance facial contouring, while targeting the depressor anguli oris and mentalis can improve marionette lines and chin dimpling. Perioral injections into the orbicularis oris are used to soften perioral rhytides and create subtle lip enhancements [3–6].

Botulinum toxin remains a cornerstone of both therapeutic and aesthetic dermatology. When administered with a precise understanding of facial anatomy and individualized treatment planning, it delivers effective, natural, and long-lasting results with minimal complications. Additionally, the integration of artificial intelligence (AI) into botulinum toxin applications is proving to be a valuable advancement, enhancing precision in dose calculation and injection site selection. AI-driven approaches improve patient safety, optimize treatment outcomes, and provide a more personalized approach to botulinum toxin therapy. By incorporating both expert technique and emerging technology, clinicians can maximize efficacy while ensuring predictable and refined aesthetic results.

15.2 Artificial Intelligence in Botulinum Toxin Therapy

15.2.1 AI-Enhanced AR for Botulinum Toxin Injection Planning

Traditionally, clinicians have relied on static anatomical diagrams depicting standardized facial structures and muscle distributions to determine injection sites. However, such diagrams may not sufficiently account for anatomical variability among individual patients, potentially compromising the accuracy of injection placement. In contrast, AI-enhanced augmented reality (AR) systems process real-time imaging and align it with pre-established anatomical markers, generating a customized overlay of critical procedural details, including standard entry points, optimal injection depths, and recommended toxin volumes. By integrating real-time anatomical visualization with virtual data overlays, AR systems enable clinicians to superimpose essential imaging modalities—such as ultrasound, computed tomography (CT), and radiographic data—directly onto a patient's facial anatomy. This advanced integration enhances the precision of injection site selection, reducing the risk of complications and optimizing clinical outcomes [7].

A controlled comparative study assessing the performance of novice injectors—individuals without prior experience in facial injections—demonstrated that practitioners using an AR application achieved a significantly lower mean deviation from expert-determined injection sites (4.60 mm) compared to those relying on conventional anatomical diagrams (6.75 mm). This increased accuracy mitigates the risk of complications such as blepharoptosis, brow ptosis, and facial asymmetry, highlighting the potential of AI-enhanced AR as an indispensable tool for clinical practice and procedural training [8].

Furthermore, deep learning-based facial recognition algorithms have refined this approach by automating the extraction of key facial landmarks, including the eyes, nose, and mouth, from images captured via standard mobile devices. These AR applications, accessible on smartphones and tablets, provide a cost-effective and widely available tool for clinicians. Once extracted, these landmarks are interconnected to generate a dynamic three-dimensional (3D) facial mesh, achieving a positional accuracy of approximately 3 mm across various facial regions. This high level of precision is particularly critical in both aesthetic and therapeutic botulinum toxin applications. By accurately mapping muscle anatomy, AR-guided injection techniques enhance clinical efficacy while minimizing the likelihood of unintended toxin diffusion or injury to adjacent structures [7].

Beyond its immediate clinical applications, the integration of AI in AR technology offers substantial educational and patient counseling benefits. Medical and dental trainees can leverage this technology to develop a deeper understanding of the intricate relationship between facial anatomy and injection techniques, thereby refining their procedural skills. Additionally, real-time, individualized visualization provided by AR assists in patient counseling by clearly illustrating treatment plans and expected outcomes, fostering informed consent and alleviating patient anxiety. As ongoing research continues to refine AI–AR integration, this technology is poised to streamline clinical workflows, enhance surgical precision in both aesthetic and functional facial procedures, and ultimately contribute to more individualized and safer patient care [7, 8].

15.2.2 AI in Predicting Immunogenicity of Botulinum Toxin

Although botulinum toxin A (BoNT-A) is widely employed in both aesthetic and therapeutic applications; its long-term effectiveness may be compromised by the development of neutralizing antibodies (NAbs), a phenomenon known as immunogenicity. Advanced machine learning (ML) techniques and Bayesian analysis have been employed in predictive modeling to evaluate immunogenic responses across FDA-approved BoNT-A products for glabellar treatments. The findings revealed that patient demographics—such as age and gender—do not significantly influence the likelihood of NAb development, indicating that treatment outcomes are broadly applicable across diverse patient populations. In contrast, treatment specifics, including dosage and frequency, emerged as significant predictors of immunogenicity. Higher dosages and more frequent treatments were associated with an increased risk of NAb formation. Moreover, the analysis differentiated the immunogenic potential among BoNT-A products, with IncobotulinumtoxinA demonstrating the lowest likelihood of inducing NAbs and ABO showing the highest risk, thereby underscoring the need for judicious treatment planning [9].

The glabellar region, commonly targeted for cosmetic applications, typically requires lower doses of BoNT-A due to its relatively simple muscle anatomy. This lower dose requirement may contribute to the absence of reported primary or secondary nonresponse in glabellar line treatments, despite the potential presence of low-titer NAbs that might not immediately affect therapeutic efficacy. The integration of AI in these predictive models offers a valuable tool for clinicians, facilitating more precise treatment planning and dosing strategies to mitigate the risk of immunogenicity. Such advanced predictive modeling not only refines our understanding of how treatment variables influence immune responses but also supports the long-term efficacy of BoNT-A therapies by guiding clinical decision-making and reducing the likelihood of resistance due to heightened immunogenic responses [9].

15.3 Fillers: Mechanisms, Applications, and Clinical Considerations

Injectable fillers have a long-standing role in dermatology, initially derived from materials such as autologous fat, liquid paraffin, and silicone oil, though some were later restricted due to complications like hypersensitivity reactions, ulcerations, and tissue necrosis. The ongoing pursuit of an ideal filler emphasizes properties such as safety, biocompatibility, nontoxicity, longevity, and ease of application. Today, an expanding range of injectable fillers is available, all classified as class III medical devices to ensure regulatory oversight in aesthetic medicine. These fillers restore volume and enhance facial contours either through direct physical filling or by stimulating collagen synthesis, with the former providing an immediate but gradually diminishing effect [10].

Dermal fillers are broadly classified into temporary, semi-permanent, and permanent categories based on their composition and duration of effect. Temporary fillers, primarily composed of hyaluronic acid, provide reversible hydration and volume restoration, making them a widely used option due to their safety and reversibility. Semi-permanent fillers, such as poly-L-lactic acid and calcium hydroxylapatite, not only restore volume but also stimulate collagen production, leading to longer-lasting effects. In contrast, permanent fillers, including polymethylmethacrylate and liquid silicone, offer sustained results but are associated with a higher risk of complications [11, 12].

An emerging advancement in aesthetic dermatology is the use of biofillers, which integrate volumization with regenerative properties to enhance both structural and functional skin rejuvenation. Biofillers, including autologous fat and plasma gel, not only restore lost volume but also stimulate collagen synthesis and angiogenesis, contributing to improved skin texture, elasticity, and longevity. These regenerative properties make biofillers a promising approach for achieving natural and sustained aesthetic outcomes [13–15].

To ensure patient safety, clinicians must have a comprehensive understanding of facial vascular anatomy, appropriate dosing protocols, and precise injection techniques. The ability to promptly recognize and manage HA filler complications with hyaluronidase is essential for minimizing risks and achieving optimal clinical outcomes [16, 17].

Facial filler injections are widely performed aesthetic procedures and are generally considered safe [18, 19]; however, complications, when they occur, can be severe. Certain anatomical regions, particularly the nasal and nasolabial fold areas, carry a higher risk due to their complex vascular networks. Inadvertent intravascular injection in these regions can lead to vascular occlusion and severe ischemic complications. To mitigate this risk, recommended strategies include aspiration before injection and administering fillers in small, controlled volumes at the periosteal layer [18].

Similarly, injections in the glabellar and periorbital regions require particular caution due to the risk of intravascular infiltration. Excessive injection force and velocity can elevate local pressure, potentially activating functionally inactive anastomoses between the external and internal carotid arteries. Increased pressure within the branches of the external carotid artery may lead to reversed blood flow through the ocular and facial vasculature, allowing filler material to migrate into the internal carotid artery. This can result in serious complications, including irreversible vision loss or cerebrovascular events [20, 21].

The choice of injection technique plays a critical role in minimizing complications. Studies indicate that using a cannula instead of a needle significantly reduces the risk of vascular occlusion, with retrospective analyses demonstrating a 77.1% lower risk. Furthermore, clinician expertise is a key factor; practitioners with more than 5 years of experience have been found to exhibit a 70.7% lower risk of vascular occlusion compared to those with less experience. These findings highlight the importance of both technique and provider skill in ensuring patient safety [18].

Given the potential severity of complications associated with facial filler injections, adherence to evidence-based techniques, careful patient selection, and timely intervention in the event of adverse outcomes are essential. In this direction, the integration of AI in filler procedures has proven to be highly beneficial. AI-driven imaging and predictive analytics help identify high-risk anatomical zones, optimize injection techniques, and enhance patient safety. Additionally, AI-assisted robotic systems and machine learning algorithms can provide real-time feedback to practitioners, reducing the likelihood of complications and improving procedural outcomes.

15.4 Artificial Intelligence in Dermal Fillers

15.4.1 ML in Hydrogel Optimization for Dermal Fillers

HA-based hydrogels, synthesized through ether crosslinking, are extensively utilized across various biomedical applications, with their primary use in aesthetic medicine as intradermal fillers. Recent research has focused on establishing precise correlations between manufacturing parameters and the resulting biophysical properties to optimize hydrogel design for specific performance outcomes. This approach aims to refine formulation techniques, enhancing the mechanical properties, durability, and overall effectiveness of hyaluronan-based fillers in both aesthetic and therapeutic applications [22].

The integration of AI and ML is further revolutionizing hydrogel development and optimization, offering advanced predictive capabilities for key properties such as swelling behavior, mechanical strength, and rheological performance. AI-driven methodologies streamline the selection of ingredients, optimize 3D printing processes, and improve performance prediction, addressing critical challenges in hydrogel manufacturing. By enabling high-throughput property measurements and refining structure–property relationships, AI and ML contribute to more precise and efficient formulation designs. Given the biocompatibility, high water content, and drug-delivery potential of hydrogels, these technological advancements pave the way for innovative applications in skincare, biomedical treatments, and the broader field of regenerative medicine [23].

15.4.2 ML-Based Predictive Modeling for Dermal Filler Volume Estimation

ML is transforming aesthetic medicine by improving the prediction and planning of dermal filler procedures. Traditionally, clinicians estimate filler volume requirements based on experience and pretreatment facial scans, which can lead to variability in treatment outcomes. ML-based predictive modeling provides a more objective and standardized approach by analyzing pre- and post-treatment 3D facial images to assess structural changes and estimate the appropriate volume of dermal filler for different facial areas (Fig. 15.1). By utilizing deep learning models designed to understand facial anatomy, ML can predict the effects of treatment before the procedure takes place, reducing uncertainty for both the patient and clinician [24].

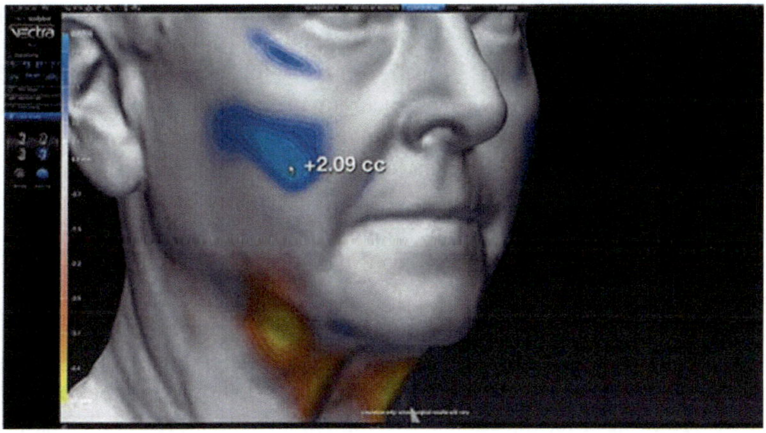

Fig. 15.1 Canfield's VECTRA H2 is a handheld 3D facial and body capture system that utilizes markerless tracking technology to objectively and precisely measure volume changes between multiple timepoints, highlighting the quantitative outcomes due to aesthetic procedures such as fillers, injections, face/body contouring, skin lifts, and others. The automatic markerless tracking uses dense correspondence algorithms to align skin surfaces and highlight differences in 3D. It has been successfully used to objectively measure treatment outcomes and demonstrate aesthetic improvement

Profilometry, a technique that measures wrinkle depth and surface characteristics, has traditionally been the most accurate method for quantifying skin aging; however, it requires physical impressions, making it impractical for routine use. ML-based systems overcome this limitation by digitally analyzing facial topography in real time, providing a noninvasive and efficient alternative. These AI-driven models rely on large datasets to improve their accuracy and generalizability. Real-world datasets, derived from actual patient scans, capture the natural anatomical diversity of facial structures, while synthetic datasets are artificially generated to expand the range of facial variations and filler volumes used in training. This dual-data approach allows AI models to better generalize across diverse patient populations, enhancing their ability to provide precise and personalized filler recommendations. These AI-driven models also address the limitations of subjective grading systems such as the Lemperle rating scale and photonumeric wrinkle assessment, which rely on visual evaluation rather than precise quantitative analysis [25].

15.4.3 Deep Learning for Wrinkle Classification and Treatment Planning

Building on this foundation, AI is increasingly being integrated into aesthetic medicine to improve the accuracy and objectivity of dermal filler assessments. One of the latest advancements in this field involves the use of deep learning models, such as the Inception model, to detect wrinkles and assess the need for filler injections in specific facial regions. The proposed AI framework utilizes a database of forehead images—both wrinkled and nonwrinkled—alongside a multitask cascaded convolutional networks (MTCNN) model for precise facial landmark detection and image preprocessing. Through a series of steps, including facial cropping and feature extraction, the Inception model is trained to classify forehead images into categories of "wrinkles" or "no wrinkles" with an accuracy of 85.3%. This AI-based classification system offers a more objective approach to evaluating wrinkle severity and assists in determining whether forehead filler injections are necessary, reducing the subjectivity associated with traditional visual assessments. However, current limitations include a lack of high-resolution image datasets and a restricted focus on forehead wrinkles, indicating the need for further advancements in AI applications across multiple facial regions [26].

To enhance AI-driven filler prediction, semantic segmentation methods can be used to label each pixel corresponding to wrinkles and fine lines, rather than simply classifying whether an area has wrinkles. This approach allows for precise mapping of facial areas requiring filler injections, offering clinicians a more detailed assessment. Additionally, AI models can compare two frontal face images of the same individual—one with a neutral expression and another with a smiling or animated expression. By analyzing these differences, the model can distinguish between transient wrinkles, which may be best treated with botulinum toxin, and static wrinkles, which require volumizing fillers such as hyaluronic acid, collagen-based substances, or body fat. This advancement essentially functions as an AI-powered cosmetic consultant, assisting practitioners in treatment planning by providing data-driven, personalized recommendations. As research progresses, integrating high-resolution datasets and expanding AI capabilities to other facial areas, such as periorbital and perioral wrinkles, will further refine the precision and applicability of AI in aesthetic medicine [26].

15.4.4 AI-Driven Facial Arterial Mapping for Vascular Safety

AI is playing a transformative role in enhancing the safety and precision of dermal filler procedures by enabling real-time visualization of the arterial anatomy of the face. Anatomical variations pose a significant challenge in aesthetic medicine, as traditional methods rely on theoretical knowledge and clinical experience rather than direct visualization of vascular structures. AI-driven AR applications, integrated with facial recognition software and magnetic resonance angiography (MRA), allow practitioners to map and visualize an individual's superficial arteries with remarkable accuracy. By capturing 68 unique facial reference points and matching them to a three-dimensional arterial network, AI technology enables precise treatment planning, minimizing the risk of inadvertent intravascular injection. This integration bridges the gap between anatomical theory and real-world clinical practice, significantly improving patient safety [27].

The accuracy of AI-generated AR images has been validated using duplex ultrasound, demonstrating an average deviation of only 0.30 mm between the projected and actual arterial locations. This high level of precision underlines AI's potential in reducing vascular complications associated with dermal filler injections, such as vascular occlusion and tissue necrosis. By processing MRA data into real-time AR visualization, AI enhances the injector's ability to navigate complex facial vasculature without requiring invasive imaging techniques. Furthermore, the ability to tailor arterial mapping to each patient's unique anatomy allows for more individualized treatment planning [27].

Taking this technology a step further, a key advantage of AI-driven AR systems is their ability to track dynamic arterial movement. Since facial arteries shift position with muscle movement and facial expressions, the AR application adjusts in real time, ensuring accuracy throughout the procedure. The process begins with MRA imaging, which captures high-resolution, radiation-free scans of the patient's facial arterial network. Unlike computed tomography angiography (CTA), MRA does not require contrast agents, making it safer for repeated use. These scans isolate superficial subcutaneous arteries, creating a detailed three-dimensional map of the patient's unique vascular structure. The MRA images are then processed through AI-driven software, which reconstructs the arterial network into a three-dimensional model, accurately mapping both the location and depth of critical arteries [28].

Once the three-dimensional arterial model is created, it is integrated into an AR application that aligns the vascular map with the patient's face in real time. By using facial recognition software, the system ensures that the visualized arteries remain precisely overlaid on the patient's anatomy, even as they move or change facial expressions. The injector can access this real-time visualization through a smartphone or AR headset, allowing for an unprecedented level of precision. Additionally, AI-enhanced features such as color-coded depth indicators or millimeter-based arterial depth readings further refine the injector's technique, reducing the likelihood of accidental intra-arterial injections. This is particularly crucial for avoiding high-risk arteries connected to the ophthalmic artery, where inadvertent occlusion could lead to retrograde embolization and central retinal artery blockage, ultimately resulting in vision loss. As AI-driven AR technology continues to advance, its role in improving safety and precision in dermal filler procedures will expand, setting new standards in aesthetic medicine [28].

15.4.5 AI-Integrated Virtual Reality for Dermal Filler Training

The integration of AI into dermal filler training represents a significant advancement in clinical education, providing an interactive and simulation-based approach to skill development. The Virtual Reality-Based Filler Injection Training System combines motion tracking technology, a three-dimensional human facial model, and a virtual reality (VR) interface to enhance procedural learning. Through the use of optical motion tracking cameras, the system monitors syringe movement in real time, offering immediate feedback on injection depth and proximity to critical anatomical structures. This interactive feedback mechanism reinforces anatomical knowledge while promoting safer injection techniques in a controlled and risk-free setting. Additionally, a structured instructional module supports clinicians in understanding proper filler injection principles and effectively navigating the VR system [29].Although the system has demonstrated promise in training applications, certain limitations must be addressed to enhance its clinical relevance. At present, the system differentiates only between bone and soft tissue, lacking the detailed anatomical stratification necessary for precise simulation of injection depths, particularly in high-risk areas such as the supra-periosteal and superficial layers. Furthermore, the system does not yet incorporate assessments of anatomical knowledge, procedural accuracy, or performance error rates, making it difficult to determine its impact on clinical proficiency. While initial usability evaluations have shown a generally positive response, variations in acceptance across different experience levels suggest the need for further refinement of the interface and training modules. Future improvements should focus on increasing anatomical accuracy, enabling individualized customization, and establishing objective outcome measures to optimize its role as a standardized educational tool in aesthetic medicine [29].

15.5 Artificial Intelligence in Neuromodulators and Dermal Fillers: AI Chatbots for Aesthetic Consultation and Risk Assessment

The integration of AI chatbots in aesthetic medicine is emerging as a valuable tool for both clinical practice and research, particularly in the administration of dermal fillers and botulinum toxin treatments. Chatbots like ChatGPT have demonstrated the ability to generate systematic review topics relevant to cosmetic procedures, including neurotoxins and soft tissue augmentation, with a measured accuracy of 55%. While reliability varies depending on topic specificity, AI's capacity to facilitate literature reviews and support evidence-based practice underscores its potential role in aesthetic medicine. Beyond research, AI-driven systems are versatile and can assist clinicians by offering procedural guidance, aiding in risk assessment, and providing insights into injection techniques. These capabilities may enhance procedural accuracy, improve safety, and support clinical decision-making [30].

In addition to research and procedural support, AI-based chatbots offer significant advantages in patient education and consultation. They can deliver structured, detailed information on the benefits, risks, and expected outcomes of dermal filler and neurotoxin treatments, enhancing patient understanding and informed decision-making. Furthermore, chatbots can streamline pretreatment assessments by addressing common patient concerns and providing postprocedure care guidance, reducing clinicians' workload while maintaining continuous patient engagement. AI's application in practice management, including patient outreach and marketing, further highlights its role in optimizing clinical workflows. As AI technology continues to advance, its integration into aesthetic medicine holds the potential to enhance provider efficiency and patient care, reinforcing its value as a complementary tool in modern cosmetic practice [30].

15.6 AI-Driven Robotics in Neuromodulator and Dermal Filler Injections

The integration of AI into robotic-assisted injections is revolutionizing aesthetic medicine by enhancing precision, standardization, and safety. LENA, a neurorobotic arm developed by NextMotion in 2023, leverages AI-driven algorithms to optimize the administration of neuromodulators and dermal fillers. By allowing clinicians to predefine injection parameters such as volume and depth, the system minimizes human variability, ensuring consistent results and reducing procedural errors. Robots offer a high level of accuracy, delivering even product distribution and controlled injection depth, which can improve aesthetic outcomes and lower complication rates. Additionally, automated injections performed at a steady, controlled pace may reduce pain and discomfort by minimizing tissue trauma [31].

AI-powered imaging and sensory technologies further enhance safety by tracking anatomical landmarks in real time, helping to mitigate risks such as vascular occlusion and asymmetry. Robots can be programmed to avoid high-risk facial zones, reducing the likelihood of complications. Moreover, their ability to replicate procedures with precision supports treatment standardization, making outcomes more predictable. The efficiency of robotic systems also has the potential to shorten treatment times and increase access to aesthetic procedures in regions with limited qualified practitioners [31].

However, despite these advantages, robotic-assisted injections have notable limitations. While robots excel in precision and consistency, they currently lack the flexibility and artistic judgment of experienced injectors, who can make real-time adjustments based on individual anatomy and patient preferences. The inability to personalize treatments beyond preprogrammed instructions may lead to suboptimal aesthetic outcomes. Additionally, robots are unable to assess patient comfort or respond to feedback during the procedure, which could impact patient satisfaction [31].

Another major barrier to widespread adoption is cost. The high expense of acquiring, maintaining, and repairing robotic systems makes them less accessible to most practitioners, potentially increasing procedure costs for patients. Ethical considerations also arise, as some patients may be hesitant to receive injections from a machine rather than a human practitioner. Ensuring transparency, patient education, and informed decision-making will be essential in integrating robotic technology into aesthetic medicine [31]. As AI and machine learning continue to evolve, future advancements may improve robotic adaptability, enabling real-time adjustments based on patient feedback and dynamic facial analysis. While robotic-assisted injections offer enhanced precision and safety, they remain a complement to, rather than a replacement for, skilled human injectors, whose expertise and artistic judgment remain critical in achieving optimal results [31].

15.7 AI-Assisted Post-treatment Evaluation of Neuromodulator and Filler Outcomes As Well as Patient Education

Post-treatment evaluation is a fundamental aspect of aesthetic medicine, ensuring that neuromodulator and filler treatments achieve optimal and natural outcomes while maintaining facial harmony. Traditional methods, such as static photography, provide a limited perspective by capturing only a fixed moment in time and failing to account for dynamic muscle activity. In contrast, customized precision facial assessment (CPFA) offers an AI-driven approach that utilizes dynamic imaging and the facial action coding system (FACS) to analyze subtle facial movements. By identifying microexpressions and quantifying changes in facial muscle activation, CPFA enables a standardized and objective assessment of treatment efficacy. This system provides clinicians with precise data regarding the reduction of negative facial expressions, facilitating a more targeted and evidence-based approach to aesthetic interventions [32].

An essential advantage of AI-assisted post-treatment evaluation is its ability to monitor facial expression scores across multiple time points, ensuring the stability and effectiveness of treatment outcomes. In a comparative study, patients who underwent CPFA-guided treatment exhibited a more significant reduction in negative facial expressions than those assessed using traditional clinical judgment. Notably, one case in the human-facilitated treatment group demonstrated initial improvement at 1 week, followed by a resurgence of negative facial expressions at 3 weeks, potentially due to inadequate neuromodulator dosing for strong muscle activity. In contrast, AI-assisted analysis allowed for precise dosing and optimized injection placement, resulting in more consistent and sustained aesthetic outcomes. Furthermore, CPFA has the potential to serve as a clinical training tool, enhancing the ability of practitioners to recognize and quantify facial expressions, ultimately refining their treatment strategies. As AI continues to advance, its role in post-treatment evaluation is expected to improve procedural accuracy, enhance reproducibility, and optimize patient satisfaction in aesthetic medicine [32].

AI has the potential to significantly improve patient education regarding the safety of botulinum toxin and facial filler injections. Despite the widespread use of these procedures, public awareness of associated risks remains limited. A survey assessing knowledge of potential complications found that while common side effects such as bruising and asymmetry were recognized by a moderate percentage of respondents, more serious risks, including vascular occlusion and blindness, were identified by only 19% and 18% of participants, respectively. AI-driven educational tools may help bridge this gap by providing patients with personalized, accessible, and evidence-based information before treatment. Interactive AI platforms can assist in explaining procedural risks, simulating expected results, and addressing patient concerns in real time, ultimately fostering informed decision-making and improving patient confidence in aesthetic treatments [33].

Beyond its role in patient education, AI can enhance procedural safety by supporting clinicians in risk assessment and injection planning. AI-assisted imaging and anatomical mapping can aid in the identification of high-risk vascular structures, guiding precise filler placement to minimize the likelihood of complications. Additionally, AI-driven monitoring systems may facilitate early detection of post-procedural adverse effects, allowing for timely intervention and improved patient outcomes. The integration of AI into both preprocedural education and clinical practice represents a significant advancement in aesthetic medicine, promoting greater patient understanding, reducing procedural risks, and enhancing the overall safety and efficacy of botulinum toxin and dermal filler treatments [33].

15.8 Conclusion

The integration of AI into aesthetic medicine holds significant potential for addressing critical challenges in the administration of neuromodulators and dermal fillers, particularly in enhancing patient safety and optimizing individualized treatment outcomes (Fig. 15.2). A major concern in contemporary aesthetic education is the oversimplification of facial anatomy, which can contribute to misconceptions regarding injection safety, an overreliance on designated "safe zones," and an increased risk of complications. AI-assisted technologies, including real-time imaging, dynamic anatomical mapping, and machine learning-based injection guidance systems, offer a means to mitigate these risks by providing personalized, data-driven insights that account for anatomical variability among patients. Furthermore, AI-enhanced educational platforms can advance practitioner training through interactive, anatomy-focused simulations and augmented reality models, which extend beyond traditional static diagrams to emphasize the complexity of facial structures.

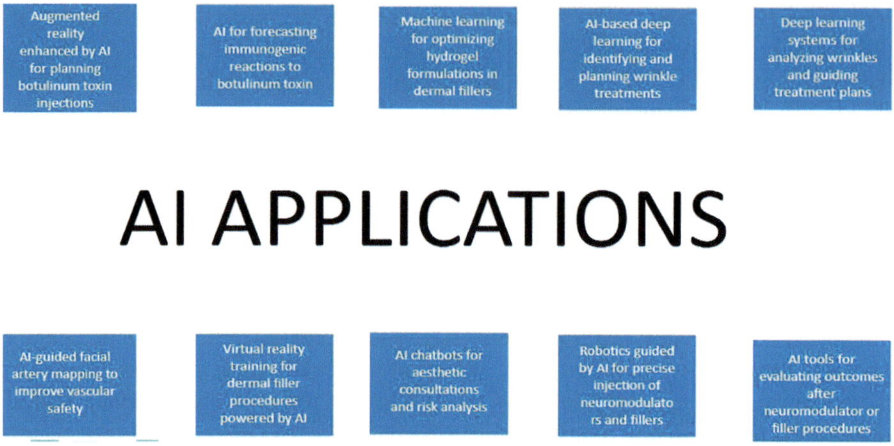

Fig. 15.2 AI applications in aesthetic medicine

The current trend toward oversimplifying anatomical education in aesthetics, often referred to as "dumbification," presents a significant risk by fostering inadequate training and promoting formulaic approaches that fail to account for the intricacies of human anatomy [34].

Beyond its role in anatomical education, AI can optimize treatment planning and procedural execution by tailoring interventions to the patient's unique facial dynamics and aesthetic requirements. The phenomenon of "alienization," in which standardized aesthetic protocols produce unnatural, homogeneous outcomes, accentuates the need for more personalized and adaptable treatment strategies in aesthetic medicine. AI-driven facial assessment tools, such as microexpression analysis and real-time injection tracking, facilitate the refinement of treatment plans to align with the patient's natural features rather than relying on rigid formulaic approaches. Additionally, AI technologies can enhance risk assessment and procedural precision through innovations such as ultrasound-guided injections, thereby reducing the likelihood of vascular complications. By integrating AI into both aesthetic education and clinical practice, the field can advance toward a model that prioritizes a comprehensive understanding of facial anatomy, individualized patient assessment, and enhanced procedural safety, ultimately leading to more natural and satisfactory outcomes in the application of neuromodulators and dermal fillers [34].

References

1. Padda IS, Tadi P. Botulinum Toxin. In: StatPearls. Treasure Island (FL): StatPearls Publishing. Copyright © 2025, StatPearls Publishing LLC.; 2025.
2. Swift A, et al. Tips and tricks for facial Toxin injections with illustrated anatomy. Plast Reconstr Surg. 2022;149(2):303e–12e. https://doi.org/10.1097/PRS.0000000000008708.
3. Yi KH, et al. Novel anatomical guidelines on botulinum neurotoxin injection for wrinkles in the nose region. Toxins (Basel). 2022;14(5) https://doi.org/10.3390/toxins14050342.

4. Durand PD, et al. Botulinum Toxin and muscle atrophy: a wanted or unwanted effect. Aesthet Surg J. 2016;36(4):482–7. https://doi.org/10.1093/asj/sjv208.
5. D'Souza A, Ng CL. Applied anatomy for botulinum Toxin injection in cosmetic interventions. Curr Otorhinolaryngol Rep. 2020;8(4):336–43. https://doi.org/10.1007/s40136-020-00308-4.
6. Meretsky CR, Umali JP, Schiuma AT. A systematic review and comparative analysis of Botox treatment in aesthetic and therapeutic applications: advantages, disadvantages, and patient outcomes. Cureus. 2024;16(8):e67961. https://doi.org/10.7759/cureus.67961.
7. Kim H, et al. Augmented reality for botulinum toxin injection. In: Concurrency and computation: practice and experience; 2019. p. 32. https://doi.org/10.1002/cpe.5526.
8. Rhee C, Jacob J, Muhammed K. Augmented reality can improve accuracy in identifying botulinum Toxin injection sites. EMJ Innov. 2022:25–32. https://doi.org/10.33590/emjinnov/21-00224.
9. Rahman E, et al. Predictive modelling of immunogenicity to Botulinumtoxin a treatments for glabellar lines. Plast Reconstr Surg. 2024; https://doi.org/10.1097/PRS.0000000000011748.
10. Guo J, Fang W, Wang F. Injectable fillers: current status, physicochemical properties, function mechanism, and perspectives. RSC Adv. 2023;13(34):23841–58. https://doi.org/10.1039/d3ra04321e.
11. Liu MH, Beynet DP, Gharavi NM. Overview of deep dermal fillers. Facial Plast Surg. 2019;35(3):224–9. https://doi.org/10.1055/s-0039-1688843.
12. Xie C, et al. Synthesis and properties of injectable hydrogel for tissue filling. Pharmaceutics. 2024;16(3) https://doi.org/10.3390/pharmaceutics16030430.
13. Vasavada A, Raggio BS. Autologous fat grafting for facial rejuvenation. In: StatPearls. Treasure Island (FL): StatPearls Publishing. Copyright © 2025, StatPearls Publishing LLC.; 2025.
14. Amiri R, et al. The innovative application of autologous biofillers in aesthetic dermatology. Ital J Dermatol Venerol. 2023;158(4):321–7. https://doi.org/10.23736/S2784-8671.23.07485-6.
15. Nanda S, et al. Platelet-rich plasma in aesthetics. Indian Dermatol Online J. 2021;12(Suppl 1):S41–54. https://doi.org/10.4103/idoj.idoj_290_21.
16. Cassuto D, Bellia G, Schiraldi C. An overview of soft tissue fillers for cosmetic dermatology: from filling to regenerative medicine. Clin Cosmet Investig Dermatol. 2021;14:1857–66. https://doi.org/10.2147/CCID.S276676.
17. Germani M, et al. High-dose pulsed hyaluronidase for managing nasal skin necrosis following hyaluronic acid treatment in nasolabial folds: a case report. J Oral Biol Craniofac Res. 2024;14(3):339–41. https://doi.org/10.1016/j.jobcr.2024.04.006.
18. Clark NW, Pan DR, Barrett DM. Facial fillers: relevant anatomy, injection techniques, and complications. World J Otorhinolaryngol Head Neck Surg. 2023;9(3):227–35. https://doi.org/10.1002/wjo2.126.
19. Almukhadeb E, et al. Dermal fillers in the treatment of acne scars: a review. Ann Dermatol. 2023;35(6):400–7. https://doi.org/10.5021/ad.22.230.
20. Yoon SS, Chang DI, Chung KC. Acute fatal stroke immediately following autologous fat injection into the face. Neurology. 2003;61(8):1151–2. https://doi.org/10.1212/wnl.61.8.1151.
21. La Padula S, et al. Nanofat in plastic reconstructive, regenerative, and aesthetic surgery: a review of advancements in face-focused applications. J Clin Med. 2023;12(13) https://doi.org/10.3390/jcm12134351.
22. La Gatta A, et al. Hyaluronan-based hydrogels via ether-crosslinking: is HA molecular weight an effective means to tune gel performance? Int J Biol Macromol. 2020;144:94–101. https://doi.org/10.1016/j.ijbiomac.2019.11.227.
23. Xin H, et al. Applications of artificial intelligence and machine learning on critical materials used in cosmetics and personal care formulation design. Curr Opin Colloid Interface Sci. 2024;73:101847. https://doi.org/10.1016/j.cocis.2024.101847.
24. Shah SAA, Bennamoun M, Molton M. A fully automatic framework for prediction of 3D facial rejuvenation. In: 2018 International Conference on Image and Vision Computing New Zealand (IVCNZ); 2018.
25. Shah S, Bennamoun M, Molton M. Machine learning approaches for prediction of facial rejuvenation using real and synthetic data. IEEE Access. 2019:1-1. https://doi.org/10.1109/ACCESS.2019.2899379.

26. Alrabiah A, Alduailij M, Crane M. Computer-based approach to detect wrinkles and suggest facial fillers. Int J Adv Comput Sci Appl. 2019:10. https://doi.org/10.14569/IJACSA.2019.0100941.
27. Waked K, et al. Visualizing the individual arterial anatomy of the face through augmented reality—a useful and accurate tool during dermal filler injections. Aesthet Surg J Open Forum. 2022;4 https://doi.org/10.1093/asjof/ojac012.
28. Mespreuve M, et al. The usefulness of magnetic resonance angiography to analyze the variable arterial facial anatomy in an effort to reduce filler-associated blindness: anatomical study and visualization through an augmented reality application. Aesthet Surg J Open Forum. 2021;3(3):ojab018. https://doi.org/10.1093/asjof/ojab018.
29. Oh SM, et al. Development and usability of a virtual reality-based filler injection training system. Aesth Plast Surg. 2020;44(5):1833–42. https://doi.org/10.1007/s00266-020-01872-2.
30. Gupta R, et al. Expanding cosmetic plastic surgery research with ChatGPT. Aesthet Surg J. 2023;43(8):930–7. https://doi.org/10.1093/asj/sjad069.
31. Kapoor KM, Kapoor A, Bertossi D. Role of robotics in neuromodulator and filler injections of face. Indian J Plast Surg. 2023;56(5):470–3. https://doi.org/10.1055/s-0043-1775867.
32. Li CW, et al. Customized precision facial assessment: an AI-assisted analysis of facial microexpressions for advanced aesthetic treatment. Plast Reconstr Surg Glob Open. 2020;8(3):e2688. https://doi.org/10.1097/gox.0000000000002688.
33. Hassell NE, et al. Perspectives on the safety of botulinum Toxin and facial filler injections: a National Survey. Ann Plast Surg. 2023;90(6S Suppl 5):S626–9. https://doi.org/10.1097/SAP.0000000000003485.
34. Harris S, Landau M, Goldust M. The dangers of oversimplifying facial anatomy in aesthetic education. Plast Reconstr Surg Glob Open. 2024;12(11):e6306. https://doi.org/10.1097/GOX.0000000000006306.

Laser Application and AI

16

Christoforos Tzermias

16.1 Introduction

Artificial intelligence (AI) is increasingly transforming both therapeutic and cosmetic domains of dermatology, offering tools that enhance diagnosis, personalize treatment, and optimize laser-based interventions across a wide range of skin conditions. Laser dermatology has experienced rapid growth in response to a growing expectation for precision, predictability, and personalization in laser interventions. In parallel, similar demands for individualized, image-guided, and efficient care are emerging across both therapeutic and cosmetic dermatology [1–3]. Traditionally, laser outcomes have been evaluated through a combination of clinical experience, patient feedback, and subjective visual assessment. While this individualized, often intuitive approach has yielded satisfactory results, it remains vulnerable to variability and bias. Additionally, when it comes to cosmetic interventions, aesthetic perceptions vary widely across age, ethnicity, gender, and cultural context, making it challenging to standardize treatment evaluation and planning [1, 4, 5].

The emergence of artificial intelligence (AI) offers new possibilities for bringing objectivity, consistency, and scalability into laser dermatology. By leveraging powerful tools such as deep learning, convolutional neural networks (CNNs), and computer vision, AI can analyze complex datasets such as high resolution skin imagery, patient demographics, and treatment history beyond the limits of human perception. These technologies allow for precise skin classification, individualized treatment planning, and dynamic tracking of treatment outcomes over time [2, 6].

Among the most promising intersections between AI and dermatology is the application of AI-enhanced laser treatments. From the selection of laser parameters based on pigment and texture analysis to predicting collagen remodeling and monitoring treatment efficacy, AI can enhance both clinical precision and patient

C. Tzermias (✉)
Intensive Quality IQ Skin Clinics, Private Dermatology One Day Clinics, Athens, Greece

E. Karampinis et al. (eds.), *Artificial Intelligence Applications in Dermatology*,
https://doi.org/10.1007/978-3-032-15614-3_16

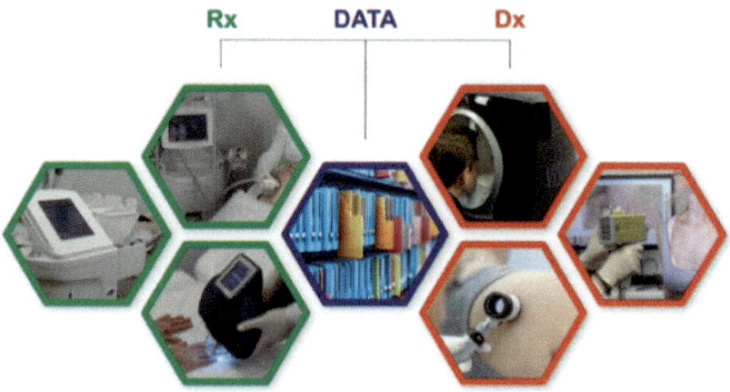

Fig. 16.1 Integration of diagnostic tools (Dx), therapeutic technologies (Rx), and patient data (DATA) in AI-driven laser platforms. AI algorithms utilize data to enhance diagnostic precision and guide personalized treatment protocols. (Designed by IQ SKIN CLINICS DESIGN DEPARTMENT—Christoforos Tzermias)

satisfaction. Moreover, innovations such as embedded imaging within laser applicators [7], real-time dermoscopic mapping [8], and adaptive control of energy delivery [8, 9] are driving a new era of integrative laser systems that combine diagnosis, therapy, and data analysis in one integrated platform [2] (Fig. 16.1). This level of integrated imaging supports adaptive treatment by enabling real-time monitoring, automatic adjustments, and personalization of the therapeutic dose based on immediate feedback effectively mimicking autonomous driving on a different scale. For example, built-in high-resolution visualization systems allow the device to detect skin contact and maintain optimal focus level, ensuring safe and effective energy delivery. During treatment, real-time dermoscopy maps are automatically generated, facilitating continuous guidance and lesion tracking. Between sessions, inter-treatment visualization provides clinicians with detailed insight into lesion placement, treatment progress, and target response. A particularly important technological advance in this context is focal point technology (FPT), a system that allows for precise control over treatment depth and injury pattern through conical thermal zones [10]. When integrated with imaging and pattern recognition software, FPT can selectively target skin structures such as pores, sebaceous glands, pigmented lesions, or vascular abnormalities, offering an additional layer of personalization and control. Its compatibility with AI-driven platforms opens new possibilities for customized treatment planning based on each patient's unique skin architecture.

This chapter aims to explore the multifaceted integration of AI into laser dermatology, with a particular emphasis on its synergy with innovative technologies. We will examine current applications, real-world tools, and future directions, offering a comprehensive overview of how AI is reshaping the landscape of laser skin care pushing the boundaries of personalization, safety, and technological sophistication.

16.2 Artificial Intelligence in Dermatologic Laser Applications

Artificial intelligence (AI) refers to a suite of computational technologies designed to replicate or enhance human cognitive functions such as pattern recognition, decision-making, and problem-solving. In laser dermatology, AI systems are increasingly employed to improve diagnostic accuracy, automate skin assessments, personalize treatment plans, and monitor patient outcomes [2]. These systems rely on methods such as machine learning (ML), deep learning (DL), artificial neural networks (ANNs), and convolutional neural networks (CNNs) [11], with applications that span both clinical practice and patient understanding. The integration of AI in this field addresses several key challenges.

First, it offers a means to reduce the subjectivity that has traditionally defined both aesthetic evaluation and treatment planning for common dermatologic conditions. For example, tools leveraging AI can detect and quantify fine lines, skin texture irregularities [12], pigmentation variations, postinflammatory erythema, and acne-related scarring with high consistency. These measurements are not only more precise but also reproducible, facilitating standardized documentation and outcome comparison across patient groups and treatment types.

Second, AI enables real-time, data-driven decision-making. Prior to administering procedures such as laser resurfacing, pigmented and vascular lesions treatment, AI can assess baseline skin conditions using image analysis, recommend the most appropriate laser parameters, and even simulate expected results [1, 2]. This facilitates greater transparency for patients and improves their engagement in the treatment planning process whether the objective is aesthetic enhancement or treatment of conditions like acne scarring and melasma. In more advanced implementations, AI systems are integrated directly into treatment devices, particularly in laser platforms, where they assist not only with pretreatment assessment, but also with live, intra-procedural analysis [8, 9]. These smart platforms detect intra-treatment skin changes and dynamically adjust settings modulating laser fluence and pulse duration in real time to ensure precise, safe energy delivery tailored to the tissue response.

AI also plays an essential role in enhancing accessibility. Mobile health applications equipped with AI-driven image analysis allow patients to conduct preliminary skin assessments from home [3], improving early detection and triage. While these applications were initially developed for medical dermatology (e.g., melanoma detection), they are now being repurposed for broader use evaluating wrinkles, pigmentation, acne lesions, and skin laxity with increasing accuracy making dermatologic screening more accessible, especially in underserved or remote populations [12].

Furthermore, AI augments clinical efficiency. Automated systems can assist in the documentation of treatment plans, monitor procedural endpoints (e.g., detecting pulsed dye laser purpura or blanching of Q-switched and pico laser or dynamic response during fractional laser), and predict treatment outcomes. This enables practitioners to focus more on patient interaction and clinical judgment, while AI handles routine assessments and follow-ups. As these systems evolve, we are witnessing the emergence of integrative AI-laser ecosystems, where diagnosis, visualization, treatment, and monitoring occur within a closed-loop, intelligent workflow. Such platforms not only enhance procedural precision but also continuously learn and improve based on cumulative patient data, paving the way for highly adaptive, self-optimizing laser dermatology interventions. Despite its early-stage development in certain areas, AI is rapidly becoming a transformative force balancing objectivity with the inherently variable nature of skin biology and perception. Its ability to analyze large, multimodal datasets positions it as a cornerstone of next-generation personalized laser dermatologic care.

16.3 AI-Enhanced Laser Applications in Dermatology

Laser technologies are foundational in modern dermatology, offering targeted interventions for a broad range of cosmetic and therapeutic skin concerns, including rejuvenation, pigmentary and vascular disorders, acne scars, and textural irregularities. AI transforms laser dermatology into a precision-guided modality, reducing variability and improving treatment reproducibility [2]. Laser systems integrated with AI can fine-tune pulse width, energy delivery, and treatment density based on real-time skin responses. By combining machine learning with dermatologic imaging, these systems are capable of offering consistently optimized outcomes [9].

(i) *AI in Pretreatment Assessment and Planning*

Before any laser therapy, a detailed skin analysis is critical for selecting appropriate laser parameters, including wavelength, fluence, pulse durations, and spot size. One of the most critical steps in ensuring successful laser treatments is an accurate understanding of a patient's skin characteristics. Traditional diagnostics rely heavily on manual inspection and the practitioner's experience. This approach, while effective, can sometimes lead to subjective results, especially for patients with more complex skin concerns or those with skin types that fall outside the typical parameters [13]. AI-based systems enhance this process by analyzing high-resolution skin imagery to detect pigmentation density, vascular irregularities, textural anomalies, and subdermal structures with far greater sensitivity than human observation alone.

Platforms like Canfield VISIA utilize cross-polarization and UV illumination mechanisms to measure both surface-level and subsurface-level skin conditions [14]. A notable example is the Canfield VISIA CR, which allows for visualization of different skin aspects, including vascularity, and has shown that using a water-absorbing wavelength instead of a traditional hemoglobin-targeting wavelength can result in deep welding of vascular structures, a remarkable finding with therapeutic implications. Utilization of this technology in clinical practice offers fine-tuned detection of distinct color characteristics that can lead to brown and red components of color concentration in conditions such as spider veins, port wine stains, and hyperpigmentation that can be then monitored more objectively and visualized more efficiently for the dermatologist to select the best treatment plan for their patient [12, 14]. The newest generation of dermoscopes includes in-built crossed polarizers, which aid in filtering out the peripheral scattered light, reducing glare, and helping in the visualization of substrata structure in the absence of linkage fluid [15]. Advanced devices, like FotoFinder, have whole-body mapping systems that help in detailed analyses and follow-up [7]. These tools offer clinically actionable data that guide laser selection and parameter optimization, while also highlighting potential risk zones, such as melanin-rich areas or regions with fragile vasculature, that may require lower energy delivery or modified technique.

Recent developments in AI-powered dermoscopy and imaging platforms allow for real-time high-resolution mapping of melanin distribution, vascular patterns, and scar topography [1]. These dynamic assessments help clinicians pre-emptively adjust treatment plans for both cosmetic procedures and dermatologic interventions, such as fractional resurfacing for acne scarring or vascular laser use in erythematous post-inflammatory lesions [2, 9]. AI not only aids in accurate skin classification (e.g., Fitzpatrick phototype), but also generates personalized heat maps of treatment priority areas, maximizing therapeutic precision while minimizing adverse effects. By translating large datasets into clinically meaningful insights within seconds, AI empowers practitioners to formulate targeted, patient-specific laser strategies, supporting both efficacy and safety before the first laser pulse is delivered.

(ii) *Real-Time Monitoring and Adaptive Laser Control*

Real-time AI analysis during laser procedures enables dynamic monitoring of treatment endpoints. For example, visual cues such as the subtle blanching effect in pigmented laser treatments can be identified and quantified by computer vision algorithms. Similarly, AI can assist in monitoring laser responses during procedures targeting acne scars or post-inflammatory erythema, ensuring uniform tissue interaction and minimizing adverse effects. Emerging AI systems also analyze thermal signatures during energy-based treatments, identifying hot spots or areas of inadequate exposure [8]. This is particularly beneficial in treating conditions such as pigmented lesions or atrophic scars, where consistent energy delivery is essential to avoid complications like postinflammatory hyperpigmentation (PIH) or insufficient collagen remodeling (Fig. 16.2).

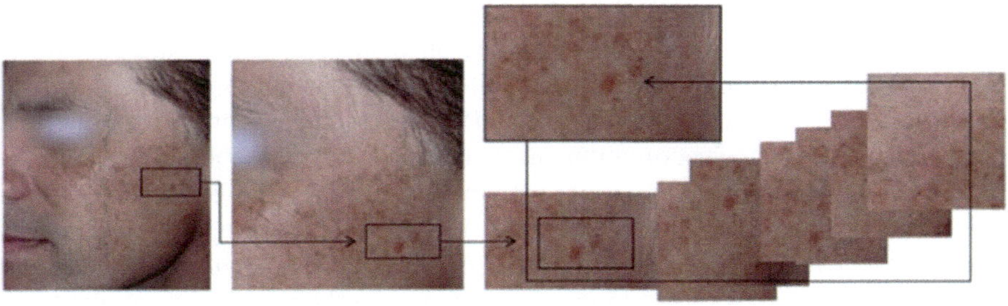

Fig. 16.2 Real-time visual dermoscopy mapping, automatically obtained, allowing clinicians to dynamically adjust laser parameters and treatment plans for optimal results. (Designed by IQ SKIN CLINICS DESIGN DEPARTMENT—Christoforos Tzermias)

In addition to monitoring, AI enables real-time adaptive control of laser parameters. Future systems, trained on thousands of treatment records, could dynamically adjust fluence and pulse duration based on intra-treatment feedback [9], such as skin temperature, moisture, or pigmentation density. These capabilities are especially important in patients with complex skin profiles or a history of pigmentary disorders. Moreover, such adaptive control helps reduce operator variability, ensuring consistency across treatments. Such intelligent platforms may eventually autonomously adapt energy output, avoiding overtreatment and improving both safety and efficacy. This represents a shift toward closed-loop AI-guided laser delivery where diagnosis, response, and adjustment are all automated.

(iii) *AI-Guided Laser Modalities and Applications*

The application of AI across various laser platforms is expanding rapidly. Laser systems, both ablative and nonablative, are increasingly being paired with convolutional neural networks (CNNs) to analyze high-resolution skin images and assist in optimizing treatment parameters [1, 10]. A key innovation supporting this evolution is focal point technology, which enables high precision in determining treatment depth. This precision can be further enhanced through AI-guided algorithms that modify laser patterning in real time, allowing for highly personalized and adaptive energy delivery based on real-time skin feedback [10]. In hair removal, long-pulsed Nd:YAG and long-pulsed Alexandrite lasers may utilize AI algorithms to adapt energy delivery based on real-time assessment of skin phototype and hair thickness, improving safety and efficacy, particularly in patients with darker skin tones [3]. Similarly, in the treatment of vascular and pigmented lesions, platforms incorporating AI models can tailor laser protocols by integrating patient-specific variables such as lesion morphology, chromophore concentration, and treatment history [2, 12]. These use cases demonstrate AI's evolving role not only as a pretreatment planning tool, but as a real-time procedural co-pilot, enhancing treatment precision, reducing operator variability, and minimizing the risk of adverse effects.

(iv) *Predictive Modeling and Outcome Simulation*

Predicting treatment outcomes is one of the most sought-after features in laser dermatologic care. AI models trained on thousands of pre- and post-treatment images can simulate expected results helping patients visualize improvements in wrinkles, skin tightening, pigmentation, vascularity, or scar remodeling. This capability enhances communication and informed consent, setting realistic expectations and improving patient satisfaction [1, 16]. Using extensive, transparent datasets from previous treatments, AI can predict not only the final results but also the expected recovery timeline [6]. This dual-layered prediction, outcome, and healing duration supports more precise scheduling, patient planning, and clinical decision-making, particularly in treatments where downtime and healing trajectory vary widely. For example, 3D simulation models can predict skin tightening treatments or estimate collagen remodeling in response to laser treatments by analyzing variations in epidermal thickness and skin texture across time [2, 9]. This level of personalization allows clinicians to fine-tune laser parameters before initiating the procedure, increasing the chances of optimal outcomes. Additionally, laser devices such as KTP (potassium titanyl phosphate) systems have been paired with machine learning algorithms that forecast individualized responses in the treatment of vascular and pigmented lesions [3, 12].

(v) *Post-treatment Monitoring and Longitudinal Data Tracking*

Traditional post-treatment evaluation has depended largely on visual inspection and photographic comparison. AI-based systems now offer objective tools to quantify laser treatment outcomes across sessions by analyzing changes in pigmentation, skin roughness, and wrinkle depth over time through standardized imaging and evaluation protocols, while in skin of color, they can additionally track progressive pigment normalization and vascular improvement across extended treatment courses [2, 3]. Such tools are particularly valuable in treatments requiring multiple sessions, including fractional laser therapy for acne scarring or skin rejuvenation. By comparing pre- and post-treatment imagery with AI models trained to recognize clinically significant changes, practitioners can monitor therapeutic progression with high precision [1]. Additionally, this data-driven tracking supports dynamic treatment plan adjustments, transforming the post-treatment phase into a feedback loop for ongoing optimization. Postcare is crucial in laser treatments, particularly in ensuring optimal results and preventing complications. AI systems are now being developed to assist in this phase as well. AI-based apps can track a patient's recovery progress by analyzing daily photographs and feedback from the patient. These systems monitor the healing process in real time, looking for signs of abnormal recovery, such as prolonged redness, swelling, or blistering [17]. By flagging potential concerns early, they can prompt timely clinical intervention and reduce the risk of adverse outcomes especially important in patients with sensitive or melanin-rich skin types.

(vi) *From Photothermolysis to AI-Assisted Laser Platforms*

The principle of selective photothermolysis, introduced in the 1980s, revolutionized laser dermatology by enabling selective targeting of chromophores like melanin and hemoglobin while minimizing damage to surrounding tissue. A major limitation of selective photothermolysis when treating targets in the dermis is that melanin in the overlying epidermis absorbs light across a broad optical spectrum, causing epidermal injury and resulting in decreased treatment efficacy. Injury to the epidermis and the dermoepidermal junction can cause potential side effects, including pain, blistering, inflammation, depigmentation, and/or postinflammatory hyperpigmentation (PIH). Various techniques for cooling the skin surface are utilized to reduce this problem, but the risk of epidermal damage remains a major limitation when treating patients with skin of color [18, 19]. To minimize the risk of adverse events, the laser fluence is often lowered, resulting in reduced efficacy for these patients [20, 21].

To improve selectivity and reduce downtime, fractional photothermolysis [22] was introduced, creating many small-scale columns of injury called microthermal treatment zones (MTZs) with intervening columns of intact skin to promote rapid healing [10, 23]. Fractional photothermolysis can be ablative or nonablative, depending on the optical absorption of that wavelength by tissue water [10]. Ablative fractional lasers (e.g., CO_2, Er:YAG) offer substantial improvements in texture and scarring but carry higher PIH risks, while nonablative systems (e.g., 1550 nm erbium-glass) are safer and better tolerated across skin types, albeit with more sessions required [24, 25]. This technology is limited by fixed tissue penetration depth, mainly dictated by wavelength and pulse energy. In darker skin types, lower energy settings increase treatment sessions and complication risks remain.

AI now introduces the next evolution, shifting from static presets to intelligent systems capable of real-time adaptation. AI-assisted fractional laser systems can assess parameters such as epidermal thickness, melanin concentration, hydration, and dermal temperature adjusting fluence, pulse duration, and treatment density accordingly [1, 8]. This dynamic modulation enhances both safety and efficacy, particularly in patients with melanin-rich skin, where conventional energy settings might lead to complications. Integrating technology, specifically the fusion of imaging, diagnostics, and machine learning, now allows for adaptive treatments with real-time monitoring and automated adjustments. Advanced systems are incorporating imaging and sensor-based modules directly into the laser handpiece, enabling visualization of skin structure, lesion targeting, and tissue response during treatment [9]. This combination of imaging to determine where energy needs to be focused allows for enhanced precision in energy delivery. This integration allows practitioners to

- Visualize thermal and structural skin changes in real time
- Track lesions and monitor endpoints dynamically
- Modify energy delivery by anatomical zone or response pattern

In the future, AI will enable practitioners to see, detect, and "shoot" specific targets with a high degree of precision. Clinical decision-making will no longer rely solely on the principle of selective photothermolysis. Instead, individual lesions can be directly targeted based on real-time feedback and image recognition, bringing to mind a level of automation and intelligence comparable to autonomous driving, but on a dermatologic scale (Fig. 16.3).

A notable advancement supporting this evolution is focal point technology (FPT), which offers precise control over treatment depth and the pattern of skin injury via a highly focused laser beam [10]. When combined with imaging and/or pattern recognition software, FPT laser system can selectively target detectable skin structures such as sweat ducts, surface features, pores, sebaceous glands, nonpigmented hair, and other traditional vascular and pigmented skin targets. The

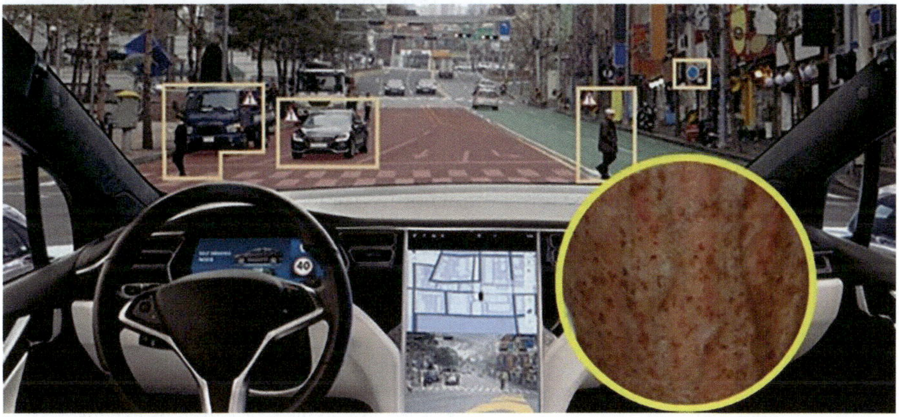

Fig. 16.3 Lesions can be accurately targeted through real-time feedback and image recognition, suggesting a level of automation and intelligence similar to that found in self-driving cars—though scaled to dermatologic applications. (Designed by IQ SKIN CLINICS DESIGN DEPARTMENT—Christoforos Tzermias)

technology provides control of lesion depth, allowing personalization of treatment based on the unique characteristics and anatomical location of the target [10]. Future enhancements to AI laser systems may enable subsurface visualization capabilities similar to optical coherent tomography or photoacoustic imaging [26]. When these are integrated with image processing algorithms, AI-enabled lasers can facilitate customizable or even fully personalized treatment plans, tailored to an individual's unique skin architecture and rare characteristics. This represents a promising step in the evolution of laser-based skin treatment. Eventually, such intelligent systems may evolve into closed-loop platforms that automatically detect, evaluate, and treat skin concerns blending diagnostic precision with therapeutic execution. This represents a new paradigm where AI laser technologies transform photothermolysis from a static procedural framework into a personalized, intelligent process advancing laser therapy toward greater adaptability and inclusivity across skin types [1, 8, 10]

16.4 AI-Guided Skin Quality Assessments for Laser Treatment Optimization

The efficacy, safety, and personalization of laser-based dermatologic interventions depend not only on lesion targeting but also on a detailed understanding of skin physiology. Factors such as hydration, oiliness, elasticity, pigmentation, and skin thickness significantly affect how laser energy interacts with tissue and thus impact treatment outcomes particularly in patients with skin of color [2, 3].

AI now plays a pivotal role in objectively quantifying these variables and converting them into optimized laser settings. AI-driven platforms can assess skin texture, pigmentation patterns, pore size, and vascular features through multispectral imaging and machine learning algorithms [12]. Multispectral imaging combined with AI classification allows precise quantification of skin texture and pigmentation variations, supporting personalized intervention strategies [2]. Moreover, some systems incorporate real-time feedback during treatment, enabling dynamic adjustment of laser parameters based on live measurements of skin response further improving safety and efficacy, especially in patients with higher risk for postinflammatory hyperpigmentation or variable dermal characteristics [9, 12].

(i) *Hydration and Barrier Function: Optimizing Energy Delivery*: The outermost layer of the skin system, known as the skin barrier, serves as a protective wall that shields the body from external hazards and maintains the body's homeostasis by regulating water loss. A traditional approach to assessing the efficacy of the skin barrier function is estimating trans epidermal water loss (TEWL), which can be time-consuming [2]. To speed up this process, a machine learning algorithm was introduced that utilizes topological data analysis to forecast skin barrier function by analyzing skin images [27]. Microscopic skin images were utilized to identify the structural characteristics of the skin through the application of topological data analysis. They found a strong correlation between the topological characteristics and the trans epidermal water loss [2]. Skin moisture and thickness can be precisely measured by noninvasive imaging methods such as touch capacitive imaging, high-resolution ultrasound imaging, and high-resolution magnetic resonance imaging. Such advancements in AI technologies provided a strong basis for creating treatment plans and the opportunity to create more specialized goods and treatments that cater to the particular demands of different skin types [2]. Real-time maps of skin hydration, melanin density, or vascularity, can influence fluence modulation [8]; post-treatment imaging helps quantify inflammation or monitor recovery, particularly in conditions like rosacea. Intra-treatment visualization via embedded imaging modules supports precise lesion targeting, endpoint detection and real-time focus or contact adjustments [7]. These AI-enhanced capabilities form the basis of closed-loop laser systems, where imaging is not merely observational but actively drives personalized and adaptive therapeutic interventions. This data-rich environment informs clinical choices such as laser modality (ablative vs. non-ablative), fluence and pulse duration settings, and post-treatment care strategies tailored to reinforce barrier recovery.

(ii) *Sebum, Pores, and Surface Texture: Informing Treatment Zones and Modalities*: Sebum production and pore structure influence energy absorption and post-treatment skin behavior. Overactive sebaceous glands may increase susceptibility to PIH, acneiform eruptions, or irritation after aggressive treatments like fractional lasers. AI-powered image analysis, using CNNs, quantifies sebum distribution, pore density and size, and roughness indices across affected skin. These inputs support protocol decisions, such as applying lower energy density in oily zones, or using nonablative/hybrid lasers. In acne-prone or seborrheic skin types, such AI insights provide safe and effective laser interventions [2].

(iii) *Elasticity, Laxity, and Collagen Mapping: Targeting Rejuvenation Zones*: Laser therapies aimed at dermal remodeling benefit from accurate mapping of elasticity and collagen architecture. AI platforms analyze wrinkle morphology, tissue deformation, and subsurface collagen distribution via imaging tools like high-frequency ultrasound or structured light. Therapeutically, these assessments assist in tracking collagen remodeling over time, helping refine protocols and enhance clinical outcomes across sessions [2].

16.5 AI-Driven Planning, Prediction, and Monitoring in Laser Cosmetic and Therapeutic Applications

Laser-based procedures in dermatology require careful planning, individualized parameter selection, and consistent follow-up. Traditionally, these elements have relied on clinical expertise and subjective visual assessment. With artificial intelligence (AI), this workflow is evolving into a data-driven, adaptive model that supports both cosmetic outcomes and treatment of skin conditions or diseases (Table 16.1).

Before treatment, AI-powered platforms integrate facial imaging, dermatoscopic data, and patient history to simulate expected results across a range of applications [3, 7, 8]. AI algorithms can analyze thousands of data points, including melanin levels, vascular structures, pore size, and skin texture in a fraction of a second. The data collected through these algorithms provides practitioners with a more objective, comprehensive understanding of a patient's skin before proceeding with laser treatments [8]. AI can also personalize treatment recommendations based on patient

Table 16.1 Traditional vs. AI-driven laser therapy

Parameter	Traditional laser therapy	AI-driven laser therapy
Treatment planning	Based on visual inspection and practitioner experience	Guided by quantified skin analysis and AI-based modeling
Parameter adjustment	Manual settings	Real-time adaptive modulation based on live feedback
Outcome prediction	Subjective estimation	Predictive simulation using pre/post datasets
Monitoring	Post-treatment only	Continuous intra- and post-treatment tracking
Safety for skin of color	Dependent on practitioner skill	Automated adjustment to minimize PIH and optimize safety
Consistency	Variable between sessions/providers	Standardized and reproducible protocols

Comparison between traditional and AI-driven approaches in laser treatments, highlighting differences in planning, safety, and precision data, including medical history, symptoms, and treatment results, enhancing diagnostic accuracy and clinical decision-making, which can significantly improve patient outcomes [3]. During treatment, AI-assisted laser platforms can dynamically analyze skin hydration, thickness, and melanin content to adjust fluence and pulse parameters in real time. This is particularly valuable in treating conditions like rosacea or port-wine stains, where vascular variability requires precise energy control [8, 9]. Similarly, in resurfacing or scar revision, AI helps minimize thermal injury and optimize coagulation zones [2]. After treatment, AI supports objective, longitudinal monitoring through standardized image capture and skin metric analysis. This includes tracking healing, pigmentation rebound, collagen remodeling, or recurrence of vascular lesions. Such systems reduce reliance on subjective grading and enhance early detection of complications such as PIH, especially in multisession therapies like fractional photothermolysis [3]. In both cosmetic and therapeutic contexts, AI enables dynamic protocol refinement based on accumulated data. As each session contributes to the algorithm's training, future treatments become more personalized, predictive, and efficient, transforming laser dermatology into a continuously improving clinical discipline.

16.6 Future Directions in AI-Driven Laser Dermatology

The integration of artificial intelligence (AI) into dermatologic laser systems represents a major advance in both cosmetic and therapeutic practice. AI enables dynamic treatment planning, intra-procedural adaptation, and longitudinal patient monitoring. However, this progress introduces significant safety and ethical considerations, particularly as AI tools gain greater autonomy and influence over clinical workflows [1, 2, 8]. Additionally, data privacy and security are critical concerns, as AI systems require access to extensive personal and biometric data, including high-resolution skin imagery, treatment histories, and demographic information to function effectively [6, 28]. Moreover, the absence of universal standards and guidelines for AI-based dermatologic tools may lead to variability in system performance and clinical outcomes. To address this, there is a growing need for standardized testing protocols and regulatory frameworks to ensure these technologies meet rigorous safety, reliability, and efficacy benchmarks before being widely adopted in clinical practice [29].

The future of AI in dermatology lies in synergistic collaboration, not replacement, between machine precision and human clinical insight. This vision of augmented aesthetic intelligence encompasses both cosmetic and therapeutic interventions, where AI serves to enhance decision-making, personalize treatments, and optimize outcomes across the spectrum of skin concerns [1, 8].Emerging AI platforms integrate multimodal data, such as high-resolution imaging, barrier function metrics, elasticity assessments, and patient-specific clinical records, to guide procedures like wrinkle reduction, pigmentation correction, and the treatment of vascular or inflammatory lesions. These AI-enhanced systems dynamically adapt to skin physiology and healing responses, enabling more accurate and safer treatments

[1, 2, 9]. Furthermore, emotional and lifestyle factors, such as anxiety or tolerance for downtime, can be incorporated into clinical decisions, supporting truly context-aware personalization [1, 2, 8]. Ultimately, this paradigm shift toward learning-enabled, adaptive systems supports a continuous feedback loop. Data from each session refines future predictions, simulates outcomes more accurately, and enhances long-term care planning across both cosmetic goals and therapeutic needs [1, 2].

Building on current advances in real-time imaging and intelligent feedback, upcoming platforms are expected to integrate high-resolution dermal scanning, thermal and hydration sensors, and automated visual endpoint detection (e.g., blanching, coagulation, microthermal zone formation). These capabilities enable on-the-fly modulation of laser fluence, pulse duration, and spot size, adjusting energy delivery in response to live skin responses [7–9]. Such functionality may support semi-autonomous workflows, where lesions are algorithmically identified, treatment boundaries are delineated, and energy application is initiated under physician supervision. Applications may include vascular lesion targeting, scar remodeling, pigmentation correction, or even early neoplastic detection, combining diagnostic and therapeutic logic in one adaptive system [7–9]. Crucially, these AI systems are trained on extensive, anonymized datasets to improve accuracy, safety, and personalization over time. However, greater autonomy also raises ethical and regulatory needs, from physician override mechanisms to validation across diverse skin types, and transparent algorithmic pathways [6, 30]. In this evolving landscape, human expertise and AI precision define the next frontier in dermatologic care.

16.7 Conclusion

The integration of artificial intelligence (AI) with laser technologies represents a pivotal evolution in dermatologic practice. What was once constrained by operator-dependent variability and generalized protocols is now transforming into a dynamic system of adaptive, data-informed care. AI enhances all stages of laser interventions: it enables individualized planning through outcome simulations, optimizes treatment parameters based on skin metrics such as phototype, hydration, and melanin density, and offers real-time procedural guidance via visual and physiological feedback mechanisms. Post-treatment, AI supports objective monitoring, ensuring consistent results and early identification of complications. Among the key innovations supporting this shift is focal point technology (FPT), which allows for highly localized control of laser energy delivery. When combined with AI-driven imaging and pattern recognition, FPT enables selective targeting of microscopic skin structures based on real-time skin analysis, improving both efficacy and safety across diverse patient populations. It exemplifies how precision hardware and intelligent software can converge to support personalized dermatologic interventions. Critically, this transformation is not about replacing clinicians, but about augmenting their judgment and capabilities. Intelligent systems provide rapid, multidimensional analysis; practitioners contribute clinical insight and human connection. Together, they create a new paradigm of augmented dermatologic intelligence where laser treatment becomes both more personal and more standardized. As these technologies evolve, they also raise ethical imperatives: ensuring fairness across skin types, maintaining transparency in algorithmic reasoning, and preserving clinician oversight. These dimensions must remain integral as AI becomes increasingly embedded into the core infrastructure of laser platforms.

References

1. Thunga S, Khan M, Cho SI, Na JI, Yoo J. AI in aesthetic/cosmetic dermatology: current and future. J Cosmet Dermatol. 2025;24:e16640. https://doi.org/10.1111/jocd.16640.
2. Vatiwutipong P, Vachmanus S, Noraset T, Tuarob S. Artificial intelligence in cosmetic dermatology: a systematic literature review. IEEE Access. 2023; Published: July 13, 2023. https://doi.org/10.1109/ACCESS.2023.3295001.
3. Fliorent R, Fardman B, Podwojniak A, et al. Artificial intelligence in dermatology: advancements and challenges in skin of color. Int J Dermatol. 2024;63:455–61.
4. Chakraborty A. Disease severity scores in dermatology: an update of the various indices. Indian J Dermatol Venereol Leprol. 2023;21:1–15. https://doi.org/10.25259/IJDVL_592_2021.
5. Humphrey S, Manson Brown S, Cross SJ, Mehta R. Defining skin quality: clinical relevance, terminology, and assessment. Dermatologic Surg. 2021;47(7):974–81. https://doi.org/10.1097/dss.0000000000003079.
6. Daneshjou R, Kittler H. Empowering the next generation of artificial intelligence in dermatology: the datasets and benchmarks track. J Invest Dermatol. 2024;144(3):437–8. https://doi.org/10.1016/j.jid.2023.11.011.
7. Jartarkar SR, Patil A, Wollina U, et al. New diagnostic and imaging technologies in dermatology. J Cosmet Dermatol. 2021;20(12):3782–7. https://doi.org/10.1111/jocd.14499.
8. Haykal D. Harnessing AI in laser aesthetic treatments: revolutionizing precision, safety, and personalization. J Cosmet Dermatol. 2024;0:e16704. https://doi.org/10.1111/jocd.16704.
9. Elder A, Ring C, Heitmiller K, Gabriel Z, Saedi N. The role of artificial intelligence in cosmetic dermatology—current, upcoming, and future trends. J Cosmet Dermatol. 2021;20(1):48–52. https://doi.org/10.1111/jocd.13797.
10. Manstein D, Chan HH, Bhawalkar J, et al. Focal point technology: controlling treatment depth and pattern of skin injury by a novel highly focused laser. J Am Acad Dermatol. 2024; https://doi.org/10.1016/j.jaad.2024.09.004.
11. De A, Sarda A, Gupta S, Das S. Use of artificial intelligence in dermatology. Indian J Dermatol. 2020;65(5):352–7. https://doi.org/10.4103/ijd.IJD_418_20.
12. Kania B, Montecinos K, Goldberg DJ. Artificial intelligence in cosmetic dermatology. J Cosmet Dermatol. 2024;23(10):3305–11. https://doi.org/10.1111/jocd.16538.
13. Haykal D, Cartier H, Maire C, Mordon S. Picosecond lasers in cosmetic dermatology: where are we now? An overview of types and indications. Lasers Med Sci. 2023;39(1):8. https://doi.org/10.1007/s10103-023-03945-5.
14. Holcomb JD. Helium plasma dermal resurfacing: VISIA CR assessment of facial spots, pores, and wrinkles-preliminary findings. J Cosmet Dermatol. 2021;20:1668–78. https://doi.org/10.1111/jocd.14106.
15. Sonthalia S, Yumeen S, Kaliyadan F. Dermoscopy a review and extra-diagnostic applications. In: Stat Pearls (internet). Stat Pearls Publishing; 2021. https://www.ncbi.nlm.nih.gov/books/NBK537131/.

16. Haykal D, Cartier H, du Crest D, Galadari H, Landau M, Haddad A. What happens when simulations get real and cosmetic dermatology goes virtual? J Cosmet Dermatol. 2023;22:2682–4. https://doi.org/10.1111/jocd.15888.
17. Hogarty DT, Su JC, Phan K, et al. Artificial intelligence in dermatology—where we are and the way to the future: a review. Am J Clin Dermatol. 2020;21(1):41–7. https://doi.org/10.1007/s40257-019-00462-6.
18. Kung K-Y, Shek SY-N, Yeung CK, Chan HH-L. Evaluation of the safety and efficacy of the dual wavelength picosecond laser for the treatment of benign pigmented lesions in Asians. Lasers Surg Med. 2019;51(1):14–22. https://doi.org/10.1002/lsm.23028.
19. Breadon JY, Barnes CA. Comparison of adverse events of laser and light-assisted hair removal systems in skin types IV–VI. J Drugs Dermatol. 2007;6(1):40–6.
20. Hu S, Atmakuri M, Rosenberg J. Adverse events of nonablative lasers and energy-based therapies in subjects with Fitzpatrick skin phototypes IV to VI: a systematic review and metaanalysis. Aesthet Surg J. 2022;42(5):537–47. https://doi.org/10.1093/asj/sjab398.
21. Handley JM. Adverse events associated with nonablative cutaneous visible and infrared laser treatment. J Am Acad Dermatol. 2006;55(3):482–9. https://doi.org/10.1016/j.jaad.2006.03.029.
22. Manstein D, Herron GS, Sink RK, Tanner H, Anderson RR. Fractional photothermolysis: a new concept for cutaneous remodeling using microscopic patterns of thermal injury. Lasers Surg Med. 2004;34(5):426–38. https://doi.org/10.1002/lsm.20048.
23. Geronemus RG. Fractional photothermolysis: current and future applications. Lasers Surg Med. 2006;38(3):169–76. https://doi.org/10.1002/lsm.20310.
24. Shamsaldeen O, Peterson JD, Goldman MP. The adverse events of deep fractional CO_2: a retrospective study of 490 treatments in 374 patients. Lasers Surg Med. 2011;43(6):453–6. https://doi.org/10.1002/lsm.21079.
25. Chan HHL, Manstein D, Yu CS, Shek S, Kono T, Wei WI. The prevalence and risk factors of post-inflammatory hyperpigmentation after fractional resurfacing in Asians. Lasers Surg Med. 2007;39(5):381–5. https://doi.org/10.1002/lsm.20512.
26. Attia ABE, Balasundaram G, Moothanchery M, et al. A review of clinical photoacoustic imaging: current and future trends. Photoacoustics. 2019;16:100144. https://doi.org/10.1016/j.pacs.2019.100144.
27. Koseki K, Kawasaki H, Atsugi T, Nakanishi M, Mizuno M, Naru E, Ebihara T, Amagai M, Kawakami E. Assessment of skin barrier function using skin images with topological data analysis. NPJ Syst Biol Appl. 2020;6(1):40.
28. Hosseini Z, Nyholm S, Le Blanc PM, Preenen PTY, Demerouti E. Assessing the artificially intelligent workplace: an ethical framework for evaluating experimental technologies in workplace settings. AI Ethics. 2023;21:1–13. https://doi.org/10.1007/s43681-023-00265-w.
29. Jobin A, Ienca M, Vayena E. The global landscape of AI ethics guidelines. Nat Mach Intell. 2019;1(9):389–99. https://doi.org/10.1038/s42256-019-0088-2.
30. Roche C, Wall PJ, Lewis D. Ethics and diversity in artificial intelligence policies. Strateg Initiat AI Ethics. 2022;6:1–21. https://doi.org/10.1007/s43681-022-00218-9.

Part V

Artificial Intelligence in Hair and Nail Disorders

Hair Disorders and Artificial Intelligence 17

Alexandros Katoulis, Stella-Maria Michelaki,
and Georgia Pappa

17.1 Introduction

Hair disorders, ranging from nonscarring types to complex scarring entities, constitute a significant part of dermatologic practice. While the majority of them do not pose a significant risk to one's overall health, they rather represent a cosmetic issue, carry a significant psychosocial burden, and negatively impact patients' quality of life [1]. Diagnosing and managing alopecia often requires a multistep approach, combining clinical examination, detailed patient history, laboratory work-up, and trichoscopy [2]. Trichoscopy has transformed our ability to assess scalp and hair pathology non-invasively, offering magnified, in vivo visualization of the hair shafts, follicular ostia, perifollicular changes, and scalp skin morphology [3]. It has become an essential component in the dermatologist's toolkit, almost like what a stethoscope is for an internist.

However, despite its diagnostic value, trichoscopy is inherently operator-dependent. Accurate interpretation requires considerable training and experience.

A. Katoulis (✉)
2nd Department of Dermatology and Venereology, Medical School, National and Kapodistrian University of Athens, Attikon General University Hospital, Athens, Greece

S.-M. Michelaki
1st Department of Dermatology-Venereology, "Andreas Syggros" Hospital for Cutaneous and Venereal Diseases, National and Kapodistrian University of Athens, Medical School, Athens, Greece

G. Pappa
2nd Department of Dermatology and Venereology, "Attikon" General University Hospital, Medical School, National and Kapodistrian University of Athens, Athens, Greece

1st Department of Dermatology-Venereology, "Andreas Syggros" Hospital for Cutaneous and Venereal Diseases, National and Kapodistrian University of Athens, Medical School, Athens, Greece

E. Karampinis et al. (eds.), *Artificial Intelligence Applications in Dermatology*,
https://doi.org/10.1007/978-3-032-15614-3_17

That is where artificial intelligence steps in. Initially used for the evaluation of pigmented and nonpigmented skin lesions (mainly to distinguish benign from malignant), it is gradually expanding into new areas, including hair disorders. By analyzing thousands of image patterns, AI can learn to detect key features of hair disorders with great consistency. For clinicians early in their training, it can serve as a second set of eyes, while for experienced dermatologists, it can help track subtle changes over time.

What makes this even more outstanding is how well AI performs in cases where visual assessment is complex or subjective. A good example comes from a study by Daniels and colleagues in 2021, which explored how AI could evaluate changes in hair following cosmetic treatments [4]. Their findings highlighted that machine learning algorithms could quantify changes in hair volume, fiber alignment, and short, unruly (flyaway) hairs (all subtle features that are really difficult to assess consistently with the naked eye). In fact, when human assessors evaluated the same images, their results only partially aligned with the AI's analysis, especially when viewing flat, two-dimensional photos [4]. The AI, on the other hand, was able to identify differences across various time points and even distinguish between treated and untreated hair with high accuracy [4].

For dermatologists, especially those treating patients for hair disorders, this kind of precision can be revolutionary. Most importantly, it opens the door to making expert-level evaluations more widely accessible, especially in settings where trichology expertise may be limited or unavailable. It also underscores the value of objective, reproducible assessment in a field where diagnosis often depends on visual interpretation and pattern recognition.

Interestingly enough, some of the earliest uses of AI in dermatology focused not on analyzing hair but rather on eliminating it [5, 6]. Hair strands interfered with the assessment of pigmented skin lesions in dermoscopic images, introducing artifacts, prompting the development of algorithms like DullRazor or E-shaver to eliminate hair and improve diagnostic clarity digitally [5, 6]. This initial focus on image enhancement laid the foundation for more advanced applications. Today, AI plays a central role in trichology. With the support of high-resolution imaging and deep learning techniques, such as convolutional neural networks (CNNs), AI now contributes to everything from diagnosing scalp conditions to assisting in robotic hair restoration. The following sections explore how AI is being applied specifically to hair disorders, shedding light on the transformative potential of these technologies in everyday dermatologic practice.

17.2 AI-Powered Diagnosis in Hair Disorders

The first true AI systems developed for hair evaluation focused on quantitative metrics. Manual hair counting had long been the standard in both research and clinical trials, but it was a really slow, copious, and imprecise procedure, marked by significant inter-observed variability. A major milestone was the introduction of TrichoScan®, developed in the mid-2000s by Hoffmann and colleagues [7]. This system was the first clinically validated, AI-powered digital trichogram, which combined epiluminescence microscopy (dermoscopy) with automated image analysis [7]. For the first time, clinicians could obtain objective data on hair density (hairs/cm^2), shaft diameter (μm), anagen-to-telogen ratio, and hair growth rate (mm/day) [7]. These parameters are crucial for diagnosing and differentiating between conditions like androgenetic alopecia and telogen effluvium, but also monitoring their progress [7]. Its intra- and inter-operator correlation was impressively high, 91% and 97%, respectively, enabling clinicians to monitor the effects of treatments like finasteride with greater accuracy and less subjectivity [7]. TrichoScan® represented a turning point, moving from subjective manual methods to digital analysis, and became particularly valuable in hair transplant planning and clinical trials due to its standardization and reproducibility [7]. Despite its strengths, TrichoScan® has several limitations: it requires hair clipping and dyeing, which introduces variability and patient discomfort; it has difficulty detecting very fine vellus hairs; and the full procedure can take up to 20 min, making it less practical for use in busy clinical settings [7].

Around the same period, flatbed scanning-based systems, like the one proposed by Vallotton and Thomas, introduced automated body hair counting and length measurement [8]. Unlike TrichoScan®, which focused on scalp hair, their system targeted sparser and finer body hair, particularly useful in assessing the results of depilatory treatments [7, 8]. A remarkable feature of this technology was the detection of linear features (i.e., hairs) even under difficult conditions, such as variations in skin texture or low contrast [8]. The system demonstrated less than 10% discrepancy compared to manual counts and could process two high-resolution images per minute [8]. However, it required trimming the hair to approximately 4 mm and relied on subjects placing a cardboard frame on flat anatomical areas [8]. Moreover, it could not reliably process overlapping or curly hairs, limiting its application to scalp trichology [8]. Despite these weaknesses, it represented a step forward in non-invasive, reproducible evaluation of hair across broader anatomical sites, using a value-based threshold, angle-dependent tracing, and segmental graph growth [8].

A few years later, Folliscope®, developed by LeadM Corp. in South Korea, took things a step further by making it possible to examine untrimmed hair [9]. Using high-resolution microscopic images (typically at 50× magnification), corresponding to a 31.07 mm^2 area, it uses AI to measure hair shaft thickness and density [9]. Each labeled square in the system can register up to four hair shafts, allowing efficient, high-resolution counting even in densely packed areas [9]. Its advantage lies in the ability to analyze hair in situ, without requiring patients to cut or dye their hair [9]. Its utility has been demonstrated in ethnically diverse populations [9, 10]. For instance, in a study conducted in the USA, Folliscope® was used to compare hair densities across Hispanic, African American, and Caucasian cohorts, highlighting its robustness in assessing various hair types and densities [10].

As hardware continued to advance and CNNs emerged dynamically, AI evolved from simple hair counting to pattern recognition and, subsequently, diagnosis. A significant leap occurred in 2015, when Shih et al. developed a 23-layer deep CNN for analyzing microscopic scalp images [11]. Their goal was to create a tool that could count hairs, measure shaft thickness and length, and even evaluate scalp oiliness from high-magnification microscope images [11]. What distinguished this system was its ability to handle real-world image imperfections, such as curly or oily hair, and overlapping strands, which often confounded simpler algorithms of the past [11]. To achieve this, the team designed a multistep process. First, they enhanced the image contrast and eliminated bright reflections caused by an oily scalp or damp hair, which can often make hairs "disappear" under the microscope [11]. Then, using a modified version of the classic Hough transform, a well-established technique originally developed to detect straight lines in images by mapping edge points into a parametric space [12], they detected hairs of varying lengths at multiple image scales [11]. To address overlapping hairs, they introduced a technique called parallel line bundling, which allowed the system to identify and reconstruct hidden hairs based on edge patterns [11]. Finally, the algorithm linked individual segments to form recognizable hair strands. This method delivered outstanding performance, achieving a precision rate of over 96% and a recall rate close to 89%, meaning the system could count most hairs accurately, even under challenging conditions [11]. It also performed excellently in measuring features like diameter and length [11]. The tool was primarily trained on dark hair, which limited its accuracy in individuals with blond or gray hair [11]. It also required high-magnification microscopy, which is not standard in most clinics. Like many deep learning models, it functioned as a black box delivering accurate results but lacked transparency, which may diminish clinical trust in subtle or complex cases. In 2018, Podlodowski et al. advanced the field by developing an ensemble of deep CNNs aimed at detecting hair follicles rather than just hair shafts [13]. Their system analyzed high-resolution scalp images by dividing them into smaller squares and examined not only the square itself but also its surrounding areas to improve accuracy near the edges [13]. Although this system performed best in the ESENSEI challenge (a competition focused on follicle detection from microscopic scalp images), it required significant computational power, making it less practical for everyday practice [13, 14]. Moreover, while it marks hair follicles, it does not account for shaft morphology, scalp inflammation, or clinical context [13].

In the years that followed, AI-integrated trichoscopy systems rapidly proliferated. One such example is HairMetrix® by Canfield Scientific (Fig. 17.1) [15]. Unlike earlier tools such as TrichoScan®, which require hair clipping and dyeing to generate reliable results, HairMetrix® embeds AI in digital dermoscopes. It analyzes trichoscopic images taken during patient visits and measures total hair count, terminal-to-vellus hair ratio, and miniaturized hair (Figs. 17.2 and 17.3) [7, 15]. This makes it especially useful for diagnosing conditions like androgenetic alopecia, planning hair transplants, and tracking how diseases progress [15].

Nowadays, the trend is to make AI-based scalp assessment tools accessible for everyone and not just for specialist clinics. AI systems, including user-friendly at-home devices, are being developed to support both specialists and patients in managing hair conditions [16]. A notable development is ScalpEye, the system introduced by Chang et al.. It combines a portable digital microscope with a mobile application that connects to a cloud-based deep learning server [17]. Users, either

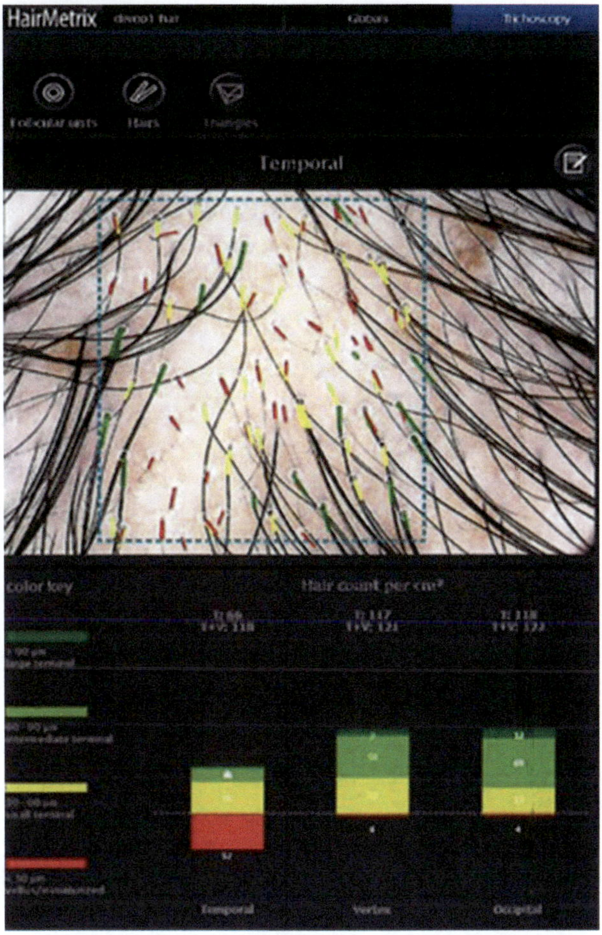

Fig. 17.1 HairMetrix scalp analysis. The system uses AI to identify and classify hair shafts by diameter and density. It provides measurements such as total hair count, terminal-to-vellus ratio, and follicular unit density in specific scalp zones

patients or clinicians, can capture close-up scalp images that are then analyzed remotely by a CNN trained on over 10,000 images labeled by dermatologists [17]. The system can distinguish between common conditions such as dandruff, folliculitis, oily scalp, and nonspecific hair loss, achieving an overall accuracy of over 95% [17].

In summary, AI is gradually transforming how we approach diagnosis in hair disorders. While each system is characterized by unique strengths, they are also accompanied by clear limitations that restrict its generalizability and extensive use. As algorithms grow more sophisticated and datasets become more inclusive, AI will probably become an integral part of clinical diagnosis.

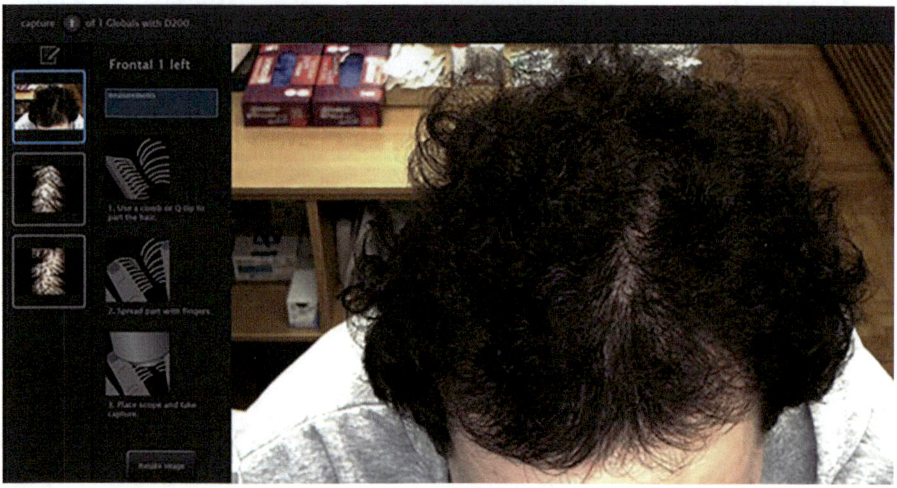

Fig. 17.2 Global scalp image showing visible thinning along the midline before treatment

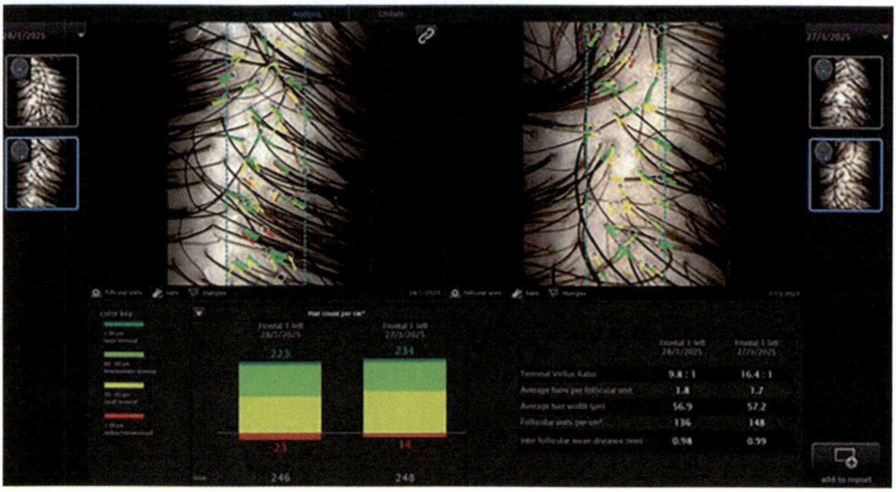

Fig. 17.3 Trichoscopic comparison before (left) and after treatment (right) of the same patient. The system enables precise analysis over time, showing improved hair density and terminal:vellus ratio post treatment

17.3 AI-Powered Staging and Prognosis in Hair Disorders

Staging hair disorders has always been an essential part of clinical practice. Establishing the severity at baseline is crucial, not only to understand the starting point of the disease, but also to assess treatment response over time [18]. Dermatologists have traditionally relied on inspection, comparison of images, and structured grading systems like the Hamilton–Norwood or Ludwig–Savin scales, in male and female pattern hair loss, respectively [19, 20]. These tools, while clinically useful, are quite subjective and limited by inter-observer variability [19, 20]. Moreover, the majority of the time, they fail to capture subtle changes in disease progression.

AI is now beginning to close that gap, as it has introduced new, objective, image-based methods for disease staging [21]. In this context, a recent study developped a support vector machine model, an algorithm that recognizes patterns and classifies data by determining the most effective boundary between categories [21]. This model uses three objective trichoscopic markers, namely the vellus hair count, the number of empty follicles, and the presence of follicular units with single hair, in order to classify patients as having either mild or moderate-to-severe androgenetic alopecia [21]. Using images from 200 patients processed through Trichoscale Pro®, the model achieved accuracy rates of 94.3% and 90.0% for the training and test sets, respectively, and areas under the curve of 0.99 and 0.95, respectively [21]. Interestingly, the algorithm also provides a probability score (from 50% to 100%) indicating the confidence of the classification, which could serve as a quantitative severity index [21].

Female pattern hair loss (FMPH) staging has also been substantially improved by computer-aided imaging systems. Hung et al. developed and validated a system that measures the central balding area (CBA) in square millimeters [22]. Their study included 38 Chinese women with FPHL, ranging from Savin stage I-2 to II-2 [22]. More specifically, the system can convert irregular balding patches into an equivalent ellipse, allowing the ellipse's width to be correlated with Ludwig–Savin scale stages [22]. The study demonstrated a clear progression in average CBA with increasing clinical severity: 3828.8 mm^2 in stage I-2; 5880.4 mm^2 in I-3; 8267.4 mm^2 in I-4; 12,999.3 mm^2 in II-1; and 15,979.7 mm^2 in II-2 [22]. All inter-stage differences were statistically significant ($p < 0.05$), and the system's measurements closely matched the Ludwig–Savin scale [22]. Importantly, exposure correction was found to affect results by 7.5% [22]. This emphasizes how important it is to maintain consistent photo conditions for accurate results. The system provides a more reliable way to assess disease severity than traditional ways, making it easier to track disease progression or treatment response. However, it needs to be evaluated in a larger population, including individuals with different hair types and ethnic backgrounds.

Furthermore, AI is gaining ground in alopecia areata (AA), where staging and monitoring also remain crucial for both clinical practice and research. The commonly used Severity of Alopecia Tool (SALT) score relies on subjective estimation and is often difficult to assess accurately, even for experienced dermatologists [23]. Any attempts to redefine the score have made it even more complicated [24]. Two major advancements have helped standardize SALT scoring. First, Lee et al. introduced a deep learning model called AloNet, trained on over 2700 standardized scalp images from 679 patients [25]. The system accurately segmented both the scalp and hair loss areas, achieving high Jaccard similarity coefficients, 0.941 for the scalp and 0.963 for alopecic regions, respectively [25]. In a validation study with eight dermatologists, AI-assisted assessments significantly reduced measurement errors and improved interrater reliability [25]. Most importantly, when the AI-generated data was used, especially with changes tracked over time (SALTtemporal), the SALT score became much better at predicting how well patients would respond to treatment [25].

In addition, Bernardis and Castelo-Soccio developed another method that uses texture analysis, examining pixel patterns in images to tell the difference between healthy hair, thinning, and alopecic areas [26]. Their algorithm was trained on images from children and young adults, aged 2–21, and could calculate SALT scores in just a few seconds, compared to the average 7 minutes it usually takes clinicians [26]. The system's results were very close to expert evaluations, with only a small error margin (0.31) and better accuracy than older methods like grayscale thresholding [26]. What makes it especially useful is that it does not just detect alopecic areas, it can also identify early hair thinning, giving a more detailed view of the severity of the hair loss [26].

Although still evolving, these early models are already changing the way we measure disease severity, plan follow-up, and define treatment response.

17.4 AI-Integrated Treatment Approach of Hair Disorders

Until recently, clinician-based diagnostic and treatment avenues have been the sole assessment and decision-making tool. AI has made way for promising new models of disease diagnosis and progression prediction, ultimately leading to personalization of treatment plans in hair and scalp disorders.

AI predictive algorithms for alopecia areata have already been developed. For instance, Alarcón-Soldevilla et al. analyzed 80 trichoscopic images and grouped them into the presence or absence of prognostic features [27]. The algorithm indicated 80% accuracy in non-responder predictions and 81% accuracy in responder predictions, which had favorable treatment outcomes [27].

Interestingly, the FDA-approved robotic system for hair restoration, the ARTAS robotic system, represents a notable advancement in hair restoration [28]. This system uses proprietary AI technology in order to analyze and detect follicular units; more specifically, their exact location, angle, and direction [28]. A robotic arm is capable of excising follicular units, with minimal scarring [28]. This innovative approach has led to the automation of follicular unit transplantation and has given surgeons a valuable tool for digital recipient sites planning, allowing for [28].

Moreover, AI-based recommendations for personalized scalp cosmetics have been explored. Kim et al. [29] developed a CNN based on the Scalp Photographic Index to objectively assess key scalp features, including dryness, greasiness, erythema, folliculitis, and dandruff, using trichoscopic images. Based on AI-defined scalp profiles, patients received personalized shampoo and serum prescriptions. This AI-guided therapeutic approach led to significant and sustained improvement in scalp health, demonstrating the potential of AI to support individualized treatment strategies [29].

Similarly, Bhardwaj et al. conducted a 6-month clinical trial demonstrating that AI can effectively support personalized treatment strategies for patients with hair loss [30]. In a 24-week study of women reporting hair thinning, participants received nonmedicated, AI-driven intervention plans aimed at improving hair quality. This approach resulted in significant improvements in hair regrowth and thickness, along with a marked reduction in hair shedding [30]. Participants also reported improved hair texture and overall scalp health, highlighting the clinical potential of AI-guided, individualized management [30].

AI has also demonstrated utility in monitoring treatment response, particularly in platelet-rich plasma (PRP) therapy for androgenetic alopecia [31]. Raymond et al., reported the use of AI-assisted imaging to objectively evaluate PRP efficacy in female patients. By providing automated quantitative data on hair density and scalp parameters, AI offered a more standardized and objective alternative to traditional assessment methods, which are largely subjective [31]. This study highlights the potential of AI-based tools to support treatment monitoring and integration into routine clinical practice [31].

Beyond current therapeutic applications, AI is also paving the way for the discovery of novel treatment strategies. In the context of drug development, AI-assisted approaches are expected to accelerate the identification of new therapeutic pathways in hair disorders. Recently, Sheikh et al. utilized machine learning in preclinical murine models to evaluate superoxide dismutase nanozyme mimics as a potential treatment for androgenetic alopecia [32]. These nanozyme mimics demonstrated a protective effect against oxidative stress–induced hair follicle damage, highlighting the promise of AI-driven drug discovery in the field [32].

Artificial intelligence is also becoming an integral part of the multifaceted field of hair disorders from the patient perspectives. Jueng et al. analyzed 102,444 social media posts related to the treatment of alopecia areata [33]. Patient Global Impression of Change scores were assigned using natural language processing and were analyzed together with underlying emotion (via Emolex) for treatment-related posts. Most treatments, including minoxidil, oral dexamethasone and prednisone, intralesional triamcinolone injections, biotin, essential oils, wigs, and JAK inhibitors, achieved positive PGIC scores in over 75% of posts [33]. On the contrary, dexamethasone was associated with a lack of improvement or even worsening of alopecia areata [33].

Effective follow-up of disease progression and treatment response is crucial to ensure optimal disease control (Figs. 17.2 and 17.3). Beyond objective clinical monitoring, AI tools are increasingly recognized for their impact on patient engagement and psychological well-being. Paiewonsky et al. investigated the effect of AI-based microphotography and automated hair counts on patients with alopecia [34]. More than half of participants reported reduced anxiety after viewing AI-analyzed images, while nearly half felt more motivated to continue or initiate treatment [34]. These findings underscore the added value of AI not only in treatment monitoring but also in improving adherence and addressing the psychosocial burden of hair loss.

17.5 Conclusions and Future Directions

AI is revolutionizing the field of hair disorders and is continuously proving to be a significant tool for both healthcare providers and patients. Advances in machine learning, deep learning, and image analysis now enable more efficient personalization of diagnosis, treatment, and follow-up. Interestingly, deep learning models have already shown accuracy that is comparable to human hair experts. From computing SALT scores to image analysis and visualization of potential condition improvements, AI has transformed incredibly the way we approach hair disorders today. Tasks that were once too time-consuming or inconsistent for humans can now be automated with high precision. This not only reduces errors but also allows for more reliable monitoring of changes over time. Despite these early steps, the clinical application of AI in hair disorders still faces important challenges. What remains lacking is a system that can recognize the full range of alopecia subtypes, especially the rarer non-scarring forms and the diverse group of scarring alopecias. This is quite surprising given that many of the diagnoses are straightforward and already follow established clinical logic. To bridge this gap, there is a clear opportunity: incorporate simple diagnostic algorithms, many of which already exist and are part of routine clinical practice, into AI training datasets [2]. By following a stepwise approach based on clinical signs and trichoscopic features (much like what is already done for skin lesions), we could guide AI systems toward much more accurate assessments in hair diseases. Given the complexity of hair and scalp diseases, it is essential for AI systems to correctly differentiate between clinically similar conditions, such as dandruff, psoriasis, or other inflammatory scalp disorders. To be truly effective in practice, these tools must also be resilient to real-world challenges, including image artifacts from hair products or treatment residues.

Looking ahead, AI is expected to improve further in the field of hair disorders. In the near future, we anticipate AI algorithms becoming synchronized with wearable devices, providing real-time monitoring of hair conditions, which will lead to early recognition and care. This could open the way to earlier detection of changes, timely intervention, and even prediction of disease progression—transforming both preventive care and long-term management. In conclusion, trichoscopy represents a "fertile ground" for the applications of AI but cannot replace the knowledge and skill of clinicians and hair experts. When integrated cautiously in daily clinical practice, together with human supervision, monitoring, and expert decision–making, it can enhance the process of patient diagnosis, treatment, as well as follow-up in hair disorders.

References

1. Moattari CR, Jafferany M. Psychological aspects of hair disorders: consideration for dermatologists, cosmetologists, aesthetic, and plastic surgeons. Skin Appendage Disord. 2022;8(3):186–94. https://doi.org/10.1159/000519817.
2. Katoulis AC, Pappa G, Sgouros D, Markou E, Kanelleas A, Bozi E, Ioannides D, Rudnicka L. A three-step diagnostic algorithm for alopecia: pattern analysis in Trichoscopy. J Clin Med. 2025;14(4):1195. https://doi.org/10.3390/jcm14041195.

3. Pirmez R. The dermatoscope in the hair clinic: Trichoscopy of scarring and nonscarring alopecia. J Am Acad Dermatol. 2023;89(2S):S9–S15. https://doi.org/10.1016/j.jaad.2023.04.033.
4. Daniels G, Tamburic S, Benini S, Randall J, Sanderson T, Savardi M. Artificial intelligence in hair research: a proof-of-concept study on evaluating hair assembly features. Int J Cosmet Sci. 2021;43(4):405–18. https://doi.org/10.1111/ics.12706.
5. Lee T, Ng V, Gallagher R, Coldman A, McLean D. DullRazor: a software approach to hair removal from images. Comput Biol Med. 1997;27(6):533–43. https://doi.org/10.1016/s0010-4825(97)00020-6.
6. Kiani K, Sharafat AR. E-shaver: an improved DullRazor(®) for digitally removing dark and light-colored hairs in dermoscopic images. Comput Biol Med. 2011;41(3):139–45. https://doi.org/10.1016/j.compbiomed.2011.01.003.
7. Hoffmann R. TrichoScan: a novel tool for the analysis of hair growth in vivo. J Investig Dermatol Symp Proc. 2003;8(1):109–15. https://doi.org/10.1046/j.1523-1747.2003.12183.x.
8. Vallotton P, Thomas N. Automated body hair counting and length measurement. Skin Res Technol. 2008;14(4):493–7. https://doi.org/10.1111/j.1600-0846.2008.00322.x.
9. Lee BS, Chan JY, Monselise A, McElwee K, Shapiro J. Assessment of hair density and caliber in Caucasian and Asian female subjects with female pattern hair loss by using the Folliscope. J Am Acad Dermatol. 2012;66(1):166–7. https://doi.org/10.1016/j.jaad.2011.04.023.
10. Birnbaum MR, McLellan BN, Shapiro J, Ye K, Reid SD. Evaluation of hair density in different ethnicities in a healthy American population using quantitative trichoscopic analysis. Skin Appendage Disord. 2018;4(4):304–7. https://doi.org/10.1159/000485522.
11. Shih H. A precise automatic system for the hair assessment in hair-care diagnosis applications. Skin Res Technol. 2015;21(4):500–7. https://doi.org/10.1111/srt.12220. Epub 2015 Jun 29
12. Duda RO, Hart PE. Use of the Hough transformation to detect lines and curves in pictures. Commun ACM. 1972;15(1):11–5.
13. Podlodowski Ł, Roziewski S, Nurzyński M. An ensemble of deep convolutional neural networks for marking hair follicles on microscopic images. In: Proceedings of the 2018 federated conference on computer science and information systems; 2018. p. 19–22. https://doi.org/10.15439/2018F389.
14. Jakubik J. Aset enhancement in hair follicle detection: ESENSEI Challenge. In: Position papers of the federated conference on computer science and information systems, vol. 16; 2018. p. 19–22. https://doi.org/10.15439/2018F388. ISSN: 2300-5963.
15. Sacha JP, Caterino TL, Fisher BK, Carr GJ, Youngquist RS, D'Alessandro BM, Melione A, Canfield D, Bergfeld WF, Piliang MP, Kainkaryam R, Davis MG. Development and qualification of a machine learning algorithm for automated hair counting. Int J Cosmet Sci. 2021;43(Suppl 1):S34–41. https://doi.org/10.1111/ics.12735.
16. Gupta A, Ivanova I, Renaud H. How good is artificial intelligence (AI) at solving hairy problems? A review of AI applications in hair restoration and hair disorders. Dermatol Ther. 2021;34(6):e14811. https://doi.org/10.1111/dth.14811.
17. Chang WJ, Chiu YC, Hsu CH, Chen LB, Chen MC, Ou YK, Chen Q. A mobile device-based hairy scalp diagnosis system using deep learning techniques. In: Proceedings of the 2020 IEEE Life Sciences Conference (LifeTech); 2020. https://doi.org/10.1109/LifeTech48969.2020.1570617332.
18. Lolli F, Pallotti F, Rossi A, et al. Androgenetic alopecia: a review. Endocrine. 2017;57(1):9–17. https://doi.org/10.1007/s12020-017-1280-y.
19. Norwood OT. Male pattern baldness: classification and incidence. South Med J. 1975;68(11):1359–65. https://doi.org/10.1097/00007611-197511000-00009.
20. Starace M, Orlando G, Alessandrini A, Piraccini BM. Female androgenetic alopecia: an update on diagnosis and management. Am J Clin Dermatol. 2020;21(1):69–84. https://doi.org/10.1007/s40257-019-00479-x.
21. Di Fraia M, Tieghi L, Magri F, et al. A machine learning algorithm applied to Trichoscopy for androgenic alopecia staging and severity assessment. Dermatol Pract Concept. 2023;13(3):e2023136.

22. Hung PK, Tsai J, Chen CM, Tsai RY. Quantitative evaluation of female pattern hair loss in Chinese women: a preliminary study. Dermatologic Surg. 2015;41(10):1171–4. https://doi.org/10.1097/DSS.0000000000000491.
23. Olsen EA, Hordinsky MK, Price VH, Roberts JL, Shapiro J, Canfield D, Duvic M, King LE Jr, McMichael AJ, Randall VA, Turner ML, Sperling L, Whiting DA, Norris D, National Alopecia Areata Foundation. Alopecia areata investigational assessment guidelines–Part II. National Alopecia Areata Foundation. J Am Acad Dermatol. 2004;51(3):440–7. https://doi.org/10.1016/j.jaad.2003.09.032.
24. Olsen EA, Canfield D. SALT II: a new take on the Severity of Alopecia Tool (SALT) for determining percentage scalp hair loss. J Am Acad Dermatol. 2016;75(6):1268–70. https://doi.org/10.1016/j.jaad.2016.08.042.
25. Lee S, Lee JW, Choe SJ, Yang S, Koh SB, Ahn YS, Lee WS. Clinically applicable deep learning framework for measurement of the extent of hair loss in patients with alopecia Areata. JAMA Dermatol. 2020;156(9):1018–20. https://doi.org/10.1001/jamadermatol.2020.2188. PMID: 32785607; PMCID: PMC7489853.
26. Bernardis E, Castelo-Soccio L. Quantifying alopecia Areata via texture analysis to automate the SALT score computation. J Invest Dermatol Symp Proc. 2018;19(1):S34–40. https://doi.org/10.1016/j.jisp.2017.10.010. Erratum in: J Invest Dermatol. 2021;141(4):947. 10.1016/j.jid.2021.02.003.
27. Alarcón-Soldevilla F, Hernández-Gómez FJ, García-Carmona JA, Campoy Carreño C, Grimalt R, Vañó-Galvan S, et al. Use of artificial intelligence as a predictor of the response to treatment in alopecia areata. iProc. 2021;7(1):e35433. https://doi.org/10.2196/35433.
28. Bernstein R, Wolfeld M, Zingaretti G. Robotic recipient site creation in hair transplantation. Hair Transplant Forum Int. 2014;24(3):95–7. https://doi.org/10.33589/24.3.0095.
29. Kim B, Kim MJ, Koo J, Choi HJ, Paik K, Kwon S, et al. Artificial intelligence-based prescription of personalized scalp cosmetics improved the scalp condition: efficacy results from 100 participants. J Dermatolog Treat. 2024;35 https://doi.org/10.1080/09546634.2024.2337908.
30. Bhardwaj V, Rodgers N, Harth O, Harth Y. Artificial intelligence-based personalization of treatment regimen for hair loss: a 6-month clinical trial. J Drugs Dermatol. 2025; https://doi.org/10.36849/JDD.8611.
31. Raymond O, Shaik J, Rypka K, Farah RS, Bellefeuille G, Hordinsky M. Use of artificial intelligence to track platelet-rich plasma treatment outcomes in females with nonscarring alopecia: a case series. JAAD Case Rep. 2024;47:103–6.
32. Sheikh H, McMullen E, Storm K, Donovan J. The future of machine learning enabled technologies for hair loss treatment. J Cutan Med Surg. 2025;24(2):e10.
33. Jueng J, Bhupalam V, Su A, Dupuis L, Infante C, Shaikh S, et al. Using artificial intelligence to analyze publicly available social media posts to understand patient perspectives toward specific treatments of alopecia areata. JAAD Int. 2022;9:102–4. https://doi.org/10.1016/j.jdin.2022.08.021.
34. Paiewonsky B, Raymond O, Bellefeuille G, Pathoulas J, Farah R, Hordinsky M. The impact and use of artificial intelligence in clinical care of scalp alopecia: a survey study assessing patient attitudes. J Am Acad Dermatol. 2023;89:AB234. https://doi.org/10.1016/j.jaad.2023.07.938.

N(AI)ls Disorders and AI

18

Ioanna Triantafillopoulou and Myrto-Maria Papadopoulou

18.1 Introduction

Nail disorders represent a diverse group of conditions that can reflect localized pathology or signal a systemic disease. As specialized appendages of the skin, nails serve protective and functional roles, and their appearance often offers critical diagnostic clues. The nail unit, comprising the matrix, nail bed, nail plate, cuticle, and nail folds, is susceptible to a wide spectrum of pathological changes—ranging from inflammatory and infectious etiologies to neoplastic and traumatic causes. With recent advancements, including the integration of artificial intelligence (AI) into dermatological diagnostics, the landscape of nail disease evaluation is rapidly evolving. AI is emerging as a valuable tool in the diagnosis and management of nail disorders, owing to its ability to detect complex patterns and subtle morphological variations. The structured, pattern-based approach of AI aligns well with the diagnostic demands of onychology. Increasingly, studies have reported the development of AI algorithms capable of identifying nuanced features in nail appearance and pathology [1].

Although AI holds significant promise in the diagnosis of nail disorders, its application faces several challenges and limitations. One major issue is the nail's structure, as its limited surface area and its curved shape make it difficult to be captured accurately in a 2D photograph. For instance, Horikawa et al. [2] reported that the detection of the fifth toenail was inconsistent across nail images when using their AI system due to the nail's small size. Another study [3] reported difficulties in accurately detecting nail thickening and subungual hyperkeratosis in certain cases of nail psoriasis. They further highlighted the necessity for precise image

I. Triantafillopoulou (✉)
Dermatology Private Practice, Optimal Dermatology, Athens, Greece

M.-M. Papadopoulou
Department of Internal Medicine, General Hospital of Karditsa, Karditsa, Greece

E. Karampinis et al. (eds.), *Artificial Intelligence Applications in Dermatology*,
https://doi.org/10.1007/978-3-032-15614-3_18

annotation, including proper labeling along the vertical axis. Furthermore, variations in nail shape and texture among individuals, along with specific areas such as those covered by nail polish or affected by other skin conditions, can complicate the algorithm's accuracy, necessitating reliable and precise feature extraction methods. Another challenge is the scarcity of large, high-quality annotated datasets focused on nail pathology, limiting the effectiveness of model training and generalizability. Most AI studies rely on small, institution-specific datasets, often lacking demographic diversity, which can lead to biased or less reliable results when applied to broader populations [4].

18.2 Onychomycosis and AI-Assisted Diagnosis

Onychomycosis is the most prevalent nail disorder worldwide, responsible for approximately 90% of toenail infections. It typically presents with nail discoloration (white, yellow, or brown), thickening, brittleness, subungual hyperkeratosis, and onycholysis. In some cases, surrounding skin may also be involved. The condition is classified based on the site and extent of infection: distal and lateral subungual, superficial, endonyx, proximal subungual, and total dystrophic onychomycosis. The distal and lateral subungual type is the most common and accounts for the classic clinical features of the disease [4].

Convolutional neural networks (CNNs) generally achieve higher accuracy with larger datasets; thus, a major limitation in medical deep learning remains the scarcity of labeled data. Han et al. [5] leveraged the high prevalence of onychomycosis to construct an extensive image database, aiming to evaluate whether AI could outperform clinicians in the clinical diagnosis of this condition. Their dataset was developed using a region-based CNN (R-CNN), which identifies and isolates nail regions from clinical photographs, along with two additional CNN models responsible for selecting appropriate images. This pipeline enabled the fully automated construction of a standardized dataset of 49,567 nail images, encompassing cases of onychomycosis, nail dystrophy, onycholysis, melanonychia, healthy nails, and other nail disorders. To achieve diagnostic classification, the study employed an ensemble model composed of two distinct CNN architectures—ResNet-152 and VGG-19—whose outputs were integrated via a two-layer feedforward neural network. This ensemble approach enhanced diagnostic robustness and accuracy by leveraging the complementary strengths of the two architectures. The AI system achieved outstanding diagnostic performance across multiple validation sets, with sensitivity ranging from 82.7% to 96.0%, specificity from 69.3% to 96.7%, and area under the curve (AUC) values between 0.82 and 0.98. Notably, when evaluated on a combined validation dataset, the AI outperformed nearly all of the 42 participating dermatologists.

In another study, Schielein et al. [6] evaluated six CNN architectures—InceptionV3, Xception, ResNet50, VGG-16, VGG-19, and MobileNetV2—for binary classification tasks across five dermatological diseases. For onychomycosis, the models achieved the highest performance, with a perfect accuracy of 1.000

across multiple architectures (notably VGG-19, InceptionV3, Xception, and ResNet50) in the initial dataset. InceptionV3 showed the best overall average accuracy and sensitivity, while Xception excelled in specificity. The authors underscored the suitability of deep CNNs, especially InceptionV3 and Xception, for accurate outlier detection in onychomycosis from clinical images.

In 2024, Agostini et al. [4] introduced an AI-powered method for diagnosing and assessing onychomycosis using the Scarletred®Vision mobile app, which captures standardized clinical images with the aid of a color calibration sticker (SkinPatch). The images are uploaded to an online platform where they undergo automated processing using CNNs to detect and segment the toenail, classify infected regions, and evaluate disease severity. The platform utilizes a combination of expert-annotated data, color space transformations, and superpixel mapping to improve diagnostic accuracy and monitor nail growth over time. At present, the application is limited to analyzing toenails using standardized clinical photographs.

Besides the use of AI in the clinical diagnosis of onychomycosis, artificial intelligence has also been applied to enhance traditional microscopic techniques such as the potassium hydroxide (KOH) preparation, a commonly used, rapid, and cost-effective method for detecting fungal elements in nail samples. Although widely accessible, KOH microscopy depends heavily on operator expertise and is limited by subjective interpretation and false negatives. In a study focused on improving the microscopic diagnosis of onychomycosis using KOH solution, Yilmaz et al. [7] developed two deep convolutional neural network models—VGG-16 and InceptionV3 (a lighter-weight architecture)—trained on grayscale patches extracted from high-resolution microscopic images. These images were captured under varied background and lighting conditions to ensure the models were not dependent on specific microscope settings.

Onychoscopy, a noninvasive dermoscopic examination of the nail unit, has become an increasingly valuable tool in the diagnosis of onychomycosis, aiding in the visualization of subtle clinical features such as streaks, discoloration, and subungual changes. The incorporation of AI into onychoscopic analysis holds promise for enhancing diagnostic accuracy, consistency, and accessibility across clinical settings. A CNN-based deep learning algorithm was developed to analyze clinical images of suspected onychomycosis, captured with a smartphone and dermatoscope by nonphysician staff in a real-world setting. In a prospective study involving 90 patients, the model demonstrated diagnostic accuracy comparable to that of dermatologists, with strong sensitivity and specificity. The publicly available algorithm shows promise for patient self-assessment and clinical use by nondermatologist healthcare providers; however, further validation across larger and more diverse populations is essential to confirm its broader applicability and reliability [8].

Expanding on this progress, Zhu et al. [9] introduced a deep learning-based model using the Faster R-CNN architecture to detect onychomycosis from dermoscopic images. The system was trained on annotated datasets incorporating hallmark dermoscopic features such as longitudinal striae, jagged edges, and cone-shaped keratosis, and employed an ensemble strategy that combined three submodels to optimize diagnostic performance. The final model achieved an accuracy of 87.5%, sensitivity of 93.0%, and specificity of 78.5%, surpassing the diagnostic performance of 54 practicing dermatologists.

Histological examination of nail clippings, particularly with periodic acid–Schiff (PAS) staining, is considered a reliable method for diagnosing onychomycosis, offering permanent slide documentation and higher sensitivity than direct microscopy. However, it is labor-intensive and requires significant expertise, making it a strong candidate for AI integration. A CNN-based deep learning algorithm was initially developed to detect onychomycosis in digitized PAS-stained nail clippings in a monocentric study [10]. Building on this foundation, a subsequent study [11] employed a CNN-based deep learning algorithm utilizing a U-Net architecture to detect fungal elements in PAS-stained whole-slide images (WSIs) of nail clippings. U-Net, a model specifically designed for biomedical image segmentation, enables pixel-level classification, allowing for precise localization of fungal structures within histological sections. This multicenter study, encompassing 664 WSIs from four laboratories, reported a sensitivity of 94% and a specificity of 77%, matching the diagnostic performance of 11 board-certified dermatopathologists. Unlike earlier models that relied on whole-image classification, the U-Net-based approach enhanced interpretability by segmenting and highlighting fungal regions directly, representing a significant advancement in AI-assisted histopathological diagnosis of onychomycosis.

18.3 Nail Psoriasis and AI-Assisted Diagnosis

The domain of nail psoriasis remains comparatively underexplored. Existing research on nail psoriasis and AI predominantly concentrates on its classification and the differential diagnosis from other nail pathologies.

Recent advancements have begun to shed light on the potential of AI in the context of nail psoriasis. In 2024, Shapiro et al. [12] assessed the capabilities of ChatGPT-4, a commercial AI tool, in interpreting unstructured electronic medical records (EMRs) of psoriasis patients, with a focus on detecting affected body regions. They reviewed EMR data from 94 individuals diagnosed with psoriasis, some of whom had nail and joint involvement. Using the ChatGPT-4 interface, the system analyzed the records to determine which body areas were impacted by the disease. These findings were then categorized and compared to evaluations made by a senior dermatologist. Nail involvement was present in 32 patients (34.0%), and ChatGPT-4 accurately identified 29 of these cases (sensitivity = 90.6%, specificity = 100%, positive predictive value = 100%). Notably, AI demonstrated strong agreement with the dermatologist's assessments, even in subtle cases—such as when nails were obscured by nail polish.

Additionally, a significant portion of the latest literature is dedicated to the evaluation of nail lesion severity in psoriasis using standardized scoring systems such as the Nail Psoriasis Severity Index (NAPSI) and the modified NAPSI (mNAPSI). NAPSI is a standardized tool used to assess the severity of nail psoriasis by dividing each nail into four quadrants and then evaluating both the nail matrix and nail bed for specific psoriatic changes. Matrix involvement includes pitting, leukonychia, red spots in the lunula, and nail crumbling, while bed involvement features oil drop discoloration, onycholysis, subungual hyperkeratosis, and splinter hemorrhages. Despite its utility, NAPSI scoring is time-consuming, and it is limited by subjectivity and interobserver variability. To address this, researchers have developed AI models to enable quicker and more accurate calculation of the NAPSI score. For instance, Horikawa et al. [2] developed an AI-based "NAPSI calculator" using deep learning techniques. The model consists of two main steps: automatic nail detection and NAPSI scoring, both implemented via CNN with a VGG-16 architecture. The system was trained and validated on a large and diverse dataset, with annotations from expert dermatologists specializing in nail diseases. The algorithm achieved a high nail detection accuracy (99.3%) and NAPSI scoring accuracy (83.9%), outperforming both nonspecialist dermatology residents (65.7%) and board-certified dermatologists without nail expertise (73.0%). It required less than one second per nail to compute the score and was capable of capturing changes over time, making it suitable for longitudinal follow-up and treatment monitoring. Although the tool struggled in a minority of complex cases and does not yet differentiate all individual psoriasis features, it provides a reliable, reproducible, and efficient method for integrating NAPSI scoring into routine clinical care.

Building on these advancements, Kemenes et al. [13] introduced and validated a deep learning photography-based model to automate scoring based on the mNAPSI, a simplified version of the NAPSI score, where pitting, crumbling, and onycholysis are scored on a semiquantitative 0–3 scale based on the severity or extent of nail involvement (0 = none, 1 = mild, 2 = moderate, 3 = severe). In contrast, splinter hemorrhages, leukonychia, red spots in the lunula, and hyperkeratosis are scored in a binary manner (0 = absent, 1 = present). The CNN developed used a transformer-based architecture and was trained on thousands of clinical nail images, including patients with psoriasis, psoriatic arthritis, and controls. In validation, the model achieved an average AUROC of 80% and a strong correlation (Pearson $r = 0.94$) with dermatologist-assigned mNAPSI scores, demonstrating its reliability in real-world, nonstandardized image settings.

References

1. Gaurav V, Grover C, Tyagi M, Saurabh S. Artificial intelligence in diagnosis and management of nail disorders: a narrative review. Indian Dermatol Online J. 2025;16:40–9. https://doi.org/10.4103/idoj.idoj_460_24.
2. Horikawa H, Tanese K, Nonaka N, Seita J, Amagai M, Saito M. Reliable and easy-to-use calculating tool for the Nail Psoriasis Severity Index using deep learning. NPJ Syst Biol Appl. 2024;10:130. https://doi.org/10.1038/s41540-024-00458-x.
3. Hsieh KY, Chen H-Y, Kim S-C, Tsai Y-J, Chiu H-Y, Chen G-Y. A mask R-CNN based automatic assessment system for nail psoriasis severity. Comput Biol Med. 2022;143:105300. https://doi.org/10.1016/j.compbiomed.2022.105300.
4. Agostini C, Ranjan R, Molnarova M, Hadzic A, Kubesch O, Schnidar V, et al. AI powered detection and assessment of onychomycosis: a spotlight on yellow and deep learning. JEADV Clin Pract. 2025;4:156–65. https://doi.org/10.1002/jvc2.577.

5. Han SS, Park GH, Lim W, Kim MS, Na JI, Park I, et al. Deep neural networks show an equivalent and often superior performance to dermatologists in onychomycosis diagnosis: automatic construction of onychomycosis datasets by region-based convolutional deep neural network. PLoS One. 2018;13:e0191493. https://doi.org/10.1371/journal.pone.0191493.
6. Schielein MC, Christl J, Sitaru S, Pilz AC, Kaczmarczyk R, Biedermann T, et al. Outlier detection in dermatology: performance of different convolutional neural networks for binary classification of inflammatory skin diseases. J Eur Acad Dermatol Venereol. 2023;37:1071–9. https://doi.org/10.1111/jdv.18853.
7. Yilmaz A, Göktay F, Varol R, Gencoglan G, Uvet H. Deep convolutional neural networks for onychomycosis detection using microscopic images with KOH examination. Mycoses. 2022;65:1119–26. https://doi.org/10.1111/myc.13498.
8. Kim YJ, Han SS, Yang HJ, Chang SE. Correction: prospective, comparative evaluation of a deep neural network and dermoscopy in the diagnosis of onychomycosis. PLoS One. 2020;15:e0244899. https://doi.org/10.1371/journal.pone.0244899.
9. Zhu X, Zheng B, Cai W, Zhang J, Lu S, Li X, et al. Deep learning-based diagnosis models for onychomycosis in dermoscopy. Mycoses. 2022;65:466–72. https://doi.org/10.1111/myc.13427.
10. Decroos F, Springenberg S, Lang T, Päpper M, Zapf A, Metze D, et al. A deep learning approach for histopathological diagnosis of onychomycosis: not inferior to analogue diagnosis by histopathologists. Acta Dermato-Venereol. 2021;101:adv00532. https://doi.org/10.2340/00015555-3893.
11. Jansen P, Creosteanu A, Matyas V, Dilling A, Pina A, Saggini A, et al. Deep learning assisted diagnosis of onychomycosis on whole-slide images. J Fungi. 2022;8:912. https://doi.org/10.3390/jof8090912.
12. Shapiro J, Baum S, Pavlotzky F, Mordehai Y Ben, Barzilai A, Freud T, et al. Application of a natural language processing artificial intelligence tool in psoriasis: a cross-sectional comparative study on identifying affected areas in patients' data. Clin Dermatol. 2024;42:480–6. https://doi.org/10.1016/j.clindermatol.2024.06.018.
13. Kemenes S, Chang L, Schlereth M, Noversa de Sousa R, Minopoulou I, Fenzl P, et al. Advancement and independent validation of a deep learning-based tool for automated scoring of nail psoriasis severity using the modified nail psoriasis severity index. Front Med (Lausanne). 2025:12. https://doi.org/10.3389/fmed.2025.1574413.

Part VI

Current Achievements, Limitations, and Future Perspectives of Artificial Intelligence in Dermatology

Artificial Intelligence Promises and Successes in Dermatology

19

Emmanouil Karampinis, Dimitrios Mantzaris, and Christoforos Tzermias

19.1 Introduction

The digitalization of human activities has transformed all sectors, including healthcare. Among the most transformative innovations is artificial intelligence (AI) in the healthcare ecosystem. Dermatology, in particular, is well suited for clinical AI applications as it is a specialty heavily dependent on visual assessment and pattern recognition. AI is revolutionizing how to diagnose, monitor, and manage skin conditions. By analyzing vast datasets and identifying complex visual patterns, AI systems offer promising solutions to long-standing challenges in dermatology.

From melanoma detection to the automated classification of rashes and lesions, AI-powered tools have demonstrated significant potential in enhancing diagnostic accuracy and accessibility, especially in underserved or remote regions. However, as with any evolving technology, integrating AI into dermatology has revealed both remarkable progress and critical limitations.

Success stories in AI dermatology have drawn considerable attention, particularly in image-based diagnostics. Convolutional neural networks (CNNs) and other deep learning models trained on thousands of dermatoscopic or macroscopic images have achieved diagnostic performances comparable to, or even surpassing, those of

E. Karampinis (✉)
Second Dermatology Department, School of Health Sciences, Aristotle University of Thessaloniki, Thessaloniki, Greece

Department of Dermatology, Faculty of Medicine, School of Health Sciences, University General Hospital of Larissa, University of Thessaly, Larissa, Greece

D. Mantzaris
Computational Intelligence and Health Informatics Lab, Nursing Department, School of Health Sciences, University of Thessaly, Larissa, Greece
e-mail: dmantzar@uth.gr

C. Tzermias
Intensive Quality IQ Skin Clinics, Private Dermatology One Day Clinics, Athens, Greece

E. Karampinis et al. (eds.), *Artificial Intelligence Applications in Dermatology*,
https://doi.org/10.1007/978-3-032-15614-3_19

experienced dermatologists in controlled settings. These advances raise expectations for faster triage, earlier detection of skin cancers, enhanced patient empowerment, and support for general practitioners in regions where specialist's care is limited.

Moreover, AI-powered mobile applications and teledermatology platforms are expanding access to skin health assessments, offering real-time feedback to patients globally. The integration of advanced AI and machine learning (ML) technologies continues to enhance the diagnosis and management of dermatological conditions, particularly skin cancers. Beyond diagnostics, AI is increasingly integrated into therapeutic dermatology, including laser-based applications where it assists in treatment planning, parameter modulation, and real-time response monitoring, leading to more personalized and precise interventions. As such, dermatology stands out as a leading specialty in showcasing AI's real-world clinical impact, and its potential to improve patient outcomes meaningfully.

19.2 The Success Story So Far: AI Applications Across the Spectrum of Dermatology

One of the greatest achievements of artificial intelligence (AI) in dermatology is its broad applicability across all domains of the specialty. AI technologies are not limited to specific, such as diagnosis, distinguishing look-alikes, assessing severity, or proposing treatment plans, but extend across the full range of dermatological conditions, including skin cancer, inflammatory diseases, hair and nail disorders, and cosmetic dermatology. AI systems, particularly CNNs with advanced attention mechanisms, have been trained on image datasets of a scale that far exceeds the clinical exposure of any individual dermatologist. Even natural language processing models like chatbots, though not fully fledged AI diagnostic tools, have been explored across many areas of dermatology [1].

The growing interest in AI's role within dermatology is evident in Fig. 19.1, which illustrates the number of publications retrieved from PubMed using the terms "Dermatology" and "Artificial Intelligence." A marked increase is noted beginning in 2014, with an ongoing upward trend. This search, conducted on May 4, 2025, suggests that research in this field is likely to grow substantially in the coming years.

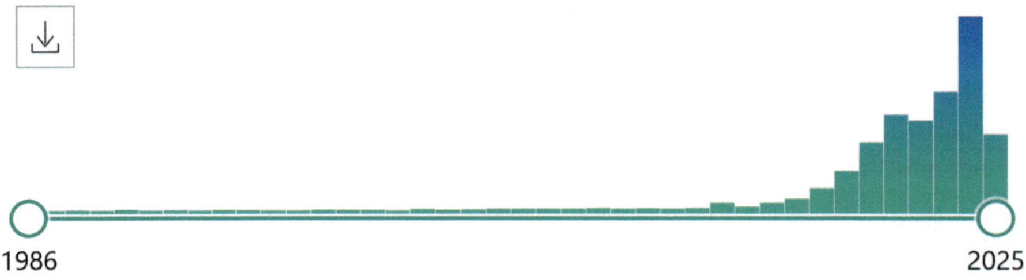

Fig. 19.1 Image displaying the growing interest and the increasing number of studies on Dermatology and Artificial Intelligence indexed in the PubMed database over time

A large proportion of AI applications in dermatology have focused on the automated diagnosis of skin lesions through image analysis, a concept explored as early as 1987 [2]. Initial efforts were aimed at simulating or supporting clinical decision-making in dermoscopy, and achieved encouraging results under controlled, conditions. However, these early systems faced limitations in generalisability and lacked external validation in real-world clinical environments. Before the breakthrough of deep learning in 2012, AI development in dermatology was hampered by limited datasets and the need for extensive manual feature engineering, extracting characteristics like color, texture, or shape. This made early models rigid and labor-intensive [3, 4].

A foundational moment came in the late 2000s with the work of Maglogiannis and Doukas [5], who introduced computer vision for noninvasive skin tumor diagnosis. Their research marked a critical step toward integrating image analysis into clinical workflows.

A landmark breakthrough occurred in 2017 when researchers from Stanford University published the results of a study showing that an AI model could match board-certified dermatologists in detecting and classifying skin cancer [6]. This study is considered a turning point for deep learning in dermatology, introducing the use of CNNs. Compared to traditional feature engineering methods, deep learning brought a transformative shift by allowing models to automatically extract the most relevant features for prediction, eliminating the need for manual input or predefined rules [3]. A major milestone in this evolution was the creation of a dataset comprising 129,450 images—two orders of magnitude larger than those used in prior studies—which was instrumental in training a CNN capable of high-performance skin lesion classification. This study marked a significant step in the application of AI to dermatology, and details of the architecture, training process, and performance of this specific implementation are presented. The researchers utilized a pretrained GoogLeNet Inception v3 architecture and applied transfer learning to fine-tune the network using a large dataset of clinical and dermoscopic images of skin lesions. For evaluation, the team curated a test set of clinical and dermoscopic images that had been histopathologically confirmed by biopsy. Twenty-one dermatologists were then asked to review the clinical and dermoscopic images—categorized as either keratinocytic or melanocytic—and make a management decision: either (i) to recommend biopsy or further intervention or (ii) to reassure the patient without further action [6].

These management decisions were used to derive a binary diagnosis of either "malignant" or "benign." Dermatologists' diagnostic performance was then mapped onto the CNN, allowing a direct comparison of classification accuracy across both dermoscopic and clinical image types. Remarkably, in both the keratinocytic and melanocytic categories, the average performance of dermatologists indicated lower diagnostic accuracy. Only one dermatologist in each category outperformed the CNN. These results suggest that, under the controlled conditions of this study, the deep learning model outperformed most of the participating dermatologists in distinguishing between benign and malignant lesions. The findings highlight the potential of CNNs to serve as highly accurate diagnostic tools in dermatology, particularly for tasks involving image-based classification [6].

After this important study, two significant "man against machine" studies followed as milestone research on the topic of dermatology and AI [7, 8]. The first study presented a well-trained CNN that outperformed dermatologists in a binary classification task distinguishing nevi from melanoma. This study was pivotal, establishing a clear performance edge for deep learning in a controlled diagnostic task. However, as with all AI model studies, there were limitations including a narrow clinical scope and a lack of real-world practice experience [7]. In the second "man against machine" study, the Moleanalyzer Pro by FotoFinder Systems was evaluated in comparison with dermatologists, who were provided with accompanying clinical information about the cases they encountered during the evaluation process. The results indicated that, under more realistic conditions that resembled daily clinical practice with a broader range of diagnoses, the CNN's performance was on par with most dermatologists [8].

After the "man against machine" studies, the focus shifted to the "man with machine" studies. In one prospective diagnostic study, dermatologists performed skin cancer screenings using both visual inspection and dermoscopy, rating suspicious melanocytic lesions based on the likelihood of malignancy and making management decisions—such as no action, follow-up, or excision. Subsequently, the same lesions were evaluated by a commercially available AI tool, the Moleanalyzer Pro (FotoFinder Systems), which also generated a malignancy score using dermoscopic images. These AI results were then shared with the dermatologists, who were asked to reassess their initial evaluations and adjust their decisions accordingly. Interestingly, dermatologists with less experience in dermoscopy showed the greatest improvement in diagnostic accuracy when working alongside the AI. This study suggests that dermatologists, particularly those with less experience, can benefit from collaborating with AI tools like the Moleanalyzer Pro. Integrating this type of human–AI partnership into routine practice could improve diagnostic accuracy and enhance patient outcomes. Moreover, the applications of AI in dermatology have expanded beyond diagnosis and skin cancer risk evaluation to include the development of AI models for other areas of dermatology [9].

Finally, on January 17, 2024, the U.S. Food and Drug Administration (FDA) approved DermaSensor, the first AI-powered medical device designed to help primary care providers detect skin cancer. It is worth mentioning that the first AI-based dermatology device to receive FDA approval was MelaFind, a multispectral spectroscopy tool authorized in 2017 through the Premarket Approval (PMA) pathway. It was specifically intended for use by dermatologists to assist in melanoma detection. However, MelaFind was eventually discontinued due to its low specificity—around 10%—which led to a high number of unnecessary biopsies [10].

Beyond skin cancer diagnosis, the study by Lee et al. focused on distinguishing between 26 common skin conditions—including various types of dermatitis, pigment disorders, alopecia, and other lesions—to assist with clinical decision-making. Unlike systems that rely solely on images, their AI system incorporated 45 types of information typically available in teledermatology, such as patient demographics and medical history. This feature is significant, as it goes beyond the AI model's dependence on image input alone. Additionally, the system was designed to handle a flexible number of input images, with the added value of using multiple photos being evaluated. While the researchers' deep learning system (DLS) primarily targeted 26 adult skin conditions commonly encountered in teleconsultations, it also provided secondary predictions from a broader set of 419 dermatological diagnoses [11].

The success of AI in dermatology is primarily attributed to the ability of deep learning models, especially those with hierarchical neural network architectures, to extract and learn abstract semantic features from visual data [4]. As digital health continues to evolve, AI is becoming an increasingly integral component of dermatological practice. Emerging evidence suggests that deep learning can not only support but, in some cases, surpass human clinical judgment in making diagnostic decisions [3].

The introduction of explainable artificial intelligence (XAI) has brought a revolution in AI-powered medicine particularly in dermatology. By making AI decisions more transparent, XAI alleviates concerns about the "black box" nature of AI, ensuring that users can trust and understand the decision-making process. This form of AI is expected to become predominant in dermatology, as it allows for human control and interaction in the diagnostic process. Efforts have been made to develop methods that enhance the transparency of AI decision-making. Diagnostic support systems need to provide clear, case-specific explanations tailored to dermatologists, enabling them to assess the reliability of AI recommendations for each individual case [12, 13].

The studies mentioned above have had a significant impact on academic dermatology. This is evident from their publication in *Nature*, one of the highest-impact journals in the scientific community, and from their high citation counts—each exceeding 1000 citations. These factors underscore the substantial influence these works have had on the advancement of dermatological research [6, 11, 12].

In parallel with skin cancer assessment, researchers have also developed deep neural network algorithms capable of distinguishing inflammatory dermatoses, such as eczema, from a range of other infectious and inflammatory skin conditions. These models not only perform well in identifying common presentations but also demonstrate the ability to classify rare skin lesions of clinical importance. Notably, the AI systems extend beyond diagnosis by offering treatment recommendations

This dual capability of accurate diagnosis and treatment guidance exemplifies the potential of AI to enhance personalized care for eczema patients, and generally for individuals with chronic inflammatory dermatoses. By using advanced computational methods, AI can assist dermatologists in tailoring management strategies to each patient's specific needs, reducing the trial-and-error approach that often characterizes eczema treatment. As AI technologies continue to evolve, their integration into dermatological care pathways is expected to transform the diagnosis, monitoring, and management of inflammatory skin conditions such as atopic dermatitis and psoriasis. These innovations promise not only greater diagnostic accuracy but also more targeted and effective treatment plans, ultimately improving both clinical outcomes and the patient experience [14]. Similar approaches using AI models have also been noted in conditions such as acne, hair disorders like alopecia areata, and nail disorders such as onychomycosis. These advancements point toward broad clinical integration and signal a potential clinical "makeover" of dermatology. The future is just around the corner!

Lastly, the applications of AI models extend to aesthetic procedures including the use of botox and dermal fillers. Machine learning is changing the way aesthetic treatments are planned. For example, machine learning models can analyze 3D facial images taken before and after treatment to track changes and help determine the optimal amount of filler for each facial area. These advanced systems, trained to understand facial anatomy, can even predict post-treatment appearance, reducing uncertainty and enhancing precision. This not only increases practitioner confidence but also offers patients greater reassurance and satisfaction [15, 16]. In addition to injectables, AI is also being integrated into laser-based dermatological treatments, where it facilitates real-time treatment optimization, lesion detection, and fluence modulation. These smart laser systems harness embedded imaging and AI-driven feedback loops to ensure personalized and effective interventions in both therapeutic and cosmetic contexts.

19.3 Objective Severity Assessment of Skin Diseases

AI models can assist in the objective severity assessment of skin diseases such as psoriasis, acne, and hidradenitis suppurativa. These models can analyze skin features, including redness, scaling, lesion types, and counts (e.g., the number of pustules or nodules on a patient's face) as well as plaque thickness and distribution in psoriasis. The measurements are performed in a consistent and quantifiable way based on how the AI model has been trained, thus minimizing human subjectivity. There are many cases where the same patient may be evaluated differently by different dermatologists. For instance, Psoriasis Area and Severity Index (PASI) score has faced criticism for being overly complex, time-consuming, and highly variable between assessments [17]. In contrast, AI models offer more consistent evaluations but may also be less sensitive in detecting changes in mild cases, and they often operate on a nonlinear scale, which can make interpretation more difficult. Unlike manual grading, which can vary between clinicians and is time-intensive, AI models can detect subtle skin changes and patterns that might be missed by the human eye or require careful examination. When it comes to severity indexes used in AI models, particularly in smartphones apps, scoring systems are often preferred over more complex ones. For example, in the case of acne, AI models tend to adopt the Investigator's Global Assessment (IGA) scale. The IGA is favored due to its simplicity and clinician-friendly structure, categorizing acne severity into a limited number of clearly defined stages. This makes it more suitable than complex systems that require detailed counting of specific lesion types across various body regions [18].

This IGA score makes it especially appropriate for automated evaluations on mobile platforms, where quick, user-accessible, and interpretable results are crucial for enhancing user engagement and supporting remote dermatological assessments (Table 19.1 and Fig. 19.2).

Table 19.1 Various studies across different skin conditions, where researchers developed or tested CNN or other AI models for disease assessment

Disease	Severity index	Study example	Main points of the study
Psoriasis	Psoriasis Area and Severity Index (PASI)	[19]	Researchers developed an automated system to assess individual components of the PASI score using CNNs. The approach involved creating separate CNN models for each body region (trunk, arms, and legs) and each PASI subscore—erythema, thickness (induration), scaling (desquamation), and area—resulting in a total of 12 specialized networks. The AI performed on par with dermatologists in scoring erythema, scaling, and thickness, and even outperformed them when it came to evaluating the affected area based on images. The CNN's performance scores in each site evaluation were scattered
Acne	Investigator's Global Assessment (IGA)	[20]	Researchers trained a system designed to automatically assign a severity score based on the IGA scale, which ranges from 0 to 4. The AI correctly identified the IGA score with an accuracy of 85.4%, and its assessments showed a very strong correlation with those made by physicians indicating excellent agreement between manual and automated evaluation
Vitiligo	Vitiligo Area Scoring Index	[21]	Researchers developed an AI system designed to evaluate the severity of facial vitiligo. To train and validate the model, they used 100 facial images of patients with vitiligo. Three expert dermatologists also rated the same 69 images, and their scores were compared with those generated by the AI to assess consistency between human and machine. The AI model achieved a great accuracy of 93%, and there was strong agreement between its assessments and those of the physicians. These findings highlight the promising potential of AI in supporting vitiligo severity evaluation
Melasma	Melasma area and severity index (MASI)	[22]	Researchers, based on a total of 1368 anonymized facial images from patients clinically diagnosed with melasma, assessed CNN architecture regarding their ability to evaluate melasma severity correctly. After preprocessing the images and labeling them based on MASI scores provided by three dermatologists, six CNN architectures were trained and evaluated. Among them, the GoogLeNet model delivered the highest accuracy, reaching 75.5%

(continued)

Table 19.1 (continued)

Disease	Severity index	Study example	Main points of the study
Hidradenitis supporativa (HS)	International Hidradenitis Suppurativa Severity Score System (IHS4)	[23]	Researchers developed an ML model to automatically assess the severity of HS using clinical images taken with smartphones. They used CNNs to classify disease severity (IHS4) on a scale from 0 to 3 and to track how the condition changed over time. To automatically detect affected skin areas, they also implemented a U-NET model. The CNNs successfully distinguished between mild and moderate-to-severe cases with an overall accuracy of 78%
Atopic dermatitis	SCORing Atopic Dermatitis (SCORAD) score	[24]	Researchers in this case gathered images from 250 atopic dermatitis patients from Indonesia, with dermatologists labeling the images as mild, moderate, severe, or none. Five pretrained convolutional neural network (CNN) architectures were tested. Among these, ResNet50 performed the best, achieving an accuracy of 89.8%
Alopecia areata	Severity of Alopecia Tool (SALT)	[25]	Researchers focused on an AI mode, which was trained on 823 head images that were labeled by trained annotators and reviewed by doctors. Hair loss severity was categorized into four levels: 0, 0.33, 0.66, and 1, with annotations based on the affected area. Following this, the system combined data from four images of each patient and calculated a single SALT score. Differences between doctors and AI assessments were mostly seen in severe cases or when patients had newly grown, short white hair—Situations where doctors rated 100% hair loss, but the AI gave slightly lower scores, with an average error of 10%
Nail psoriasis	Nail Psoriasis Severity Index (NAPSI)	[26]	Researchers, based on a dataset of 7054 individual fingernail images, perform annotations of each image with the 8-point NAPSI scores and trained a deep learning model based on YOLOv7 with this data. In 98.6% of the images, the NAPSI score predicted by the deep learning algorithm AI model was very close to the score given by experts—specifically, it differed by approximately 2 points. The results showed that the algorithm could assess NAPSI scores both quickly and accurately

As indicated by the examples presented in Table 19.1, the choice between CNN classifiers and models like YOLO depends on the specific goals of the researchers whether they aim to classify the severity of a condition or to locate and identify specific areas of concern on the skin using those identifications to calculate an assessment score. For example, in the case of melasma assessment, the researchers' goal was to evaluate the severity of melasma using the MASI score, which provides a regional severity rating rather than requiring pinpoint accuracy for

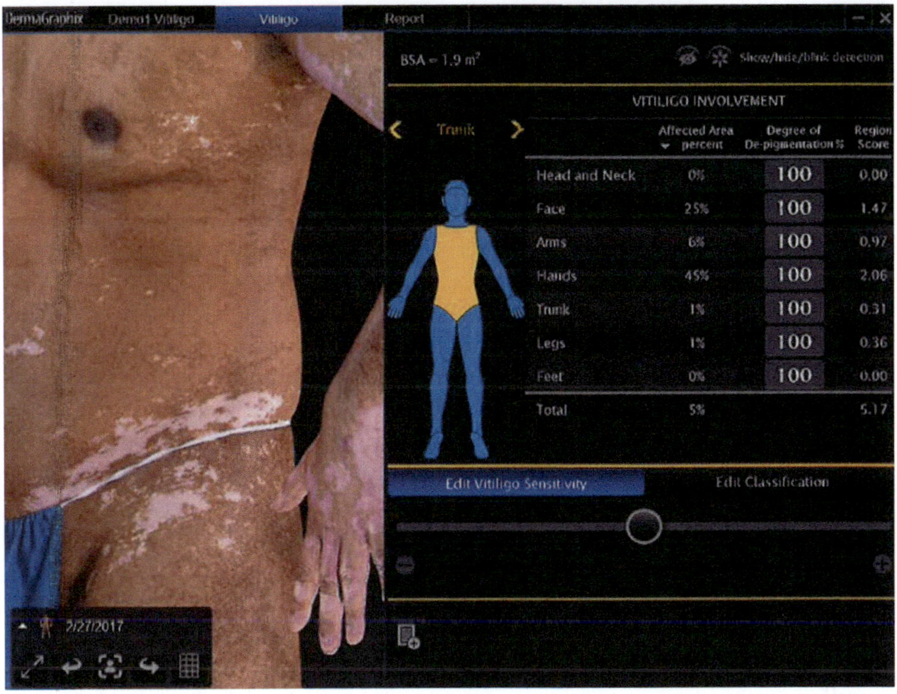

Fig. 19.2 Canfield's vitiligo module uses AI to segment areas of vitiligo in 3D or 2D total body images. By providing an objective, quantitative detection, the percentage of vitiligo-affected body surface area (BSA) can be obtained in a more repeatable and robust way compared to traditional (and subjective) human-based assessment. (Reproduced with permission from Canfield © All rights retained)

each individual patch. For this type of task, GoogLeNet, a deep learning model designed for image classification, is an appropriate choice, as it analyzes the image as a whole and outputs a single severity score, rather than detecting individual lesion locations [22].

Apart from assessing inflammatory dermatoses, objective assessment is also crucial in cosmetic procedure outcomes. One of the primary challenges in evaluating post-treatment results—such as those following filler injections or sensitive skincare regimens—is the high degree of subjectivity involved. These assessments often rely on patient self-reports and subjective descriptions of their experiences and perceived changes. The development and integration of AI applications that can highlight post-treatment facial modifications offer a clear and objective feedback. This approach can improve communication between patients and clinicians, provide transparent documentation, and build trust through measurable outcomes. AI-supported tools can serve as visual evidence of treatment results, helping to move the evaluation process away from subjective impressions and toward explainable, quantifiable tracking—enhancing clinical practice across both medical and aesthetic dermatology.

19.4 AI as an Easily Accessible Tool

The development of AI-driven dermatological systems aims to apply their application in everyday clinical practice, serving as valuable tools for specialists in the diagnosis and treatment of patients with skin diseases. In laser-based procedures, artificial intelligence is increasingly utilized to enhance diagnostic precision and optimize treatment parameters, such as fluence, and pulse duration, based on lesion characteristics and patient-specific skin features. By integrating real-time image analysis, AI systems help tailor laser settings, leading to improved clinical outcomes, especially in the management of vascular lesions, pigmentation disorders, and acne scarring.

Modern computing systems possess the processing power required to support and execute artificial intelligence applications. In particular, smartphones have become an integral part of our daily lives and are widely recognized for their processing capabilities. This has led AI systems experts to adapt applications to run on smartphones, making them accessible to both specialists and the general public.

The rise of mobile apps aimed at assisting with skin conditions offers both opportunities and challenges. However, these apps vary significantly in performance, and none have yet received approval from the U.S. Food and Drug Administration. Research on smartphone apps for assessing skin cancer risk has revealed inconsistent accuracy and sensitivity, with most apps performing poorly overall.

Some of these applications are presented in Table 19.2 and Fig. 19.3. In his comprehensive review, Wongvibulsin highlighted that four apps were targeted at clinicians and five apps were designed for both clinicians and patients. In terms of platform availability, 12 apps were Android-exclusive, 13 were Apple-exclusive, and 16 were available on both platforms (Table 19.2). As shown in the table, the primary purposes of these apps included skin cancer detection, skin disease diagnosis, and/or identification of skin or hair conditions, mole tracking, acne diagnosis, treatment and monitoring, management of atopic dermatitis, and sun protection [27]. Of these, five apps were supported by peer-reviewed journal articles, and only one was part of a multicenter prospective clinical trial, authored by W. Menzies et al. [28].

Aysa, for example, is an AI-powered symptom-checker app developed by VisualDx. This AI app uses a problem-focused clinical search with a well-organized medical image library that includes over 120,000 images representing 200 skin conditions across all Fitzpatrick skin types. It adjusts its results based on the user's medical history, offering a more personalized experience. In a recent study, evaluating Aysa's performance, users completed a patient profile by describing each lesion's appearance, mapping its location on a body diagram, and entering information about duration and associated symptoms. Aysa then generated eight possible diagnoses, which were compared to the patients' actual clinical diagnoses. The app performed well, accurately identifying most of the skin conditions [29].

In a recent study, researchers tested the ability of six online skin cancer diagnosis applications— Aysa, Skin-Check, Dermos, Scanoma,

Table 19.2 Available apps based on AI tasks and dermatology available on Android, Apple, or both

Available only on Android	
Acne Doc	Acne management
AI Skin Disease Detection	Diagnosis of skin conditions
AI Tool for Skin Problems	Tracking skin conditions
Blemish Types, Skin Cancer ID	Skin cancer detection, mole tracking
Derma AI	Skin cancer detection
DermoApp: SkinCancer Detection	Skin cancer detection
DermObserver: Dermatology Scan	Skin cancer detection
Emdee Skin	Skin cancer detection
FaceDia—Acne Diagnostic Scan	Acne diagnosis and treatment
Human Disease Checker With AI	Diagnosis of skin conditions
Medgic—AI Skin Analysís	Identification of skin conditions
Medic Scanner-Skin Analyze	Skin cancer detection
Medic Scanner-Skin Analyze	Skin cancer detection
Available only on Apple	
Atopic Dermatitis	Atopic dermatitis management
Cube-Check Ur Birthmark Easlly	Identification of skin conditions
iHairium: Hair & Skin Heatıh	Diagnosis of hair conditions
MatchLab AI	Tracking skin conditions
Melatect	Skin cancer detection
MetisAI+	Identification of skin conditions
Mole Checker Skin Dermaıotogy	Skin cancer detection
Piel	Skin cancer detection
Rash ID—Rash Identifier	Diagnosis of skin conditions
SkinChange.AI	Mole tracking
Skin-Check	Skin cancer detection, mole tracking
Skinner: Analyze Your Skin	Identification of skin conditions
UV Safe-Sun Protection	Skin cancer detection, sun protection
Available on both applications	Mole tracking, visual search for similar images
Acno	Acne management
AI Dermatologist: Skin Scanner	Skin cancer detection, mole tracking, identification of skin conditions
Aysa	Identification of skin conditions
DermEngine	Identification of skin conditions
EczemaLess	Eczema tracking and management
Kara AI Skin Expert Assistant	Tracking skin conditions
MDAcne	Acne treatment and monitoring
Miiskin Skin & Dermatology	Mole tracking, acne tracking
Model Dermatology	Identification of skin conditions
Proton Health: Acne & Eczema	Identification of skin conditions
Scanoma—Mole Check	Skin cancer detection
Skin Bliss: Skincare Routines	Tracking skin conditions
SkinIO	Skin cancer detection, mole tracking
Skinlog I Skin Diary, Analysis	Tracking skin conditions
Sun Index-Vitamin D & UV	Tracking skin conditions, sun protection
VisualDx	Identification of skin conditions

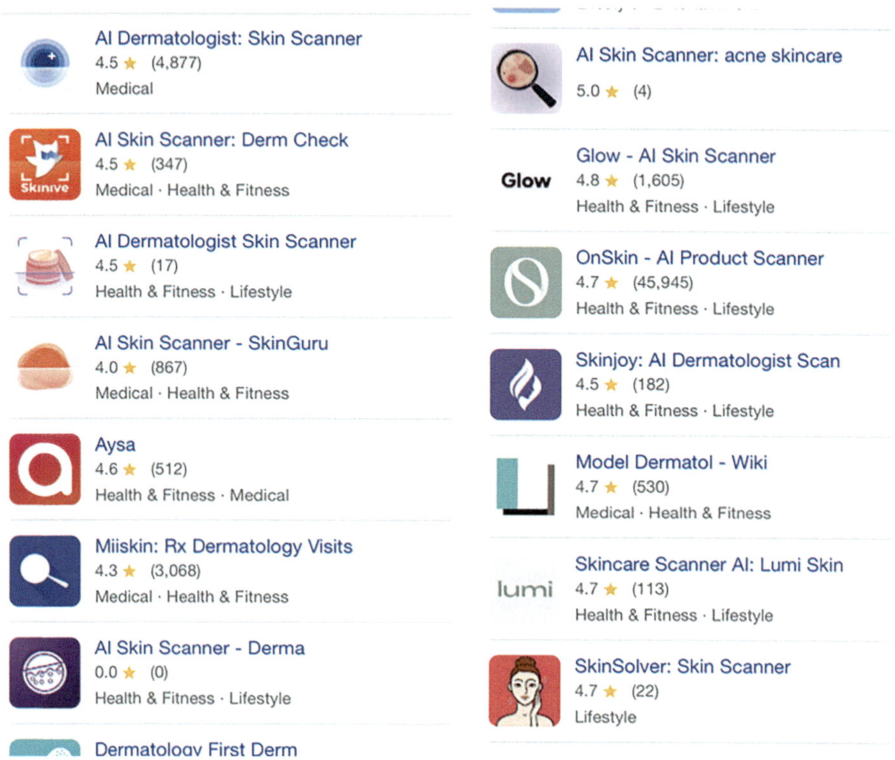

Fig. 19.3 Image showing some of the AI apps in dermatology available to both dermatologists and patients, ranging from skin care apps to skin cancer detectors and diagnosis providers

AIDermatologist, and Skinner—and two AI chatbots, ChatGPT-4 and Microsoft Copilot, to correctly diagnose images of melanoma and seborrheic keratosis (SK), used with permission from VisualDx.com These two conditions were selected due to their clinical similarity, which often poses diagnostic challenges for nonspecialists. AI chatbots and apps varied widely in performance, but overall performed better at diagnosing melanoma (average, 67.5%; 20–95%) than SK (average, 56.3%; 10–80%). Among the applications, Skinner and AI Dermatologist demonstrated the highest diagnostic accuracy for both conditions. Microsoft Copilot showed 30% higher performance than ChatGPT-4 in identifying these two conditions. Conversely, Aysa showed substantially lower performance in diagnosing melanoma compared to the chatbots, AI dermatologist, and Skinner. Notably, the two fee-based platforms, Skinner and AI Dermatologist, consistently yielded the most reliable diagnostic results across all image types [30].

Of course, the clinical use of these apps raises unresolved questions regarding legality, ethics, privacy, and responsibility. Moreover, their "black box" decision-making process leads many users to hesitate before placing full trust in them.

19.5 Let's ChatGPT About Dermatology!

When OpenAI launched ChatGPT in November 2022, this chatbot quickly became the fastest-growing online application in history, gaining 100 million users within just 2 months, an impressive milestone! Thanks to its advanced language capabilities, ChatGPT allows anyone with internet access to receive tailored responses to a wide range of questions—including those related to dermatology.

ChatGPT is becoming increasingly influential in dermatology for several key reasons. First, ChatGPT and other large language models (LLMs) are widely accessible and easy to use, making them strong candidates for exploring how AI can support medical fields. Secondly, numerous studies have confirmed its usefulness in dermatology settings, showing that ChatGPT can pass dermatology board-style exams, educate patients, and assist with medical documentation. Its use in dermatology spans from patient education to supporting clinical decisions, highlighting its practical value [31].

Moreover, because ChatGPT frequently features in discussions around AI ethics, it also serves as a useful case study for exploring the ethical and legal challenges of integrating AI into dermatology. As one of the most well-known chatbots, its functionalities are understandable by a broad audience, making it particularly relevant to these discussions. Thirdly, ChatGPT's ability to generate clear, well-written content, sometimes nearly indistinguishable from human-written reports, has sparked both excitement and concern among medical professionals and academics [32].

ChatGPT has also shown promise in assisting dermatologists by suggesting possible diagnoses using clinical and dermoscopic information. This suggests it could be a helpful tool alongside standard dermatology practices particularly in settings where patient communication and education are essential. In addition to supporting clinicians, chatbots like ChatGPT can also assist patients directly, providing quick answers to common questions about their condition, such as possible triggers like diet or medications (Fig. 19.4). However, it is important to note that ChatGPT bases its answers on preexisting data, which means it may not always reflect the most current medical updates. Additionally, when patients ask vague or incorrect questions, it can be challenging for ChatGPT to interpret

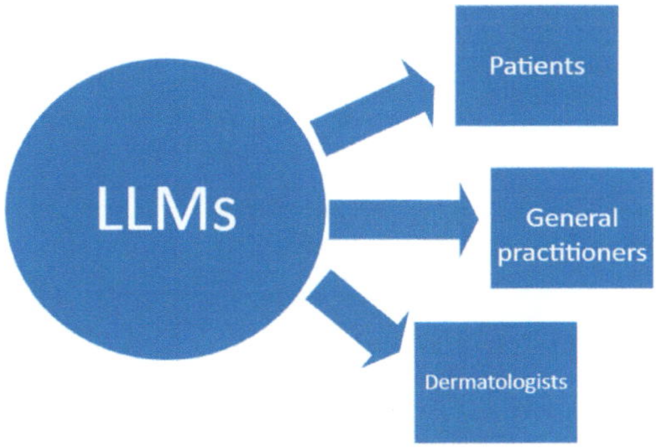

Fig. 19.4 It is important to note that LLMs in dermatology are not limited to dermatologists, but they can also be used by patients and general practitioners (GPs), changing the specialist–GP–patient relationship dynamics

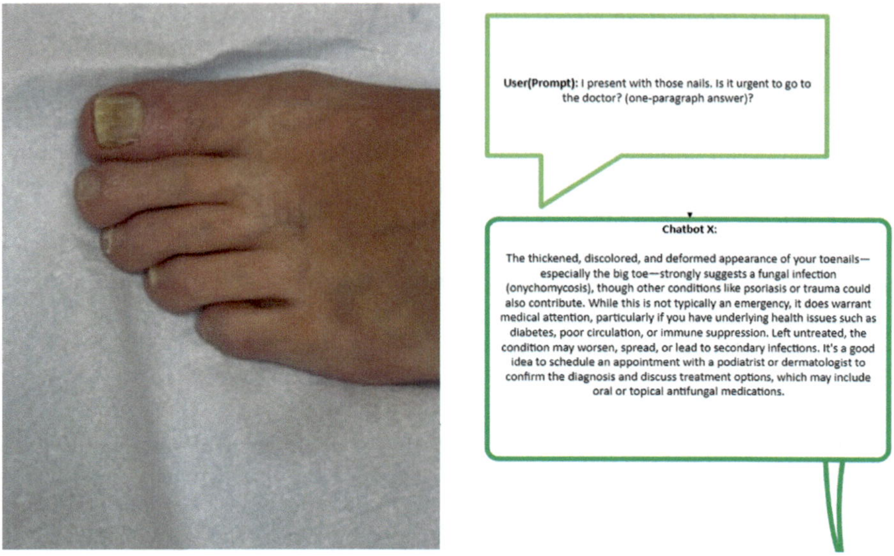

Fig. 19.5 A screenshot of chatbot answer to patient questions about their nail lesions and if it is urgent to ask for medical help. The chatbot's answer is quite satisfactory as it adequately provides the main differential diagnosis and possible triggering factors. However, the dermatologist evaluation remains irreplaceable

them accurately and provide useful responses [33, 34] (Figs. 19.5 and 19.6). There have also been studies comparing ChatGPT's performance with other chatbots. These concluded that ChatGPT provided the most accurate and relevant answers to patient questions. However, its responses were generally written at a college reading level, which could make them less accessible to the general public (Tables 19.3, 19.4 and 19.5).

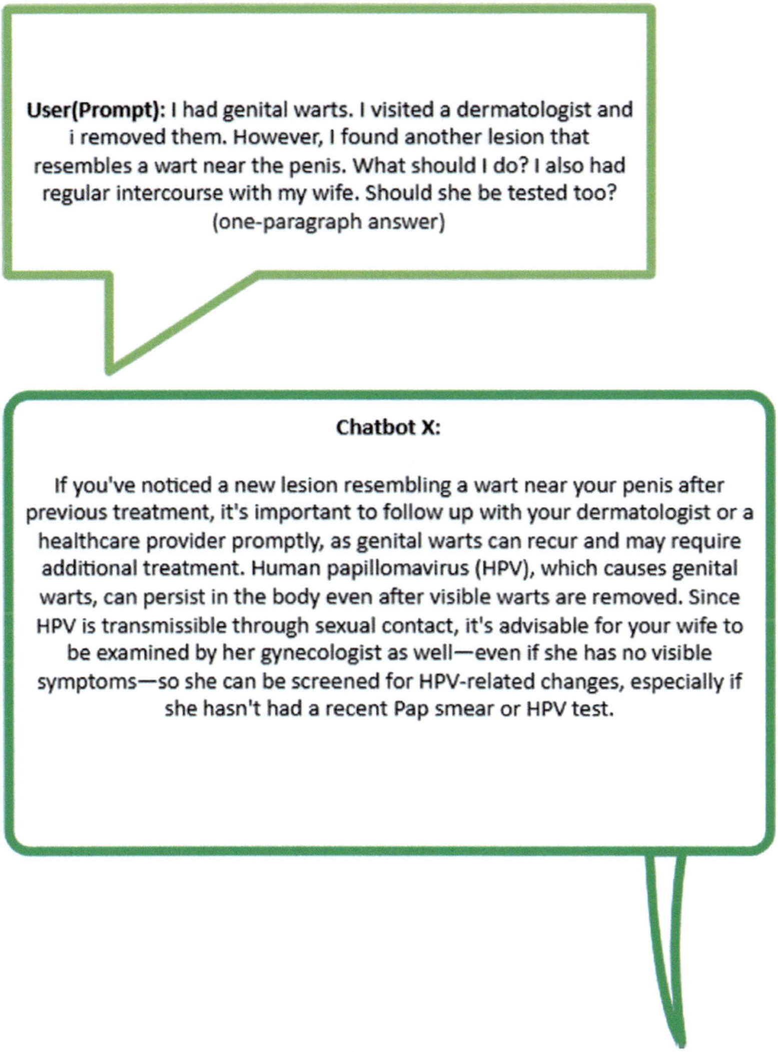

Fig. 19.6 Screenshot of a chatbot, with an anxious patient asking information about his condition and thc next steps. The presence of warts and general genital lesions can cause intense stress to patients who may seek info and advice from chatbots

Table 19.3 Examples with studies focusing on chatbot assistance to clinicians

Skin disease	Chatbot	Study	Scope of study
Skin cancer	ChatGPT Vision	[35]	A random selection of dermoscopy images from the ISIC database was used to test ChatGPT Vision. The model assessed 100 melanocytic lesions (50 melanomas and 50 benign nevi). When only the top diagnosis from ChatGPT was considered, it achieved a sensitivity of 32%, and when the correct diagnosis was counted as correct if it appeared within the top three suggested differentials, the sensitivity improved to 56%
	ChatGPT-3.5	[36]	Chatbot provided satisfactory differential diagnosis proposals in case a dermoscopy description was provided. The descriptions provided included both BCC, melanoma, and SCC. According to the authors, the least adequate answer was given for SCC dermoscopy description
Psoriasis	ChatGPT-4	[37]	Clinicians used ChatGPT-4 to convert unstructured data on anatomic regions involved in psoriasis patients into structured data, with applications for follow-up and research

Table 19.4 Examples of chatbots contributing to patient understanding across various areas, from preventive care to lifestyle choices and their impact on disease progression

Skin disease	Chatbot	Study	Scope of study
Melanoma	ChatGPT-3.5	[38]	Patients can question the chatbot's advice for preventive skin cancer. The chatbot proved to be a great educational tool for informing patients about skin cancer prevention. The users on the question were characterized as satisfied or very satisfied regarding the chatbot answers
Warts	VaxBot-HPV	[39]	A chatbot designed to enhance understanding of health topics and encourage HPV vaccination by offering information and responding to users' questions about the vaccine
Psoriasis	ChatGPT-3.5-turbo, mode	[40]	ChatGPT can provide useful information and advice regarding psoriasis disease to patients. However, that advice cannot be replaced with those given by experts
Acne	ChatGPT (not specified version)	[41]	Chatbots as ChatGPT can create interesting conversations with acne patients, providing useful advice for skin care
Rosacea	ChatGPT-3.5	[42]	ChatGPT-3.5 proves to be highly reliable and clinically useful when answering typical patient questions about rosacea

Table 19.5 Examples of how ChatGPT has contributed to aesthetic medicine research and practice

ChatGPT has been used to evaluate the results of botulinum toxin treatments by analyzing before-and-after images [43]
ChatGPT can offer accurate clinical information about common cosmetic procedures [44]
Plastic surgeons are encouraged to use ChatGPT as a helpful tool during patient consultations, for ongoing support, and in marketing [45]
The chatbot also offers useful guidance for both patients and clinicians on more complex procedures like rhinoplasty, blepharoptosis repair, and breast reconstruction [46–50]
Additionally, ChatGPT shows strong potential in helping triage concerns that arise after aesthetic surgeries [51]
ChatGPT has also been used to create consent form for aesthetics procedures in a study that was the first one to present a case in which a chatbot was used to create bioethics material [52]

19.6 Combinations of AI with Other Technologies in Dermatology

Artificial intelligence can not only be integrated into many aspects of dermatology but can also be combined with other technologies to create powerful tools in the hands of dermatologists.

19.6.1 Combination with Teledermatology

Telehealth, as defined by the World Health Organization (WHO), is the use of information and communication technologies to deliver health services at a distance. It involves the secure exchange of accurate medical information for purposes such as the diagnosis, treatment, and prevention of illness and injury, the conduct of research and evaluation, and the support of continuing education for health professionals. The ultimate goal of telemedicine is to improve the health and well-being of individuals and communities, regardless of geographical barriers. The use of telemedicine has significantly improved access to healthcare, especially for people in remote or underserved regions with limited access to healthcare providers or transportation. In addition to bridging geographical barriers, telemedicine has proven to be a cost-effective alternative to traditional face-to-face consultations, helping to reduce overall healthcare costs for patients [53].

The combination of AI and teledermatology has led to many innovative applications. The focus of certain applications of AI in technology was to assess the quality of image used for the process. Jaloboi et al. developed an AI-powered tool based on CNNs to assess image quality and detect potential issues. The tool performed comparably to dermatologists in identifying image quality problems [54]. In another study, Montilla et al. emphasized the importance of image quality in teledermatology and demonstrated the key role AI plays in determining whether an image is suitable for remote evaluations [55].

In synchronous teledermatology consultations, where the dermatologist and patient interact in real time, AI can facilitate more detailed and personalized data collection. A notable example is Dermbot, an AI-powered chatbot integrated with the patient's electronic medical record. Dermbot begins by analyzing that record and initiates a chat-based conversation to gather further information. It asks targeted questions based on clinical knowledge, then prompts the patients to upload images of their skin condition. Using AI analysis, it may ask follow-up questions, provide a preliminary differential diagnosis, suggest further tests, and outline a treatment plan. Finally, Dermbot generates a detailed consultation summary for review and finalization by a human dermatologist, who assumes responsibility for the medical advice given [56].

It is important to note that AI-powered teledermatology must clearly address medical-legal, ethical, and reimbursement-related issues to ensure safe and effective implementation.

19.6.2 Combination with Virtual Reality

Augmented reality (AR) has also been combined with AI, and this examination has been tested in certain studies. Augmented reality is a subset of virtual reality (VR), where users are fully immersed in a digitally created space, without visibility of the real world. AI has shown significant potential when integrated with VR, especially for body surface reconstruction. A notable example is the Canfield® Vectra WB360 system, which uses 2D images from 46 stereo-vision pods to create a comprehensive, interactive 3D model of the body. This model can be rotated and examined in detail. The system also applies machine learning algorithms to segment and classify skin features, such as naevi and other skin lesions, evaluating their potential malignancy. Each lesion is precisely mapped and tracked over time through repeated imaging, facilitating the early detection of new melanomas [57].

AI combined with virtual reality offers promising support for inflammatory dermatosis management, especially during follow-up. Virtual "before-and-after" simulations help build patient trust and improve adherence to treatment. Interactive VR tools can also guide users through proper skincare routines and suggest lifestyle changes like healthier eating habits. By delivering educational content in a more engaging and relatable format, these tools help boost motivation and encourage long-term commitment to treatment. In a recent study, Goldust highlights platforms such as Viveport Human Skin VR, which allow users to explore detailed 3D models of skin anatomy and acne conditions, which are beneficial for both patient education and professional training [58].

19.6.3 The "Internet of Things": The Ultimate Dermatology Combination (Devices, AI, and Teledermatology)

A typical Internet of Things (IoT) ecosystem in healthcare includes sensors, intelligent algorithms, communication networks, and cloud-based platforms. The resulting ecosystem includes a wide range of applications, with telemedicine being a key

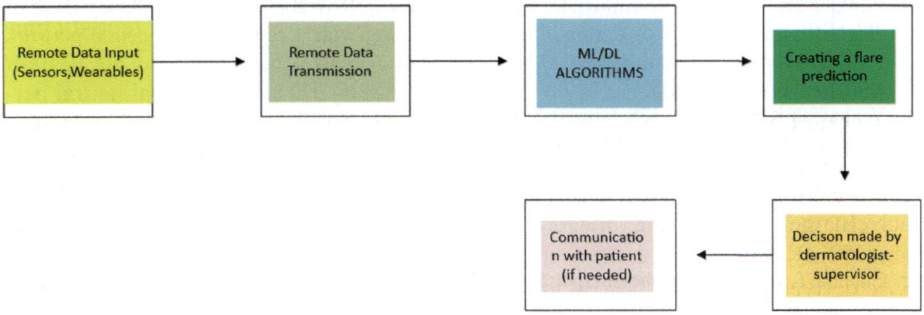

Fig. 19.7 Schematic representation demonstrating the architecture of the IoT module in dermatology

driver behind IoT's expansion in the medical field. IoT enables patients to receive high-quality, personalized care with equal access, regardless of geographic or socio-economic barriers, all while safeguarding their privacy (Fig. 19.7). In dermatology, IoT has the potential to support remote monitoring, more accurate diagnoses, timely treatment, and individualized care. One of the fastest-growing areas in this space is IoT-based skin condition monitoring, fueled by rising patient numbers and a shortage of dermatologists—particularly in underserved or rural areas [59].

References

1. Omiye JA, Gui H, Daneshjou R, Cai ZR, Muralidharan V. Principles, applications, and future of artificial intelligence in dermatology. Front Med (Lausanne). 2023;10 https://doi.org/10.3389/fmed.2023.1278232.
2. Cascinelli N, Ferrario M, Tonelli T, Leo E. A possible new tool for clinical diagnosis of melanoma: the computer. J Am Acad Dermatol. 1987;16:361–7. https://doi.org/10.1016/S0190-9622(87)70050-4.
3. Stadelmann T, Tolkachev V, Sick B, Stampfli J, Dürr O. Beyond ImageNet: deep learning in industrial practice. In: Applied data science. Cham: Springer International Publishing; 2019. p. 205–32. https://doi.org/10.1007/978-3-030-11821-1_12.
4. Rajpara SM, Botello AP, Townend J, Ormerod AD. Systematic review of dermoscopy and digital dermoscopy/artificial intelligence for the diagnosis of melanoma. Br J Dermatol. 2009;161:591–604. https://doi.org/10.1111/j.1365-2133.2009.09093.x.
5. Maglogiannis I, Doukas CN. Overview of advanced computer vision systems for skin lesions characterization. IEEE Trans Inf Technol Biomed. 2009;13:721–33. https://doi.org/10.1109/TITB.2009.2017529.
6. Esteva A, Kuprel B, Novoa RA, Ko J, Swetter SM, Blau HM, et al. Dermatologist-level classification of skin cancer with deep neural networks. Nature. 2017;542:115–8. https://doi.org/10.1038/nature21056.
7. Haenssle HA, Fink C, Schneiderbauer R, Toberer F, Buhl T, Blum A, et al. Man against machine: diagnostic performance of a deep learning convolutional neural network for dermoscopic melanoma recognition in comparison to 58 dermatologists. Ann Oncol. 2018;29:1836–42. https://doi.org/10.1093/annonc/mdy166.
8. Haenssle HA, Fink C, Toberer F, Winkler J, Stolz W, Deinlein T, et al. Man against machine reloaded: performance of a market-approved convolutional neural network in classifying a broad spectrum of skin lesions in comparison with 96 dermatologists working under less artificial conditions. Ann Oncol. 2020;31:137–43. https://doi.org/10.1016/j.annonc.2019.10.013.

9. Winkler JK, Blum A, Kommoss K, Enk A, Toberer F, Rosenberger A, et al. Assessment of diagnostic performance of dermatologists cooperating with a convolutional neural network in a prospective clinical study. JAMA Dermatol. 2023;159:621. https://doi.org/10.1001/jamadermatol.2023.0905.
10. Venkatesh KP, Kadakia KT, Gilbert S. Learnings from the first AI-enabled skin cancer device for primary care authorized by FDA. NPJ Digit Med. 2024;7:156. https://doi.org/10.1038/s41746-024-01161-1.
11. Liu Y, Jain A, Eng C, Way DH, Lee K, Bui P, et al. A deep learning system for differential diagnosis of skin diseases. Nat Med. 2020;26:900–8. https://doi.org/10.1038/s41591-020-0842-3.
12. Chanda T, Hauser K, Hobelsberger S, Bucher T-C, Garcia CN, Wies C, et al. Dermatologist-like explainable AI enhances trust and confidence in diagnosing melanoma. Nat Commun. 2024;15:524. https://doi.org/10.1038/s41467-023-43095-4.
13. Bradshaw TJ, McCradden MD, Jha AK, Dutta J, Saboury B, Siegel EL, et al. Artificial intelligence algorithms need to be explainable—or do they? J Nucl Med. 2023;64:976–7. https://doi.org/10.2967/jnumed.122.264949.
14. Alowais SA, Alghamdi SS, Alsuhebany N, Alqahtani T, Alshaya AI, Almohareb SN, et al. Revolutionizing healthcare: the role of artificial intelligence in clinical practice. BMC Med Educ. 2023;23:689. https://doi.org/10.1186/s12909-023-04698-z.
15. Li R, Chen X, Sun H, Hao L, Luo S. Application of 3-dimensional technology for evaluating muscular type and muscle-fat pad mixed-type nasolabial folds with botulinum Toxin-A treatment. Aesthet Surg J. 2023;43:NP271–82. https://doi.org/10.1093/asj/sjac341.
16. Tabaru A, Kapusuz Gencer Z, Öğreden Ş, Akyel S, Özum Ö, Bayram İ. Enhancing facial filler training with 3D-printed models: a prospective observational study on medical student competence. Med Sci Monit. 2024;30 https://doi.org/10.12659/MSM.945074.
17. Leonardi C, See K, Gallo G, McKean-Matthews M, Zhang Y, Goldblum O, et al. Psoriasis severity assessment combining physician and patient reported outcomes: the optimal psoriasis assessment tool. Dermatol Ther (Heidelb). 2021;11:1249–63. https://doi.org/10.1007/s13555-021-00544-6.
18. Bae IH, Kwak JH, Na CH, Kim MS, Shin BS, Choi H. A comprehensive review of the acne grading scale in 2023. Ann Dermatol. 2024;36:65. https://doi.org/10.5021/ad.23.094.
19. Schaap MJ, Cardozo NJ, Patel A, de Jong EMGJ, van Ginneken B, Seyger MMB. Image-based automated psoriasis area severity index scoring by convolutional neural networks. J Eur Acad Dermatol Venereol. 2022;36:68–75. https://doi.org/10.1111/jdv.17711.
20. Melina A, Dinh NN, Tafuri B, Schipani G, Nisticò S, Cosentino C, et al. Artificial intelligence for the objective evaluation of acne investigator global assessment. J Drugs Dermatol. 2018;17:1006–9.
21. Hillmer D, Merhi R, Boniface K, Taieb A, Barnetche T, Seneschal J, et al. Evaluation of facial vitiligo severity with a mixed clinical and artificial intelligence approach. J Invest Dermatol. 2024;144:351–357.e4. https://doi.org/10.1016/j.jid.2023.07.014.
22. Zhang J, Jiang Q, Chen Q, Hu B, Chen L. Deep learning-based multiclass framework for real-time Melasma severity classification: clinical image analysis and model interpretability evaluation. Clin Cosmet Investig Dermatol. 2025;18:1033–44. https://doi.org/10.2147/CCID.S508580.
23. Tzellos T. First steps into AI-supported hidradenitis suppurativa severity assessment. J Eur Acad Dermatol Venereol. 2024;38:456–7. https://doi.org/10.1111/jdv.19785.
24. Maulana A, Noviandy TR, Suhendra R, Earlia N, Bulqiah M, Idroes GM, et al. Evaluation of atopic dermatitis severity using artificial intelligence. Narra J. 2023;3:e511. https://doi.org/10.52225/narra.v3i3.511.
25. Nguyen H, Gazeau L, Wolfe J. Using artificial intelligence to compute severity of alopecia tool scores. JAAD Int. 2025;18:101–2. https://doi.org/10.1016/j.jdin.2024.04.003.
26. Paik K, Kim BR, Youn SW. Automatic evaluation of nail psoriasis severity index using deep learning algorithm. J Dermatol. 2024;51:1310–7. https://doi.org/10.1111/1346-8138.17313.

27. Wongvibulsin S, Yan MJ, Pahalyants V, Murphy W, Daneshjou R, Rotemberg V. Current state of dermatology Mobile applications with artificial intelligence features. JAMA Dermatol. 2024;160:646. https://doi.org/10.1001/jamadermatol.2024.0468.
28. Menzies SW, Sinz C, Menzies M, Lo SN, Yolland W, Lingohr J, et al. Comparison of humans versus mobile phone-powered artificial intelligence for the diagnosis and management of pigmented skin cancer in secondary care: a multicentre, prospective, diagnostic, clinical trial. Lancet Digit Health. 2023;5:e679–91. https://doi.org/10.1016/S2589-7500(23)00130-9.
29. Marri SS, Albadri W, Hyder MS, Janagond AB, Inamadar AC. Efficacy of an Artificial Intelligence App (Aysa) in dermatological diagnosis: cross-sectional analysis. JMIR Dermatol. 2024;7:e48811. https://doi.org/10.2196/48811.
30. Zhang Y, Chung J, Chen R, Malhotra S, Nguyen D, Levin NA. Testing the ability of artificial intelligence chatbots and dermatologic diagnosis mobile applications to diagnose melanoma and seborrheic keratosis. J Am Acad Dermatol. 2025;92:161–3. https://doi.org/10.1016/j.jaad.2024.08.077.
31. Chakraborty C, Pal S, Bhattacharya M, Dash S, Lee S-S. Overview of Chatbots with special emphasis on artificial intelligence-enabled ChatGPT in medical science. Front Artif Intell. 2023;6 https://doi.org/10.3389/frai.2023.1237704.
32. Kim Y-H, Zhang MZ, Vidal NY. ChatGPT offers an editorial on the opportunities for chatbots in dermatologic research and patient care. Dermatol Online J. 2024;29 https://doi.org/10.5070/D329662990.
33. Al-Ashwal FY, Zawiah M, Gharaibeh L, Abu-Farha R, Bitar AN. Evaluating the sensitivity, specificity, and accuracy of ChatGPT-3.5, ChatGPT-4, Bing AI, and bard against conventional drug-drug interactions clinical tools. Drug Healthc Patient Saf. 2023;15:137–47. https://doi.org/10.2147/DHPS.S425858.
34. Abu-Haifa M, Etawi B, Alkhatatbeh H, Ababneh A. Comparative analysis of ChatGPT, GPT-4, and Microsoft copilot Chatbots for GRE test. Int J Learn Teach Educ Res. 2024;23:327–47. https://doi.org/10.26803/ijlter.23.6.15.
35. Shifai N, van Doorn R, Malvehy J, Sangers TE. Can ChatGPT vision diagnose melanoma? An exploratory diagnostic accuracy study. J Am Acad Dermatol. 2024;90:1057–9. https://doi.org/10.1016/j.jaad.2023.12.062.
36. Karampinis E, Toli O, Georgopoulou K-E, Kampra E, Spyridonidou C, Roussaki Schulze A-V, et al. Can artificial intelligence "hold" a Dermoscope?—the evaluation of an artificial intelligence Chatbot to translate the Dermoscopic language. Diagnostics. 2024;14:1165. https://doi.org/10.3390/diagnostics14111165.
37. Shapiro J, Baum S, Pavlotzky F, Mordehai YB, Barzilai A, Freud T, et al. Application of a natural language processing artificial intelligence tool in psoriasis: a cross-sectional comparative study on identifying affected areas in patients' data. Clin Dermatol. 2024;42:480–6. https://doi.org/10.1016/j.clindermatol.2024.06.018.
38. De Luca E, Cappilli S, Coscarella G, Chiricozzi A, Peris K. ChatGPT for skin cancer prevention: high patients' satisfaction to educational material. JEADV Clin Pract. 2024;3:1283–7. https://doi.org/10.1002/jvc2.383.
39. Tao C, Li Y, Li J, Li M, Yu E, Amith M, et al. VaxBot-HPV: a GPT-based Chatbot for answering HPV vaccine-related questions. Res Sq. 2024; https://doi.org/10.21203/rs.3.rs-4876692/v1.
40. Huang C, Hong D, Chen X. ChatGPT in medicine: evaluating psoriasis patient concerns. Skin Res Technol. 2024;30 https://doi.org/10.1111/srt.13680.
41. Deoghare S. An interesting conversation with ChatGPT about acne vulgaris. Indian Dermatol Online J. 2024;15:137–40. https://doi.org/10.4103/idoj.idoj_77_23.
42. Yan S, Du D, Liu X, Dai Y, Kim M-K, Zhou X, et al. Assessment of the reliability and clinical applicability of ChatGPT's responses to patients' common queries about rosacea. Patient Prefer Adherence. 2024;18:249–53. https://doi.org/10.2147/PPA.S444928.
43. Ali R, Cui H. Leveraging ChatGPT for enhanced aesthetic evaluations in minimally invasive facial procedures. Aesth Plast Surg. 2025;49:950–61. https://doi.org/10.1007/s00266-024-04524-x.

44. Rames MM, O'Hern K, Rames JD, Tooley AA, Hausauer AK, Munavalli GS, et al. ChatGPT as a resource for patient education in cosmetic dermatological procedures: a boon or a bane? J Cosmet Dermatol. 2024;23:1085–6. https://doi.org/10.1111/jocd.16166.
45. Gupta R, Park JB, Bisht C, Herzog I, Weisberger J, Chao J, et al. Expanding cosmetic plastic surgery research with ChatGPT. Aesthet Surg J. 2023;43:930–7. https://doi.org/10.1093/asj/sjad069.
46. Meyer MKR, Kandathil CK, Davis SJ, Durairaj KK, Patel PN, Pepper J-P, et al. Evaluation of Rhinoplasty information from ChatGPT, Gemini, and Claude for readability and accuracy. Aesth Plast Surg. 2024; https://doi.org/10.1007/s00266-024-04343-0.
47. Xie Y, Seth I, Hunter-Smith DJ, Rozen WM, Ross R, Lee M. Aesthetic surgery advice and counseling from artificial intelligence: a Rhinoplasty consultation with ChatGPT. Aesth Plast Surg. 2023;47:1985–93. https://doi.org/10.1007/s00266-023-03338-7.
48. Shiraishi M, Tomioka Y, Miyakuni A, Ishii S, Hori A, Park H, et al. Performance of ChatGPT in answering clinical questions on the practical guideline of Blepharoptosis. Aesth Plast Surg. 2024;48:2389–98. https://doi.org/10.1007/s00266-024-04005-1.
49. Shiraishi M, Tanigawa K, Tomioka Y, Miyakuni A, Moriwaki Y, Yang R, et al. Blepharoptosis consultation with artificial intelligence: aesthetic surgery advice and counseling from chat generative pre-trained transformer (ChatGPT). Aesth Plast Surg. 2024;48:2057–63. https://doi.org/10.1007/s00266-024-04002-4.
50. Li W, Lu W, Gong Z. Harnessing the potential of ChatGPT in breast reconstruction: a revolution in patient communication and education. Aesth Plast Surg. 2024;48:35–40. https://doi.org/10.1007/s00266-023-03490-0.
51. Mac O, Ayre J, Bell K, McCaffery K, Muscat DM. Comparison of readability scores for written health information across formulas using automated vs manual measures. JAMA Netw Open. 2022;5:e2246051. https://doi.org/10.1001/jamanetworkopen.2022.46051.
52. Patel I, Om A, Cuzzone D, Garcia Nores G. Comparing ChatGPT vs surgeon-generated informed consent documentation for plastic surgery procedures. Aesthet Surg J Open Forum. 2024;6 https://doi.org/10.1093/asjof/ojae092.
53. Gajarawala SN, Pelkowski JN. Telehealth benefits and barriers. J Nurse Pract. 2021;17:218–21. https://doi.org/10.1016/j.nurpra.2020.09.013.
54. Jalaboi R, Winther O, Galimzianova A. Explainable image quality assessments in Teledermatological photography. Telemed E-Health. 2023;29:1342–8. https://doi.org/10.1089/tmj.2022.0405.
55. Hernández Montilla I, Mac Carthy T, Aguilar A, Medela A. Dermatology Image Quality Assessment (DIQA): artificial intelligence to ensure the clinical utility of images for remote consultations and clinical trials. J Am Acad Dermatol. 2023;88:927–8. https://doi.org/10.1016/j.jaad.2022.11.002.
56. Shapiro J, Lyakhovitsky A. Revolutionizing teledermatology: exploring the integration of artificial intelligence, including Generative Pre-trained Transformer chatbots for artificial intelligence-driven anamnesis, diagnosis, and treatment plans. Clin Dermatol. 2024;42:492–7. https://doi.org/10.1016/j.clindermatol.2024.06.020.
57. Marchetti MA, Nazir ZH, Nanda JK, Dusza SW, D'Alessandro BM, DeFazio J, et al. 3D whole-body skin imaging for automated melanoma detection. J Eur Acad Dermatol Venereol. 2023;37:945–50. https://doi.org/10.1111/jdv.18924.
58. Goldust M. AI-powered virtual reality in acne vulgaris. J Cosmet Dermatol. 2025;24 https://doi.org/10.1111/jocd.70104.
59. Mathew NT, Mathachan SR. Internet of medical things in dermatology: a step toward next-generation patient care. J Cosmet Dermatol. 2024;23:3058–9. https://doi.org/10.1111/jocd.16367.

Artificial Intelligence Failures, Bias, and Limitations in Dermatology

20

Emmanouil Karampinis and Dimitrios Mantzaris

20.1 Introduction

The integration of advanced artificial intelligence (AI) and machine learning (ML) technologies has been demonstrated to enhance the diagnosis and management of dermatologic conditions, particularly skin cancers. Dermatology has emerged as a leading medical specialty where AI is demonstrating transformative potential, real-world clinical impact and meaningful improvements in patient outcomes.

However, as with any emerging technology, the integration of AI into clinical practice is accompanied by both advantages and limitations. While previous sections have highlighted the accomplishments and potential of AI in dermatology, it is equally important to critically assess the challenges that hinder its optimal implementation and performance [1].

The integration of AI within the field of dermatology raises several critical issues, including issues of access to and utilization of patient data, transparency in AI-driven decision-making processes, automation of clinical procedures, and algorithmic bias, as well as broader ethical and societal concerns [2].

E. Karampinis (✉)
Second Dermatology Department, School of Health Sciences, Aristotle University of Thessaloniki, Thessaloniki, Greece

Department of Dermatology, Faculty of Medicine, School of Health Sciences, University General Hospital of Larissa, University of Thessaly, Larissa, Greece

D. Mantzaris
Computational Intelligence and Health Informatics Lab, Nursing Department, School of Health Sciences, University of Thessaly, Larissa, Greece
e-mail: dmantzar@uth.gr

E. Karampinis et al. (eds.), *Artificial Intelligence Applications in Dermatology*,
https://doi.org/10.1007/978-3-032-15614-3_20

20.2 The Issue of Input Image Quality

The most frequent reasons for poor image quality include

(i) Improper framing, where the lesion is not centered or partially cut off especially in case of large lesions that cannot fit properly in just one image.
(ii) Inadequate lighting, causing shadows, glares, or uneven skin tone appearance.
(iii) Blurriness, often due to camera shake or poor focus.
(iv) Low resolution, which reduces the clarity of skin texture or lesion border. This phenomenon is especially frequent in case of smartphone images.
(v) Incorrect distance, where the camera is either too far, causing detail loss or too close causing distortion (Fig. 20.1).
(vi) Presence of noise due to unwanted visual distortion that interferes with the clarity or accuracy of the image. This can manifest as color distortions or the presence of artifacts such as hair or ink (Fig. 20.2). The presence of noise may mask important features in the image, modifying the input and creating diagnostic risks [1, 3].

The importance of image quality has become especially evident in the past years, as teledermatology has seen a surge in use due to the COVID-19 pandemic and related global lockdowns [4]. Therefore, it is important to estimate the image quality of the images input as well as the quality and parameters of the images that the model used has been trained with. The performance of object detection algorithms such as You Only Look Once (YOLO) is expected to degrade when low-quality images are used as input. Similarly, convolutional neural networks (CNNs) like ResNet and EfficientNet, as well as vision transformers, are also sensitive to image quality. This holds true for segmentation models used in skin lesion analysis, such as U-Net, DeepLab, and Mask R-CNN, where both training and testing performance can be significantly impacted by the quality of the input images [5].

Therefore, in case of different quality images, how dermatologists' and CNNs' accuracy actually differ? In a study, 18 dermatology clinicians evaluated 303 images of 101 skin lesions, which were divided into three categories based on image quality: low quality (LQ), high quality (HQ), and enhanced quality (EQ), the latter created using an HDR-style technique. Clinicians outperformed the CNN model in binary classification for LQ and EQ images, though their performance matched the models on HQ images. However, in multiclass classification, the CNN model significantly exceeded clinician performance on HQ images ($p < 0.01$) [6].

Nevertheless, the absence of standardization in image characteristics, including but not limited to lighting conditions, patient positioning, and resolution, poses a substantial challenge. This variability restricts the comparability of images across datasets and highlights the consistency required for reliable machine learning applications [7]. However, the obstacle of quality can be overpassed, as indicated by certain studies. A recent work demonstrated that deep learning can still be highly effective in dermatology, even under practical and often challenging real-world conditions. By using consumer-grade cameras like the iPhone 11, working with small

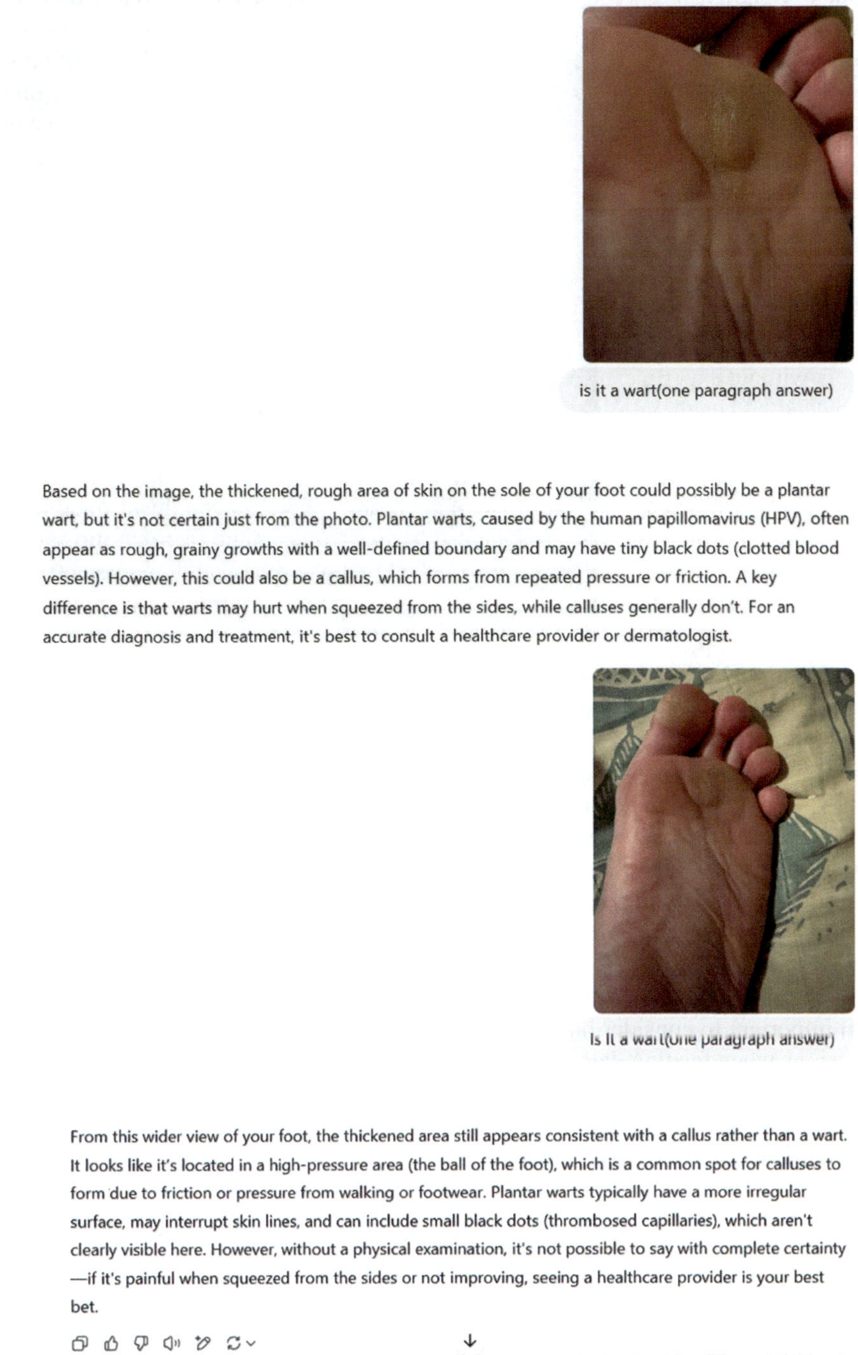

Fig. 20.1 Image illustrating the significance of image distance in influencing AI-generated responses. In the first scenario, a close-up of the plantar lesion prompts the chatbot (ChatGPT-4, OpenAI) to suggest it might be a plantar wart. However, in the second scenario, where a wider view of the entire plantar area is provided, the response leans more toward identifying the issue as a callus

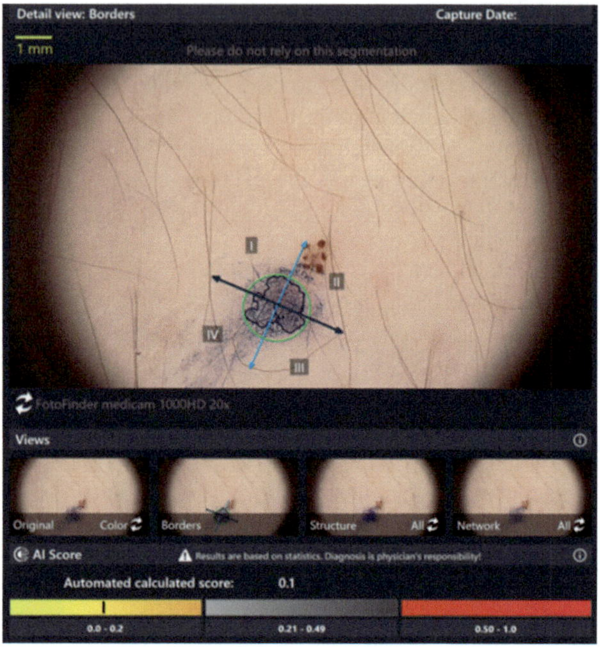

Fig. 20.2 A screenshot of FotoFinder Moleanalyzer AI assistant (FotoFinder Systmen GmbH) showing that the AI algorithm by taking into account the ink measurements on the skin and calculating the risk assessment based on the ink itself even blue, rather than the nearby nevi dermoscopy

or imperfect datasets, and accounting for variations in lighting and skin appearance, the model developed by Bernhard et al. proves that high diagnostic performance is achievable without relying on idealized inputs. This makes their approach especially valuable for applications in teledermatology and at-home assessments, where controlled conditions are not guaranteed [8]. Also, there are many CNNs used to improve the image qualityby removing the noise [9].

In addition to the image quality, the content of the image provided to the CNN is also crucial. For instance, the presence of a large lesion, widespread eruption, or skin lesions distributed across multiple sites can significantly impact the analysis. Such factors can affect how the model interprets and classifies the condition, making it important to consider both the visual quality and the extent or distribution of the lesions when feeding data into the neural network [3].

20.3 Bias in Training Data

The field of artificial intelligence (AI) holds immense potential in reducing human error and cognitive bias in clinical decision-making. Nevertheless, in spite of its considerable potential, AI has the capacity to unwittingly mirror and even amplify the biases inherent in its training data. As highlighted in the extant literature, concerns have emerged about AI's potential to perpetuate discrimination in subtle or opaque ways, particularly in relation to legally protected attributes such as gender, ethnicity, age, and disability.

The reliability, accuracy, and fairness of AI algorithms are fundamentally dependent on the quality, diversity, and representativeness of the training data from which they learn [10]. This is especially salient in the context of deep learning models, which necessitate substantial and diverse datasets to yield outputs that are both generalizable and clinically reliable. However, in the context of healthcare, training datasets frequently exhibit a paucity of representation of minority populations. This imbalance can result in algorithms that inadvertently perpetuate or amplify existing healthcare disparities by producing systematically biased outputs that disproportionately affect underrepresented groups [11].

It is important to note that algorithmic bias is not solely a function of data distribution. It can also be embedded in the model architecture, the practices involved in the labeling of data, and the implicit assumptions of developers. This reinforces the subjective viewpoints and cultural norms of the individuals and institutions involved in the design of AI systems [12].

When models are trained on datasets that are not inclusive of or that are demographically skewed toward a specific group, and these models are then deployed in populations that are ethnically diverse, there is a significant increase in the risk of diagnostic error. The manifestation of clinical conditions varies across racial and ethnic groups; therefore, it is essential for AI systems to be trained on representative image and clinical data. This is especially critical for improving diagnostic accuracy and health equity in Black, Indigenous, and People of Color (BIPOC) communities [13].

For instance, psoriasis in individuals with darker skin types may present as violaceous plaques with an ash-gray scale, in contrast to the erythematous and silvery appearance commonly observed in lighter skin. Such variations in clinical presentation are also seen across a range of other dermatologic conditions, including eczema, melanoma, cellulitis, and vitiligo. It is imperative to acknowledge these variations in training data to ensure accurate diagnoses, thereby enhancing the clinical utility and ethical deployment of AI in dermatology.

In addition to the technical inconsistencies mentioned above, there is a critical issue of representational bias. Many existing dermatology AI models are trained on datasets that disproportionately include lighter skin types, resulting in underrepresentation of darker skin tones [14]. This has the potential to compromise the generalizability and clinical efficacy of these models in diverse populations, particularly in regions where darker-skinned individuals are predominant. This imbalance risks exacerbating existing disparities in dermatologic care and diagnostic accuracy (Table 20.1). Apart from skin of color issues, a model trained, for example, only on skin lesions of adults may not perform adequately in case of a lesion in a child patient due to different patterns that are consistent with age. To this end, enhancing algorithmic equity necessitates the

Table 20.1 Examples of image datasets with race-specific characteristics

Race/ethnicity specific	Examples of datasets
Asian	XiangyaDerm, DIET-AI, Acne04 [15–17]
African	CASIA-Face-Africa, PASSION derm 2024 dataset [18]
Hispanics	PAD-UFES-20 [19]
Mixed	Fitzpatrick 17k [20]

diversification of development team composition and the incorporation of fairness as a fundamental design consideration from the outset.

Apart from selection bias, there are also other bias regarding the training data (Table 20.2) and can be detected in multiple AI techniques such as transfer learning.

Table 20.2 Bias in training models in dermatology and examples of those bias

Bias in training models	Terminology	Examples
Selection bias	The data used to train AI models might not be representative of the entire population. This might result in poor performance in underrepresented populations such as skin of color patients and children [21]	In case of an AI model that is trained primarily on images of young, fair-skinned individuals with acne, due to sampling bias, the AI may misidentify or fail to detect acne lesions or acne cases and misevaluate acne severity in individuals with darker skin tones, where postinflammatory hyperpigmentation may be more prominent than redness or pustules
Sampling bias	If the dataset consists primarily of certain skin conditions or diagnoses in the dataset, the model might perform poorer when other less represented conditions [22]	When an AI dermatology model is trained on a dataset consisting of 1000 acne cases and only 50 rosacea cases, it develops a significant sampling bias due to the overwhelming dominance of acne examples. This imbalance causes the model to become highly attuned to identifying acne while lacking sufficient exposure to rosacea's varied presentations. As a result, the AI tends to overdiagnose acne and underrecognize or misclassify rosacea, especially in cases where the symptoms overlap, such as facial redness and pustules
Recall or labeling bias	AI systems rely on labeled data for training. In case the labeling process is wrong or inconsistent, the model will learn from biased labels [23]	Incorrect diagnoses or categorizations from annotators can influence the model's performance. For example, if the annotators label early-stage alopecia areata (with patchy hair loss) correctly, while others mistakenly label it as tinea capitis, the resulting AI model would learn incorrect association
Data augmentation bias	AI models often use techniques like data augmentation to create more training data from the available samples. If augmentation methods are applied incorrectly, it can introduce bias	For example, if images of dermatofibromas, which typically present as small, firm nodules, are artificially rotated, flipped, and/or brightened in order to create more data in terms of data augmentation techniques, key features of the lesions such as color uniformity may be distorted and the resulting performance of the model is poor
Overfitting bias	AI might develop a tendency to "confirm" and diagnose patterns that it has already seen and examined in the training data. Therefore, in case of new or atypical images of the same disease are presented, its performance is anticipated to drop [23, 24]	An AI model trained on classic cases of psoriasis, such as well-defined plaques with silvery scale on elbows and knees, may present limited accuracy in case of psoriasis plaques without the presence of silvery scale

20.4 The Limitation of CNNs

CNNs have emerged as the dominant architecture in image and video processing, thanks to their ability to extract hierarchical spatial representations from input data. Although they offer significant performance in a variety of applications, they have some significant drawbacks that limit their general usability and reliability (Table 20.3).

As observed in Fig. 20.3, both the tendency of CNNs to overfit and the resulting confirmation bias present in the training data represent significant drawbacks. As indicated by Fig. 20.3, to understand better the overfitting bias, the user can imagine a dense, tightly packed cluster of dots representing skin images of a certain diagnosis with a pack of features as edges, textures, colors, and other visual cues. This method represents the training data that the model has memorized perfectly. In case a handful of stray dots scattered well outside that cluster, representing the new cases (yellow triangles)—the new images—the new, unseen examples on which the model will struggle because it has not learned to generalize beyond its familiar cluster. To confront overfitting, dropout randomly "removes" some of the neurons in the network that are responsible for detecting certain patterns. For example, during training, the network might rely on particular features like color or shape to recognize a lesion. But with dropout, certain features are masked, forcing the model to rely on a broader range of features rather than memorizing specific patterns. Dropout in overfitting can mirror the process of meiosis. Through meiosis, the fusion of gametes recombines genetic material, and, as a result, the offspring exhibits novel traits absent from either parent's genome. This inherent randomness enables populations to adapt more effectively to their surroundings—a process we call evolution. In much the same way, dropout in neural networks and meiosis in biology both inject diversity into a system, preventing overreliance on any fixed set of parameters and leaving room for continuous improvement [33].

Overfitting limitation is particularly crucial in dermatology due to the high variability present in the images that neural networks are required to analyze. In addition to dropout layer, methods to deal with overfitting include applying data augmentation, a technique where images are altered to add variability that can occur during image acquisition (different colors, rotations, or scales) [34].

CNNs are one of the most important achievements of modern artificial intelligence. However, they are not without limitations. Their drawbacks, both technical and interpretative, require careful evaluation. Understanding and addressing these issues is essential for their safe, fair, and effective use in practice.

The need for large amounts of labeled data for training is a significant limitation in AI-powered dermatology, particularly when dealing with rare skin conditions or common skin diseases that have atypical features. Methods to address this limitation of CNNs include data augmentation techniques and transfer learning. According to transfer learning terminology, knowledge gained from one task trained with a huge dataset is leveraged to enhance performance on a different but related task based on training on a more limited dataset. In transfer learning, pretrained models are those that have been trained on extensive datasets and can be adapted for specific

Table 20.3 Limitations of CNNs

Computational resource and training time	Computational resource and training time requirements CNNs, especially deep and complex models such as ResNet or Inception, require significant computational resources for training and extracting predictions. The convolutional process involves multiple filters, pooling layers, and nonlinear activations, which makes the processing time-consuming and energy-intensive. The need for graphics processing units (GPUs) or tensor processing units (TPUs) increases the cost and limits access to smaller groups. Furthermore, the use of artificial neural networks (ANNs) is generally not appropriate in cases where efficient mathematical or algorithmic methods for solving the problem exist. In such cases, the time and resources required to design and train an ANN are not justified compared to the simpler alternative [25]
Lack of contextual awareness	While CNNs perform exceptionally well at recognizing local features, they lack the inherent ability to understand the overall context of the image. Small-scale filters that are applied locally often do not capture information that depends on the layout or environment of the object. This limitation has led to the development of new architectures, such as vision transformers [26]
Sensitivity to noise and input alterations	CNNs are vulnerable to small modifications of the input data, which can drastically alter the network's output [27]. So-called adversarial attacks, i.e., the deliberate introduction of minimal distortions to the image, can lead the network to make incorrect predictions [28]. This weakness raises serious concerns for applications in security or medicine
Limited interpretability and decision justification	Like all deep networks, CNNs operate as black box. Their decisions are based on thousands of parameters, making their predictions difficult to interpret. Although techniques such as class activation maps (Grad-CAM) and saliency maps allow for a degree of visualization interpretability remains limited and is a subject of research. Particularly problematic is the difficulty of explaining why an ANN reaches a particular solution and not another. This lack of transparency makes it difficult to accept the model in critical domains, such as healthcare or legal evaluation, where justification for each decision is essential [29]
Need for large volumes of labeled data training	CNN requires large amounts of labeled data, dermatology images, especially for classification applications. Labeling is time-consuming and often requires human intervention. In specialized domains, such as medicine, this data is limited, which negatively affects the performance of the model [30]
Overfitting and poor generalization	CNNs often exhibit the phenomenon of overfitting, especially when the dataset is small or the network is overly complex. In such cases, the model learns very well on the training data, but fails to generalize to new data. Although techniques such as dropout and data augmentation attempt to mitigate this problem, the balance remains fragile [31]
Specialization on structured image data	CNNs are designed to handle two-dimensional image data, where spatial arrangement is important. However, they have difficulty processing unstructured or heterogeneous data, such as graphs or multimodal information, limiting their usefulness in such cases [32]

tasks. They are commonly used as a foundation to accelerate training and improve the effectiveness of deep learning models. Typically, just the weights in convolutional layers are copied, rather than the entire network including the fully connected layers [35].

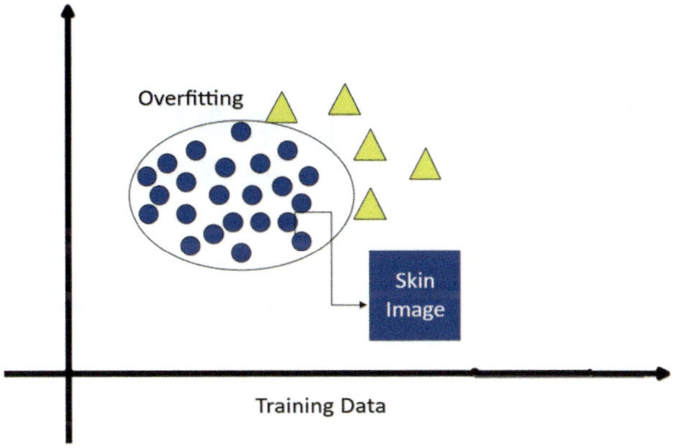

Fig. 20.3 A schematic representation of overfitting—with the elliptic circle covering the cluster of image dataset (blue circles) and the new cases (yellow triangles) not being included in the cluster

In a comprehensive study, the authors assessed the potential of using fine-tuned CNNs for medical image analysis as an alternative to training deep CNNs from scratch. The analysis was performed with both large and smaller training datasets. When using full datasets, the authors found that shallow fine-tuning of pretrained CNNs generally resulted in lower performance compared to CNNs trained from scratch. Feature extraction with shallow transfer learning involves freezing all the pretrained layers and only train the new layers that are added. On the contrary, the fine-tuning (deep transfer learning) includes unfreezing some (or all) of the pretrained layers and continue training them on the dataset. In the same study, CNNs with deeper fine-tuning, performed accordingly, and in some cases exceeded, that of CNNs trained from scratch. As the training datasets became smaller, the performance gap between deeply fine-tuned CNNs and those trained from scratch increased. This led us to conclude that fine-tuned CNNs should always be the preferred choice, regardless of the available size of the training sets [36].

Data augmentation techniques include modifying existing data (data warping) or generating new examples (oversampling). Data warping involves altering images in ways that maintain their original labels, using techniques such as geometric and color shifts, random erasing, and adversarial or crafted examples. On the other hand, oversampling methods introduce new, synthetic samples into the dataset through techniques such as image mixing, transformations in feature space, or the use of generative adversarial networks. Machine learning models process data (like images) are often converted from the raw data into a set of numerical features. This "feature space" is where each image is represented by a vector and by modifying or combining these feature vectors rather than changing the original images can help to confront overfitting [37, 38].

Notably, data warping and oversampling are not mutually exclusive as those techniques can be combined. In Agarwal's study, to address overfitting in a model designed to distinguish acne from rosacea, an augmented data warping approach was applied. This led to an improvement in the model's specificity for acne, increasing from 0.9 to 0.95. Overall, the performance metrics for all the conditions

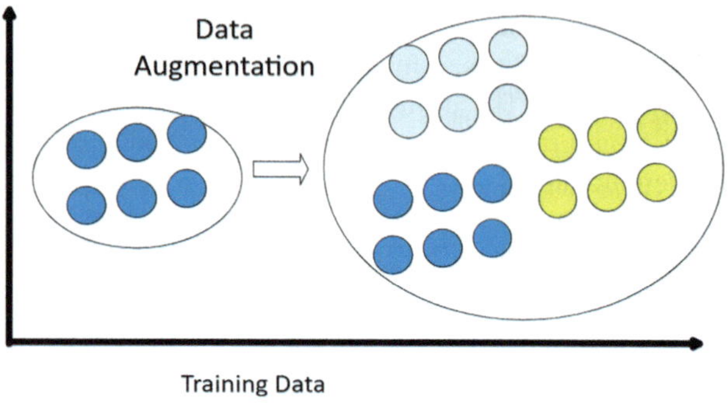

Fig. 20.4 A schematic representation of data augmentation with data wrapping (including color shift) creating a wider area of training data

examined either improved or stayed consistent following data augmentation [39] (Fig. 20.4).

20.5 Lack of Explainability

A critical and as yet unresolved challenge in the deployment of AI systems in healthcare is the opacity of their decision-making processes. In many cases, it is either difficult or entirely infeasible to determine the rationale underlying the outputs produced by AI models. This dearth of transparency emanates from numerous sources. In some cases, the algorithms are proprietary and thus deliberately concealed from scrutiny [40]. In other cases, the complexity of the models, particularly in the context of deep learning architectures, makes them uninterpretable to humans. These models frequently function as "black boxes," generating predictions without a clear, traceable chain of reasoning [41].

Machine learning systems, in particular those employing deep neural networks, have been shown to exacerbate this issue due to their dynamic nature. As these models are trained, they continuously modify their internal parameters in response to new data, thereby obscuring the rules and patterns driving their behavior. This adaptive learning process makes the validation of outputs as well as the identification of systematic errors within the decision logic particularly challenging.

In clinical contexts, this absence of interpretability poses significant limitations. Neural networks (NNs), which are extensively utilized in medical AI applications, are particularly opaque and their internal operations frequently escape human comprehension, as the specific features or data points that influence their predictions remain largely unknown. This has given rise to criticism, as these models have the potential to generate unanticipated outputs that are challenging to clinicians to comprehend or predict. This has led to the characterization of neural networks as "blackbox" systems, a term that emphasizes their potential to malfunction in ways that are both unpredictable and difficult to recognize [41] (Fig. 20.5).

Chanda et al. demonstrated a strong alignment between explainable artificial intelligence (XAI) outputs and dermatologists' clinical reasoning. Their study showed that dermatologists' confidence in their diagnoses and trust in the AI

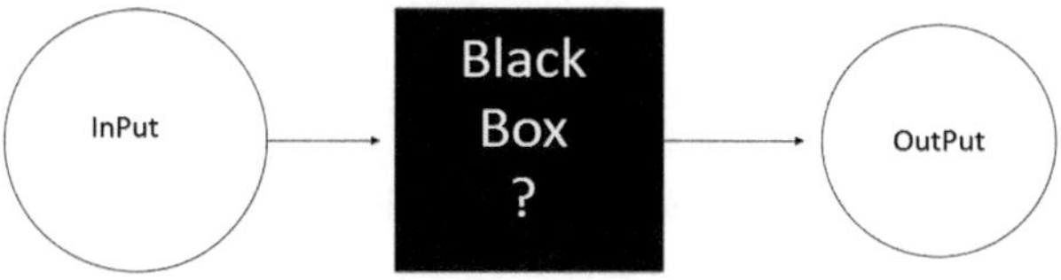

Fig. 20.5 Image showing the understanding and observation of the inputs and outputs, but due to black box (complicated model such as CNNs) the internal logic or decision-making process is not fully understood

support system significantly increased when using XAI compared to conventional "black-box" AI. These findings underscore dermatologists' willingness to adopt XAI-driven systems, supporting their potential integration into future clinical practice [42].

Nevertheless, the field of explainable AI (XAI) is advancing rapidly. Innovative statistical methodologies and interpretability frameworks are being developed to elucidate how complex models reach their conclusions. These techniques aim to provide clinicians and developers with greater insight into the behavior of models, with the ultimate aim of bridging the gap between high-performance AI and the level of transparency required in medical decision-making. Continued research in this area has the potential to develop AI systems that are more accountable and trustworthy [43].

Due to their complexity and frequent lack of robustness, DNNs often operate as "black boxes," making their decision-making processes difficult to interpret. In clinical settings, however, it is crucial for healthcare professionals to understand how much they can trust the outputs of diagnostic support systems in each individual case. In dermatology, XAI methods commonly address this phenomenon by either presenting images that resemble the one being analyzed or by highlighting specific image regions that significantly influenced the classification [44].

In XAI, a heatmap is a common way of visually showing which parts of an input, such as an image, the AI model focused on to make its decision. The heatmaps can be described plainly as the shining of a light on the areas that caught the model's attention the most to make its decision. Regions highlighted in hotter colors like red or orange indicate parts the model considered important, meaning they had a major influence on the final outcome and consequently the output. On the other hand, cooler colors like blue point indicated areas that mattered less and influenced minimally the model's decision [45]. An XAI method refers to which parts of its decision-making process an AI model is based on and should explain, revealing the underlying algorithm or technique that generates the output. Common examples include class activation maps such as Grad-CAM and Integrated Gradients (see Table 20.3). Each of these methods has its own way of analyzing the model's "thought process" and determining which inputs' features had the most influence on the final prediction. On the other hand, the form of explanation such as heatmap is how the output of these methods is actually presented to clinicians [46]. Given the potentially severe consequences of false negatives in diagnostic tasks especially in case of melanoma, it is crucial to verify whether the decision-making rules learned by deep neural networks in these life-threatening situations are supported by medical science.

Local Interpretable Model-Agnostic Explanations (LIME) is designed to explain the predictions of various ML and DL models, regardless of their complexity or structure. The term "model-agnostic" is used to characterize techniques used to interpret AI models functioning. LIME helps in revealing which features most influenced a particular decision made by the ML or DL model. For LIME to be truly effective in healthcare settings, it is important that its outputs are easily interpretable by especially clinicians. Thanks to its flexibility, LIME can be used across many ML approaches, including deep neural networks, random forests, and gradient boosting models [47]. Nigar et al. applied LIME to develop a skin lesion classification system, accurately distinguishing between eight types of skin lesions using the ISIC 2019 dataset. By incorporating LIME-generated visual explanations, the model supports dermatologists in making more informed decisions. Their approach combined transfer learning with a ResNet-18 architecture, demonstrating how ML tools can facilitate earlier detection, lower healthcare costs, and enhance patient outcomes. Additionally, the study proposed that LIME could aid dermatologists in identifying new lesion patterns and improving existing datasets, emphasizing the importance of continuous data quality improvement to ensure high-performing ML models [48] (Fig. 20.6).

SHapley Additive exPlanations (SHAP) is an approach that brings improved interpretability to a wide range of ML and DL models. In medical imaging as in dermatology, however, there is a stronger emphasis on LIME's explanations over SHAP's. This is because LIME creates quick, local approximations of any black-box model—giving clear, on-the-spot insights into individual predictions—whereas SHAP delivers both local and global explanations at the cost of greater computational overhead, making it less immediately practical in this domain [51].

Class activation maps (CAMs) give a fixed explanation after the model makes a prediction. It highlights which areas of the image were most important for a particular class, but it does not show how attention is applied throughout the entire process. On

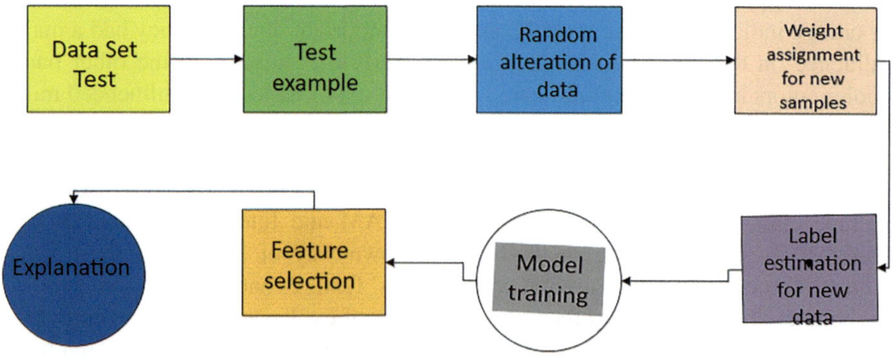

Fig. 20.6 Image presenting the workflow presented in LIME studies

the other hand, visual attention provides a more dynamic view, showing how the model focuses on different parts of the image or data at each step of its decision-making process. It gives insight into how the model shifts its attention over time as it works through the input (Table 20.4). Other forms of explanatory AI include integrated gradients, according to which an assignment is made to the contribution to each input feature based on how it affects the final prediction. This helps us understand why the model made a certain decision and it calculates how the model's output changes as the inputs are modified from a baseline, for example, a blank image [52].

Table 20.4 Examples of XAI methods that have been used and associated studies in dermatology

XAI method	Functions	Study example	Work
Local Interpretable Model-Agnostic Explanations (LIME)	Reveals which features most influenced a particular decision	Nigar et al. [48]	The model successfully classifies eight different types of skin lesions—including dermatofibroma, squamous cell carcinoma, benign keratosis, melanocytic nevus, vascular lesion, actinic keratosis, basal cell carcinoma, and melanoma—with high classification accuracy. The authors used LIME framework, which provides visual explanations that align with established prior knowledge and follow best practices for interpretability
Content-Based Image Retrieval (CBIR)	Finds similar images from a database based on specific visual features	Sadeghi et al. [44]	Presentation of the design and assessment of a CBIR examining how accurately users classify dermoscopy images. CBIR allows beginners to classify a new skin lesion image with much greater accuracy, distinguishing it into one of four commonly observed categories: Nevus, seborrheic keratosis, basal cell carcinoma, and malignant melanoma
Backpropagation	Traces backward the model's output and work the way back to "see" which parts of the image played the biggest role in the AI model's output	Winkler et al. [49]	Observation that skin markings had a notable impact on the CNN's ability to accurately diagnose nevi, leading to higher melanoma probability scores and, as a result, an increased false-positive rate
Class activation maps (GradCAM)	Highlights the image regions that contributed the most to an output	Chowdhury et al. [50]	Conduction of visual analysis to determine if the activation maps of deep models show any similarity to the segmentation maps used for extracting clinical features (ABCD features) of skin lesions

The question of explainability has also been a point of interest for regulatory bodies. The European Union's General Data Protection Regulation (GDPR) is a case in point as it explicitly addresses the rights of individuals subjected to automated decision-making. Article 22 of the GDPR establishes a right not to be subject to decisions based solely on automated processing—including profiling—that produce legal or similarly significant effects. Furthermore, the regulation mandates that data controllers provide "meaningful information about the logic involved," as well as the potential consequences of such processing. These provisions impose a legal imperative for algorithmic transparency and accountability [53].

In contrast, the regulatory landscape in the United States is characterized by greater fragmentation. The Food and Drug Administration (FDA) has issued guidance suggesting that until AI-based clinical decision tools are supported by robust clinical trial data, their outputs should be considered "AI-guided" rather than "AI-determined." In this regulatory framework, the onus of clinical responsibility and liability remains firmly with the healthcare provider, as opposed to being allocated to the AI system. This cautious regulatory stance is indicative of the prevailing concerns surrounding the safety, reliability, and ethical use of AI in clinical practice [54].

20.6 Hallucinations

Apart from the limitations implemented into image-based AI models, there are many biases regarding the use of large language models. While many researchers have explored the positive effects of those models on different aspects of dermatology practices [55], growing concerns have also emerged around AI hallucination. For example, in studying ChatGPT's role in dermatologists or patient's advisory, researchers have warned about its potential to produce hallucinatory answers, stressing the importance of using such AI tools with caution. Some researchers have even created mathematical models to better understand both the hallucination tendencies and creative aspects of ChatGPT models. They argue that hallucination is an inherent feature of ChatGPT and that trying to completely eliminate it without sacrificing the model's high performance is nearly impossible. Tackling AI hallucination is a major challenge: while reducing its negative impacts is critical, fully eradicating it seems unlikely [56].

Despite the ongoing attention AI hallucination receives in academic discussions, there is still no consensus among researchers about what exactly the term means. While some scholars use "hallucination" to describe the irrational outputs of AI systems, others are dissatisfied with this label. In fact, "AI hallucination" has yet to settle into a universally accepted definition, and researchers continue to interpret it differently. Some define AI hallucination as instances where a chatbot invents false, inaccurate, or baseless information when answering questions [57]. One study even proposed classifying hallucinations in large language models (LLMs) into three types: input-conflicting, context-conflicting, and fact-conflicting hallucinations (Table 20.5) [56]. Finally, errors due to hallucinations are frequently observed in reference reporting.

Table 20.5 Types of hallucination with examples

Type of hallucination	Chatbot response based on alopecia areata	Hallucination type
Input-conflicting	Input: a clinical image showing well-demarcated, round patches of hair loss typical of alopecia areata AI output: "*The lesion appears to be consistent with tinea capitis due to the presence of scaling and inflammation.*"	There is no scaling or inflammation presented in the image uploaded in the chatbot, contrary to the AI description
Context-conflicting	Case context: *A 35-year-old woman with a family history of autoimmune disorders and sudden onset of patchy scalp hair loss* AI output: "*This presentation is most likely due to age-related androgenetic alopecia.*"	The context clearly supports a different etiology hair loss disease that has a different pattern and onset
Fact-conflicting hallucinations	AI output: "*Alopecia areata is caused by a fungal infection and is highly contagious.*"	This statement is factually incorrect

20.7 Skin Cancer Overdiagnosis

Integrating AI into current clinical workflows remains major challenges. AI has the potential to automate routine tasks, freeing healthcare professionals to concentrate on more complex, patient-centered care. However, if images of nevi are uploaded alongside AI-generated risk scores, there is a risk that clinicians—particularly less experienced dermatologists who heavily rely on AI outputs—may be overly influenced. Out of fear of missing a melanoma diagnosis, they might opt to excise any atypical nevi for histopathological examination. This could lead to the overdiagnosis of skin cancer, increasing healthcare costs and subjecting patients to unnecessary procedures and tests [58].

20.8 Limitations Concerning Social Aspects of AI Integration into Dermatology

20.8.1 The Matter of Cost

Furthermore, the performance of AI systems is not uniform. Substantial disparities exist in terms of diagnostic accuracy, sensitivity, and multimodal capabilities. A compelling illustration of this variation can be observed in the progression from GPT-3.5 to GPT-4. While GPT-3.5, trained on 17 gigabytes of data, scored in the bottom 10% on the US bar exam, GPT-4, trained on 45 gigabytes and equipped with multimodal capabilities, scored in the top 10%. While these advancements represent significant breakthroughs, they also come with increased computational and financial costs, raising ethical questions around equitable deployment.

In environments where resources are limited, there is a tangible risk that lower-cost, less capable AI models will be used disproportionately, further exacerbating disparities in care access and quality. It is therefore vital to ensure that under-resourced communities are not marginalized by the deployment of outdated or underperforming AI technologies [59].

20.8.2 Security and Privacy

The advent of artificial intelligence (AI) in the field of healthcare has precipitated a paradigm shift toward a new era of data-driven clinical decision-making, diagnosis, and patient management. AI systems, in particular those that employ ML and Dl models, are dependent on substantial volumes of data for the training and validation of their predictive algorithms. In the domain of dermatology, for instance, where the analysis of images is a fundamental component of clinical practice, the application of AI holds particular promise. However, this potential is accompanied by significant challenges, particularly concerning data privacy, regulatory compliance, and ethical considerations [60].

The inherent reliance of AI systems in healthcare on the acquisition, storage, and processing of sensitive and often personally identifiable health data is a matter of particular concern. This data is subject to stringent legal frameworks designed to safeguard patient confidentiality and prevent misuse. In the United States, for instance, the Health Insurance Portability and Accountability Act of 1996 (HIPAA) governs the handling of protected health information (PHI), including any data that can be used to identify an individual, either directly or indirectly. These legal safeguards, while essential, impose significant constraints on the ability of AI developers to access and use real-world clinical data, particularly at the scale required for high-performance machine learning models [61].

In the field of dermatology, these challenges are particularly evident. It is commonplace for clinical images to contain identifiable anatomical features, including but not limited to facial characteristics, tattoos, and other unique skin markings. This raises significant concerns regarding patient privacy. Despite efforts to anonymize such images, advancements in image analysis and facial recognition technologies may still enable their re-identification [60]. This poses significant ethical challenges, as obtaining informed consent from patients for the collection and utilization of such images in AI development is ethically intricate [62].

Moreover, the field of dermatology is characterized by a paucity of universally accepted standards for the capture, processing, transmission, and storage of clinical images. This is in stark contrast to fields like radiology, which have long benefited from the use of structured and standardized imaging protocols. The Digital Imaging and Communications in Medicine (DICOM) standard, a widely adopted framework in radiology, ensures that images are consistently formatted and embedded with metadata such as patient demographics, acquisition parameters, and timestamps. Systems such as Picture Archiving and Communication Systems (PACS) further streamline the secure storage and retrieval of medical images across healthcare networks [63]. Despite the efforts to adapt DICOM standards for use in dermatology, these adaptations have yet to achieve widespread implementation or consensus among clinical practitioners [64].

Beyond the structured clinical data, AI systems are increasingly drawing upon unconventional data sources, such as social media activity, search engine histories, and consumer health applications. While not inherently clinical, such data can offer insights into a person's health behaviors, symptomatology, or mental health status. However, this raises additional privacy concerns, particularly regarding the secondary use of data that users may not have intended for health-related analysis. The convergence of AI, big data, and digital surveillance has given rise to a new ethical debate, where the boundaries between informed consent, privacy, and public health benefit are often indistinct [65].

Concerns have been raised regarding the potential for covert surveillance and unauthorized health screening through the use of AI. Technologies capable of analyzing motor behavior—such as keystroke patterns—or tracking mobility through smartphones can infer sensitive health information without the individual's knowledge or consent. These capabilities introduce significant risks to personal privacy and challenge the ethical boundaries of health data collection and usage.

In addition to privacy concerns, AI can be weaponized to conduct cyberattacks at unprecedented scale and reduced cost. Machine learning algorithms have the capacity to automate system exploitation, dynamically adapt to security defenses, and orchestrate complex attacks with minimal human intervention. The implications for healthcare systems, which are already vulnerable due to their reliance on vast and often under-secured digital infrastructure, are particularly severe [66].

20.8.3 Accountability

These issues give rise to fundamental questions concerning accountability in the field of AI-driven healthcare. In circumstances where an AI system contributes to a clinical error or adverse outcome, the determination of responsibility becomes a complex undertaking. The question of liability, therefore, becomes a crucial one and must be addressed through a thorough examination of the various parties involved: namely, the developer, the healthcare institution, and the clinician who utilize the tool [67]. Moreover, the absence of legal and institutional clarity surrounding redress mechanisms for individuals adversely affected by algorithmic decisions constitutes a pressing challenge. As AI continues to expand its role in healthcare, it is imperative to address these ambiguities to ensure trust, ethical deployment, and the protection of patient rights [68].

These risks have prompted an increasing number of calls for proactive governance measures. It is incumbent upon policymakers, engineers, and researchers to collaborate in order to address the potential for AI to be misused through the establishment of robust regulatory frameworks, ethical design standards, and cross-sector collaboration. The establishment of safeguards to ensure transparency, auditability, and accountability in the deployment of AI systems is imperative, particularly in sensitive domains such as healthcare [69].

It is imperative to acknowledge that the recognition and preparation for the malicious use of AI is not a discretionary matter; rather, it is a fundamental responsibility in the era of intelligent systems.

20.9 Conclusions

In general, there is an urgent requirement for regulatory frameworks that are specifically tailored to the unique challenges posed by AI in dermatology and broader healthcare contexts. These frameworks must encompass a range of issues, including but not limited to data ownership, consent models, liability in the event of AI-driven misdiagnosis, and transparency in algorithmic decision-making.

Stakeholder engagement is critical to ensuring the responsible and equitable deployment of AI in dermatology [70]. This encompasses not only clinicians and technologists but also ethicists, legal experts, patient advocacy groups, and representatives from diverse communities. Inclusive governance structures have the potential to ensure that AI tools are aligned with societal values, clinical needs, and the rights of individuals.

References

1. Li Z, Koban KC, Schenck TL, Giunta RE, Li Q, Sun Y. Artificial intelligence in dermatology image analysis: current developments and future trends. J Clin Med. 2022;11:6826. https://doi.org/10.3390/jcm11226826.
2. Grzybowski A, Jin K, Wu H. Challenges of artificial intelligence in medicine and dermatology. Clin Dermatol. 2024;42:210–5. https://doi.org/10.1016/j.clindermatol.2023.12.013.
3. Liopyris K, Gregoriou S, Dias J, Stratigos AJ. Artificial intelligence in dermatology: challenges and perspectives. Dermatol Ther (Heidelb). 2022;12:2637–51. https://doi.org/10.1007/s13555-022-00833-8.
4. Jalaboi R, Winther O, Galimzianova A. Explainable image quality assessments in Teledermatological photography. Telemed E-Health. 2023;29:1342–8. https://doi.org/10.1089/tmj.2022.0405.
5. Al-hammuri K, Gebali F, Kanan A, Chelvan IT. Vision transformer architecture and applications in digital health: a tutorial and survey. Vis Comput Ind Biomed Art. 2023;6:14. https://doi.org/10.1186/s42492-023-00140-9.
6. Oloruntoba AI, Asghari-Jafarabadi M, Sashindranath M, Ingvar Å, Adler NR, Vico-Alonso C, et al. Assessment of image quality on the diagnostic performance of clinicians and deep learning models: cross-sectional comparative reader study. J Eur Acad Dermatol Venereol. 2024; https://doi.org/10.1111/jdv.20462.
7. Scheinfeld N. Photographic images, digital imaging, dermatology, and the law. Arch Dermatol. 2004;140 https://doi.org/10.1001/archderm.140.4.473.
8. Bernhard R, Bletterer A, Le Caro M, García Álvarez E, Kostov B, Herrera ED. Automatic acne severity grading with a small and imbalanced data set of low-resolution images. Dermatol Ther (Heidelb). 2024;14:2953–69. https://doi.org/10.1007/s13555-024-01283-0.
9. Schaefferkoetter J, Yan J, Ortega C, Sertic A, Lechtman E, Eshet Y, et al. Convolutional neural networks for improving image quality with noisy PET data. EJNMMI Res. 2020;10:105. https://doi.org/10.1186/s13550-020-00695-1.

10. Rashid D, Hirani R, Khessib S, Ali N, Etienne M. Unveiling biases of artificial intelligence in healthcare: navigating the promise and pitfalls. Injury. 2024;55:111358. https://doi.org/10.1016/j.injury.2024.111358.
11. Aquino YSJ. Making decisions: bias in artificial intelligence and data-driven diagnostic tools. Aust J Gen Pract. 2023;52:439–42. https://doi.org/10.31128/AJGP-12-22-6630.
12. Nazer LH, Zatarah R, Waldrip S, Ke JXC, Moukheiber M, Khanna AK, et al. Bias in artificial intelligence algorithms and recommendations for mitigation. PLOS Digital Health. 2023;2:e0000278. https://doi.org/10.1371/journal.pdig.0000278.
13. Al Kuwaiti A, Nazer K, Al-Reedy A, Al-Shehri S, Al-Muhanna A, Subbarayalu AV, et al. A review of the role of artificial intelligence in healthcare. J Pers Med. 2023;13:951. https://doi.org/10.3390/jpm13060951.
14. Bhat Y, Jha A. Dermatoscopy of inflammatory diseases in skin of color. Indian Dermatol Online J. 2021;12:45. https://doi.org/10.4103/idoj.IDOJ_613_20.
15. Li H, Zhang P, Wei Z, Qian T, Tang Y, Hu K, et al. Deep skin diseases diagnostic system with Dual-channel image and extracted text. Front Artif Intell. 2023;6 https://doi.org/10.3389/frai.2023.1213620.
16. Xie B, He X, Zhao S, Li Y, Su J, Zhao X, et al. XiangyaDerm: a clinical image dataset of Asian race for skin disease aided diagnosis. Springer; 2019. p. 22–31. https://doi.org/10.1007/978-3-030-33642-4_3.
17. Trivedi NK, Maheshwari H, Tiwari RG, Gautam V, Agarwal AK, Sharma M. Deep acne: advancing automated acne identification through deep neural networks. In: 2024 1st international conference on Advanced Computing and Emerging Technologies (ACET). IEEE; 2024. p. 1–5. https://doi.org/10.1109/ACET61898.2024.10730442.
18. https://passionderm.github.io. n.d.; Last accessed on 29 Apr 2025.
19. Pacheco AGC, Lima GR, Salomão AS, Krohling B, Biral IP, de Angelo GG, et al. PAD-UFES-20: a skin lesion dataset composed of patient data and clinical images collected from smartphones. Data Brief. 2020;32:106221. https://doi.org/10.1016/j.dib.2020.106221.
20. Proceedings of the IEEE/CVF Conference on Computer Vision and Pattern Recognition; 2021. pp. 1820–28.
21. Chen Z. Ethics and discrimination in artificial intelligence-enabled recruitment practices. Hum Soc Sci Commun. 2023;10:567. https://doi.org/10.1057/s41599-023-02079-x.
22. Ferrara E. Fairness and bias in artificial intelligence: a brief survey of sources, impacts, and mitigation strategies. Science. 2023;6:3. https://doi.org/10.3390/sci6010003.
23. Belenguer L. AI bias: exploring discriminatory algorithmic decision-making models and the application of possible machine-centric solutions adapted from the pharmaceutical industry. AI Ethics. 2022;2:771–87. https://doi.org/10.1007/s43681-022-00138-8.
24. Ravishankar P, Mo Q, McFowland E III, Neill DB. Provable detection of propagating sampling bias in prediction models. Proc AAAI Conf Artif Intell. 2023;37:9562–9. https://doi.org/10.1609/aaai.v37i8.26144.
25. He K, Zhang X, Ren S, Sun J. Deep residual learning for image recognition. In: 2016 IEEE conference on computer vision and pattern recognition (CVPR). IEEE; 2016. p. 770–8. https://doi.org/10.1109/CVPR.2016.90.
26. Mitrea CA, Lee CKM, Wu Z. A comparison between neural networks and traditional forecasting methods: a case study. Int J Eng Bus Manage. 2009;1 https://doi.org/10.5772/6777.
27. An Image is Worth 16x16 Words: Transformers for Image Recognition at Scale. n.d.
28. Szegedy C, Liu W, Jia Y, Sermanet P, Reed S, Anguelov D, et al. Going deeper with convolutions. In: 2015 IEEE conference on computer vision and pattern recognition (CVPR). IEEE; 2015. p. 1–9. https://doi.org/10.1109/CVPR.2015.7298594.
29. Bradshaw TJ, McCradden MD, Jha AK, Dutta J, Saboury B, Siegel EL, et al. Artificial intelligence algorithms need to be explainable—or do they? J Nucl Med. 2023;64:976–7. https://doi.org/10.2967/jnumed.122.264949.
30. Jeong HK, Park C, Henao R, Kheterpal M. Deep learning in dermatology: a systematic review of current approaches, outcomes, and limitations. JID Innov. 2023;3:100150. https://doi.org/10.1016/j.xjidi.2022.100150.

31. Charilaou P, Battat R. Machine learning models and over-fitting considerations. World J Gastroenterol. 2022;28:605–7. https://doi.org/10.3748/wjg.v28.i5.605.
32. LeCun Y, Bengio Y, Hinton G. Deep learning. Nature. 2015;521:436–44. https://doi.org/10.1038/nature14539.
33. Li H, Weng J, Mao Y, Wang Y, Zhan Y, Cai Q, et al. Adaptive dropout method based on biological principles. IEEE Trans Neural Netw Learn Syst. 2021;32:4267–76. https://doi.org/10.1109/TNNLS.2021.3070895.
34. Liang Y, Niu C, Yan P, Wang G. Flipover outperforms dropout in deep learning. Vis Comput Ind Biomed Art. 2024;7:4. https://doi.org/10.1186/s42492-024-00153-y.
35. Hao R, Namdar K, Liu L, Haider MA, Khalvati F. A comprehensive study of data augmentation strategies for prostate cancer detection in diffusion-weighted MRI using convolutional neural networks. J Digit Imaging. 2021;34:862–76. https://doi.org/10.1007/s10278-021-00478-7.
36. Tajbakhsh N, Shin JY, Gurudu SR, Hurst RT, Kendall CB, Gotway MB, et al. Convolutional neural networks for medical image analysis: full training or fine tuning? IEEE Trans Med Imaging. 2016;35:1299–312. https://doi.org/10.1109/TMI.2016.2535302.
37. Alomar K, Aysel HI, Cai X. Data augmentation in classification and segmentation: a survey and new strategies. J Imaging. 2023;9:46. https://doi.org/10.3390/jimaging9020046.
38. Sanchez S, Vallez N, Bueno G, Marrugo AG. Data augmentation via warping transforms for modeling natural variability in the corneal endothelium enhances semi-supervised segmentation. PLoS One. 2024;19:e0311849. https://doi.org/10.1371/journal.pone.0311849.
39. Aggarwal St Lt P. Data augmentation in dermatology image recognition using machine learning. Skin Res Technol. 2019;25:815–20. https://doi.org/10.1111/srt.12726.
40. Price WN. Big data and black-box medical algorithms. Sci Transl Med. 2018;10 https://doi.org/10.1126/scitranslmed.aao5333.
41. Wadden JJ. Defining the undefinable: the black box problem in healthcare artificial intelligence. J Med Ethics. 2022;48:764–8. https://doi.org/10.1136/medethics-2021-107529.
42. Chanda T, Hauser K, Hobelsberger S, Bucher T-C, Garcia CN, Wies C, et al. Dermatologist-like explainable AI enhances trust and confidence in diagnosing melanoma. Nat Commun. 2024;15:524. https://doi.org/10.1038/s41467-023-43095-4.
43. Linardatos P, Papastefanopoulos V, Kotsiantis S. Explainable AI: a review of machine learning interpretability methods. Entropy. 2020;23:18. https://doi.org/10.3390/e23010018.
44. Sadeghi M, Chilana PK, Atkins MS. How users perceive content-based image retrieval for identifying skin images. In: Understanding and interpreting machine learning in medical image computing applications. Springer; 2018. p. 141–8. https://doi.org/10.1007/978-3-030-02628-8_16.
45. Giavina-Bianchi M, Vitor WG, Fornasiero de Paiva V, Okita AL, Sousa RM, Machado B. Explainability agreement between dermatologists and five visual explanations techniques in deep neural networks for melanoma AI classification. Front Med (Lausanne). 2023:10. https://doi.org/10.3389/fmed.2023.1241484.
46. Hauser K, Kurz A, Haggenmüller S, Maron RC, von Kalle C, Utikal JS, et al. Explainable artificial intelligence in skin cancer recognition: a systematic review. Eur J Cancer. 2022;167:54–69. https://doi.org/10.1016/j.ejca.2022.02.025.
47. Hassan SU, Abdulkadir SJ, MSM Z, Al-Selwi SM. Local interpretable model-agnostic explanation approach for medical imaging analysis: a systematic literature review. Comput Biol Med. 2025;185:109569. https://doi.org/10.1016/j.compbiomed.2024.109569.
48. Nigar N, Umar M, Shahzad MK, Islam S, Abalo D. A deep learning approach based on explainable artificial intelligence for skin lesion classification. IEEE Access. 2022;10:113715–25. https://doi.org/10.1109/ACCESS.2022.3217217.
49. Winkler JK, Fink C, Toberer F, Enk A, Deinlein T, Hofmann-Wellenhof R, et al. Association between surgical skin markings in Dermoscopic images and diagnostic performance of a deep learning convolutional neural network for melanoma recognition. JAMA Dermatol. 2019;155:1135. https://doi.org/10.1001/jamadermatol.2019.1735.
50. Selvaraju RR, Cogswell M, Das A, Vedantam R, Parikh D, Batra D. Grad-CAM: visual explanations from deep networks via gradient-based localization. In: 2017 IEEE international

conference on computer vision (ICCV). IEEE; 2017. p. 618–26. https://doi.org/10.1109/ICCV.2017.74.
51. Ponce-Bobadilla AV, Schmitt V, Maier CS, Mensing S, Stodtmann S. Practical guide to SHAP analysis: explaining supervised machine learning model predictions in drug development. Clin Transl Sci. 2024;17 https://doi.org/10.1111/cts.70056.
52. Majdandzic A, Rajesh C, Koo PK. Correcting gradient-based interpretations of deep neural networks for genomics. Genome Biol. 2023;24:109. https://doi.org/10.1186/s13059-023-02956-3.
53. van Kolfschooten HB. A health-conformant reading of the GDPR'S right not to be subject to automated decision-making. Med Law Rev. 2024;32:373–91. https://doi.org/10.1093/medlaw/fwae029.
54. Hanassab S, Abbara A, Yeung AC, Voliotis M, Tsaneva-Atanasova K, Kelsey TW, et al. The prospect of artificial intelligence to personalize assisted reproductive technology. NPJ Digit Med. 2024;7:55. https://doi.org/10.1038/s41746-024-01006-x.
55. Karampinis E, Toli O, Georgopoulou K-E, Kampra E, Spyridonidou C, Roussaki Schulze A-V, et al. Can artificial intelligence "hold" a Dermoscope?—the evaluation of an artificial intelligence Chatbot to translate the Dermoscopic language. Diagnostics. 2024;14:1165. https://doi.org/10.3390/diagnostics14111165.
56. Sun Y, Sheng D, Zhou Z, Wu Y. AI hallucination: towards a comprehensive classification of distorted information in artificial intelligence-generated content. Hum Soc Sci Commun. 2024;11:1278. https://doi.org/10.1057/s41599-024-03811-x.
57. Aljamaan F, Temsah M-H, Altamimi I, Al-Eyadhy A, Jamal A, Alhasan K, et al. Reference hallucination score for medical artificial intelligence Chatbots: development and usability study. JMIR Med Inform. 2024;12:e54345. https://doi.org/10.2196/54345.
58. Semsarian CR, Ma T, Nickel B, Scolyer RA, Ferguson PM, Soyer HP, et al. Do we need to rethink the diagnoses melanoma *in situ* and severely dysplastic naevus? Br J Dermatol. 2022;186:1030–2. https://doi.org/10.1111/bjd.21010.
59. Karakaş Ü, Özdemir V. Artificial intelligence and environmental impact: moving beyond humanizing vocabulary and anthropocentrism. OMICS. 2025;29:2–4. https://doi.org/10.1089/omi.2024.0197.
60. Yadav N, Pandey S, Gupta A, Dudani P, Gupta S, Rangarajan K. Data privacy in healthcare: in the era of artificial intelligence. Indian Dermatol Online J. 2023;14:788–92. https://doi.org/10.4103/idoj.idoj_543_23.
61. Marks M, Haupt CE. AI Chatbots, health privacy, and challenges to HIPAA compliance. JAMA. 2023;330:309. https://doi.org/10.1001/jama.2023.9458.
62. Harishbhai Tilala M, Kumar Chenchala P, Choppadandi A, Kaur J, Naguri S, Saoji R, et al. Ethical considerations in the use of artificial intelligence and machine learning in health care: a comprehensive review. Cureus. 2024; https://doi.org/10.7759/cureus.62443.
63. Caffery LJ, Clunie D, Curiel-Lewandrowski C, Malvehy J, Soyer HP, Halpern AC. Transforming dermatologic imaging for the digital era: metadata and standards. J Digit Imaging. 2018;31:568–77. https://doi.org/10.1007/s10278-017-0045-8.
64. Larobina M. Thirty years of the DICOM standard. Tomography. 2023;9:1829–38. https://doi.org/10.3390/tomography9050145.
65. Murdoch B. Privacy and artificial intelligence: challenges for protecting health information in a new era. BMC Med Ethics. 2021;22:122. https://doi.org/10.1186/s12910-021-00687-3.
66. Khalid N, Qayyum A, Bilal M, Al-Fuqaha A, Qadir J. Privacy-preserving artificial intelligence in healthcare: techniques and applications. Comput Biol Med. 2023;158:106848. https://doi.org/10.1016/j.compbiomed.2023.106848.
67. Da Silva M, Horsley T, Singh D, Da Silva E, Ly V, Thomas B, et al. Legal concerns in health-related artificial intelligence: a scoping review protocol. Syst Rev. 2022;11:123. https://doi.org/10.1186/s13643-022-01939-y.
68. Wang X, Wu YC, Ji X, Fu H. Algorithmic discrimination: examining its types and regulatory measures with emphasis on US legal practices. Front Artif Intell. 2024;7 https://doi.org/10.3389/frai.2024.1320277.

69. Jassar S, Adams SJ, Zarzeczny A, Burbridge BE. The future of artificial intelligence in medicine: medical-legal considerations for health leaders. Healthc Manage Forum. 2022;35:185–9. https://doi.org/10.1177/08404704221082069.
70. Ling Kuo RY, Freethy A, Smith J, Hill R, C J, Jerome D, et al. Stakeholder perspectives towards diagnostic artificial intelligence: a co-produced qualitative evidence synthesis. EClinicalMedicine. 2024;71:102555. https://doi.org/10.1016/j.eclinm.2024.102555.

Artificial Intelligence and Special Populations: Age Considerations

21

Emmanouil Karampinis and Olga Toli

21.1 Pediatric Dermatology: Can the Adult Medicine-Based Artificial Intelligence Be Integrated Normally Into Pediatric Dermatology?

Pediatric dermatology encompasses a wide range of different skin entities ranging from birthmarks and infantile hemangiomas to different types of dermatitis such as napkin dermatitis and atopic dermatitis with different distributions. Questions arise whether artificial intelligence (AI) models with convolutional neural networks (CNNs) trained on images and data derived from the adult population should be used in the case of a child patient. Pediatric dermatology often involves distinct clinical characteristics and skin conditions. Firstly, there are many inflammatory dermatoses that have different distributions between children and adults, such as atopic dermatitis. In the case of children, there is a higher prevalence of dermatitis in the eyelid, auricular area, and ventral wrist while hand eczema tends to be localized to the dorsal hands and ventral wrists, presenting with acute or subacute lesions. On the contrary, adults with atopic dermatitis usually present with chronic lesions on the dorsal hands, including dorsal lichenoid papules, lichenification, and knuckle dermatitis [1]. In the AI field of atopic dermatitis, there are many examples of studies that evaluated the severity of the disease. A recent study evaluated deep learning models for automated atopic dermatitis severity scoring using a dataset of Indonesian individuals. The dataset of clinical images was collected from 250 patients and

E. Karampinis (✉)
Second Dermatology Department, School of Health Sciences, Aristotle University of Thessaloniki, Thessaloniki, Greece

Department of Dermatology, Faculty of Medicine, School of Health Sciences, University General Hospital of Larissa, University of Thessaly, Larissa, Greece

O. Toli
Department of Dermatology, Oncoderm Center One Day Clinic, Ioannina, Greece

E. Karampinis et al. (eds.), *Artificial Intelligence Applications in Dermatology*,
https://doi.org/10.1007/978-3-032-15614-3_21

labeled by dermatologists as mild, moderate, severe, or none based only on adult atopic dermatitis patients. Five pretrained CNN architectures were evaluated, namely ResNet50, VGGNet19, MobileNetV3, MnasNet, and EfficientNetB0. Among the models, ResNet50 emerged as the most proficient in terms of precision, sensitivity, and specificity [2]. Consequently, this model is not anticipated to achieve the same high performance when images with atopic children are presented due to the abovementioned clinical differences. Also, this example outlines that dermatologists should know and understand exactly the way an AI model that they use is trained to avoid malpractice.

Additionally, differences can also be detected among dermoscopy images. For example, dermoscopy of nevus patterns varies with age. Childhood is a dynamic phase for nevus development, during which new nevi emerge, grow, and eventually regress. In children, common nevi often exhibit peripheral dots and clods, which tend to disappear over time as the lesions enlarge. Also, other nevus types can be found in children. Halo nevi initially display a central globular pattern, gradually fading during follow-up. The globular pattern is the most prevalent dermoscopic pattern in childhood, with nevi transitioning from a globular to a reticular pattern over the years [3]. Research by Zalaudek et al. identified the globular pattern as the most frequent, followed by complex, reticular, and homogeneous patterns. Furthermore, the dermoscopic characteristics of nevi are influenced by factors such as body location, phenotype, melanoma risk, and age [3], and those parameters should be considered as well when using an AI model. The lack of further classification regarding those parameters in the training of CNNs may lead to overgenerosity and, finally, to false predictions.

Another challenging nevus type that needs to be considered in the child population is the Spitz nevus. A younger age is generally associated with Spitz nevi, which tend to exhibit benign behavior. Spitz tumors typically arise between ages 10 and 20, and their differentiation from melanoma is heavily influenced by the patient's age. Pigmented Spitz nevi, also known as Reed's nevi, present distinct dermoscopic patterns, most commonly the starburst or globular pattern (Fig. 21.1). The starburst pattern features diffuse blue-to-black pigmentation extending into radial streaks at

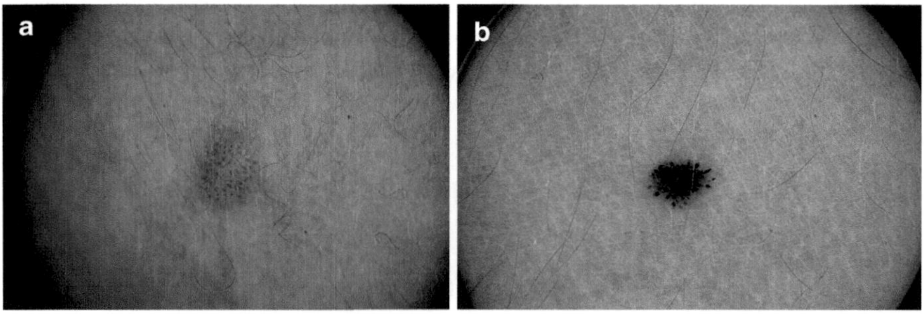

Fig. 21.1 Image presenting Spitz nevus dermoscopy. (**a**) A predominantly light brown color with a distinct reticulated (net-like) pattern. (**b**) A Spitz nevus characterized by a prominent globular pattern. The center of the lesion displays a dense cluster of dark brown to black globules

the periphery, creating a stellate appearance. In contrast, the globular pattern is marked by prominent brown to gray-blue pigmentation, surrounded by a peripheral rim of discrete pigment globules [4].

Apart from diagnosis and severity assessment, AI models that provide treatment guidance must adopt their recommendations according to the suggested guidelines respecting the age-specific physiological differences, such as metabolism, organ development, and hormonal changes in the child patient. The importance including pediatric images of lesions was indicated in the study by Mehta et al. In this study, the researchers trained one model exclusively on adult lesions and another on both adult and pediatric image lesions, adding to the previous dataset of images and also images from pediatric patients. The two AI models were compared with both adult and child images not used for training. The addition of images from the pediatric population did not impact performance in adults while it improved its efficacy when used in the case of a child patient. Such a strategy is very important as the use of a dataset in improving automated diagnostic performance adding specific population images without changing algorithm can maintain performance on the original dataset and make other diagnostic improvements [5].

21.2 AI and Skin Diseases in the Elderly Populations

The impact of AI in dermatology for aged patients is evident in numerous studies that highlight the high performance of different AI models in various aspects of skin diseases, including skin cancer and mimickers, autoimmune blistering diseases like bullous pemphigoid, and skin aging processes. However, managing these conditions in elderly patients can be further complicated by the presence of multiple comorbidities, the use of numerous medications, and socioeconomic pressures [6]. Age is a piece of information that represents an important input in the AI model. In examples of texts to large language models, different age reports in the same clinical scenarios and lesion descriptions give different differential diagnoses. Karampinis et al. combined dermoscopic image descriptions with additional patient characteristics such as age, phototype, or immune status. More precisely, the descriptions also included comparisons between patients aged 20 and 70, those with lighter and darker skin types, and immunocompetent individuals versus those under immunosuppression. The differential diagnosis is modified to reflect the lesion types relevant to each group. For example, in elderly patients, the differential diagnosis included more skin cancer subtypes and lesions like seborrheic and actinic keratosis, which are common in this population. Additionally, atypical Spitz nevus, often found in younger patients, was also included. In the third scenario, the chatbot-generated list remained unchanged for both young and elderly patients [7].

According to Valencia Long, the challenges of dermatology in elderly patients can be divided into three sections: life expectancy and treatment to benefit, preexisting comorbidities, and functional status of elderly patients and prescription practices [8]. Regarding the first parameter, doctors should consider whether it is appropriate to biopsy or excise or follow up a lesion in an older patient, taking into account the possible complications in each procedure. The AI-promoted personalized treatment is quite promising in this field, as well as predictive models that would help in the prognosis of the lesion. For example, if you ask a large language model how you approach an elderly patient with BCC who is taking antiplatelet medication compared to one who do not, the chatbot answer would highlight that surgery is linked with a high bleeding risk, the coordination with the cardiologist, preop planning with possible blood thinner hold, as well as preferred option being Mohs excision, topical treatment, and radiation. The info provided is correct, but, in clinical practice, more medical history needs to be considered such as the site of cancer, BCC subtype, and preferences of the patient. An AI model trained on the correlations between elderly patient treatment planning and outcome would be extremely helpful in the management of those patients. However, in terms of healthcare systems, this approach can be rather challenging.

In the study of AljoHani, the researcher used fuzzy logic technique; more precisely, they converted numbers and accuracy scores into linguistic categories such as "very poor," "poor", "fair," "good," "very good," and "excellent" statements to handle inaccuracies and personal views. Then, they used matrices in the categories of efficacy, safety, and cost and utilized VIKOR fuzzy method with these linguistic categories to construct a max–max normalization category (maximization of the value of positive criteria) and max–min normalization category (minimization of the value of negative criteria). The balanced comparison that occurred was used to select the most optimal treatment considering both benefits and drawbacks [9]. Another example of the importance of AI-calculated prognosis in elderly patients is actinic keratosis, which are potential precursors to squamous cell carcinomas that can be self-resolved in about 25% of cases. In cases of elderly patients with numerous actinic keratoses, clinicians may use AI-assisted prognosis tools to monitor these lesions, expecting self-resolution in some cases and choosing more effectively that need further intervention [10].

Elderly patients may have comorbidities and mobility limitations that impact both their treatment options and overall disease risk. Caregivers may use AI to get instructions on how to take images of specific sites of interest and when it is appropriate to ask for further medical assistance. Telemedicine with further AI integrations can also be utilized by elderly patients; however, the need for technological equipment should be considered. The clinician should confirm that the patient has understood how to use a certain application and that the decision to incorporate such technology in their care serves the goal of better medical practice and patient health improvement well. AI in prescribing systems can modify the medication management cycle. In the past, identifying new comorbidities or medications was more time-consuming with paper-based records. However, an AI-organized system by combining telehealth, billing, scheduling, reporting, and e-prescriptions would change healthcare for the better, saving elderly patients time with fewer delays and better outcomes. AI-enabled systems also automatically flag potential drug–drug interactions, aiding dermatologists in safer prescribing. By predicting the interactions between drugs and specific proteins, AI systems can provide guidance for the design and discovery of new drugs for the elderly [11].

Drug interactions are a common and complex challenge in elderly patients. Regarding studies on AI contributions to this topic, sequence model-based methods have been used. Those machine learning tools were built to understand patterns in ordered data such as drug administration, timing, and content such as age and disease. Drug–target interaction was studied with the use of the Intermolecular Graph Transformer (IGT), a model that better correlates how chemical bonding patterns, ring structures, and polarity interactions of molecules interact by using a specialized transformer design, which captures complex, nonlinear relations. It significantly outperforms existing methods in predicting how well and how accurately drugs bind to their targets, even when only sequence information is used [12–14]. There are also deep learning models that specialize in graph-structured data of drugs through graph neural network (GNN) to predict their interactions. Deep generative models such as variational autoencoders (VAEs) (AI models that learn to compress and reconstruct data while they can generate similar new data based on their training), generative adversarial networks (GANs) (models that use two networks, a generator and a discriminator, that "compete" to produce realistic new samples), and diffusion models (models that generate data by reversing a noise-adding process, producing outputs). Mixed models were also used. Those models would not only give more flexibility to multimedication patients and also lead to the creation of new treatments [15].

Drug interactions have also been evaluated by more accessible AI tools such as online large language models. Performance metrics of various AI tools, including Microsoft Bing AI, ChatGPT-3.5, ChatGPT-4, and Bard, are compared to drugs.com as a benchmark. Bing AI demonstrated the highest accuracy, surpassing Google's Bard, ChatGPT-3.5, and ChatGPT-4. The results emphasize the considerable potential of these AI tools to transform patient care; however, their limitations should always be considered. Also, drug-specific interaction accuracy was reported. For example, ChatGPT-4 demonstrated better results in the case of interactions regarding azithromycin rather than clarithromycin [16].

An example of an AI app that controls specific drug interactions is Warfa-Check. Warfa-Check is a bilingual AI-powered web application designed for both Arabic and English speakers. It assists users in identifying possible drug interactions related to warfarin through an easy-to-use interface that supports text, image, or voice inputs. The AI model was developed using Python and Flask, Warfa-Check integrates OpenAI's GPT-4 API and advanced natural language processing tools, enabling accurate interpretation of warfarin-related interactions. The code and all programming scripts can be accessed through https://github.com/Xor01/warfa-check. Figure 21.2 A shows the app's front page containing the name of the app (Warfa-Check) and a title describing its features. The user can choose file upload and use a picture of their medication to check if there are possible harmful interactions [17]. Indeed, studies have shown that quercetin and curcumin can cause food–drug interactions with warfarin, and the combination of multiple compounds in a "cocktail effect" can further amplify these interactions, increasing the risk of adverse outcomes [18].

Fig. 21.2 A 69-year-old man with atrial fibrillation on stable warfarin therapy asks about taking a curcumin supplement for psoriasis as he read the anti-inflammatory effects of this supplement in an article online. The clinician can check the possible interaction between the drug and the supplement on the AI app as shown in the figure

A AI-Check
Check if the medicine or herb affects your blood clotting medication
Upload a photo of the medicine or herb:
Enter the name of the medicine or herb:
Start talking:
Use your voice:

B Result for: Curcumin

Curcumin, yes, it affects blood clotting. Risk level: high

References

1. Özcelik S, Kulac I, Yazici M, Ocal E. Distribution of childhood skin diseases according to age and gender, a single institution experience. Turk Pediatri Ars. 2018;53:105–12. https://doi.org/10.5152/TurkPediatriArs.2018.6431.
2. Maulana A, Noviandy TR, Suhendra R, Earlia N, Bulqiah M, Idroes GM, et al. Evaluation of atopic dermatitis severity using artificial intelligence. Narra J. 2023;3:e511. https://doi.org/10.52225/narra.v3i3.511.
3. Zalaudek I, Catricalà C, Moscarella E, Argenziano G. What dermoscopy tells us about nevogenesis. J Dermatol. 2011;38:16–24. https://doi.org/10.1111/j.1346-8138.2010.01141.x.
4. Sainz-Gaspar L, Sánchez-Bernal J, Noguera-Morel L, Hernández-Martín A, Colmenero I, Torrelo A. Nevo de Spitz y otros tumores spitzoides en la infancia. Parte 1: aspectos clínicos, histológicos e inmunohistoquímicos. Actas Dermosifiliogr. 2020;111:7–19. https://doi.org/10.1016/j.ad.2019.02.011.
5. Mehta PP, Sun M, Betz-Stablein B, Halpern A, Soyer HP, Weber J, et al. Improving artificial intelligence–based diagnosis on pediatric skin lesions. J Invest Dermatol. 2023;143:1423–1429.e1. https://doi.org/10.1016/j.jid.2022.08.058.
6. Linos E, Chren M-M, Covinsky K. Geriatric dermatology—a framework for caring for older patients with skin disease. JAMA Dermatol. 2018;154:757. https://doi.org/10.1001/jamadermatol.2018.0286.
7. Karampinis E, Toli O, Georgopoulou K-E, Kampra E, Spyridonidou C, Roussaki Schulze A-V, et al. Can artificial intelligence “hold” a dermoscope?—the evaluation of an artificial intelligence chatbot to translate the dermoscopic language. Diagnostics. 2024;14:1165. https://doi.org/10.3390/diagnostics14111165.
8. Long V. Is artificial intelligence useful in the practice of geriatric dermatology? Clin Dermatol. 2024;42:443–6. https://doi.org/10.1016/j.clindermatol.2024.06.012.
9. Aljohani A. AI-driven decision-making for personalized elderly care: a fuzzy MCDM-based framework for enhancing treatment recommendations. BMC Med Inform Decis Mak. 2025;25:119. https://doi.org/10.1186/s12911-025-02953-5.

10. Balcere A, Konrāde-Jilmaza L, Pauliņa LA, Čēma I, Krūmiņa A. Clinical characteristics of actinic keratosis associated with the risk of progression to invasive squamous cell carcinoma: a systematic review. J Clin Med. 2022;11:5899. https://doi.org/10.3390/jcm11195899.
11. Bajwa J, Munir U, Nori A, Williams B. Artificial intelligence in healthcare: transforming the practice of medicine. Future Healthc J. 2021;8:e188–94. https://doi.org/10.7861/fhj.2021-0095.
12. Liu S, Wang Y, Deng Y, He L, Shao B, Yin J, et al. Improved drug–target interaction prediction with intermolecular graph transformer. Brief Bioinform. 2022;23 https://doi.org/10.1093/bib/bbac162.
13. Asfand-e-yar M, Hashir Q, Shah AA, Malik HAM, Alourani A, Khalil W. Multimodal CNN-DDI: using multimodal CNN for drug to drug interaction associated events. Sci Rep. 2024;14:4076. https://doi.org/10.1038/s41598-024-54409-x.
14. Wang W, Liang S, Yu M, Liu D, Zhang H, Wang X, et al. GCHN-DTI: predicting drug-target interactions by graph convolution on heterogeneous networks. Methods. 2022;206:101–7. https://doi.org/10.1016/j.ymeth.2022.08.016.
15. Lopez-Alvis J, Laloy E, Nguyen F, Hermans T. Deep generative models in inversion: the impact of the generator's nonlinearity and development of a new approach based on a variational autoencoder. Comput Geosci. 2021;152:104762. https://doi.org/10.1016/j.cageo.2021.104762.
16. Al-Ashwal FY, Zawiah M, Gharaibeh L, Abu-Farha R, Bitar AN. Evaluating the sensitivity, specificity, and accuracy of ChatGPT-3.5, ChatGPT-4, Bing AI, and bard against conventional drug-drug interactions clinical tools. Drug Healthc Patient Saf. 2023;15:137–47. https://doi.org/10.2147/DHPS.S425858.
17. Alsultan MA, Alabdulmuhsin M, AlBunyan D. Development of an artificial intelligence-enhanced warfarin interaction checker platform. PLOS Digit Health. 2025;4:e0000756. https://doi.org/10.1371/journal.pdig.0000756.
18. Burkina V, Zamaratskaia G, Rasmussen MK. Curcumin and quercetin modify warfarin-induced regulation of porcine CYP1A2 and CYP3A expression and activity *in vitro*. Xenobiotica. 2022;52:435–41. https://doi.org/10.1080/00498254.2022.2089932.

22 Artificial Intelligence and Special Populations: Skin of Color Considerations

Nkechi Anne Enechukwu and Divinefavour Echezona Malachy

22.1 Current AI Tools and Their Performance in Skin of Color

Skin of color (SoC), also known as ethnic skin, traditionally refers to that of persons of African, Asian, Native American, Middle Eastern, and Hispanic backgrounds. The color of the skin matters to the artificial intelligence (AI) for two main reasons. Firstly, convolutional neural networks (CNN) start off by converting the images into numerical data based on color and pixel densities; hence, the background color of the skin affects how the AI interprets the image it is presented with. Secondly, persons with Fitzpatrick skin phototypes IV–VI typically belong to particular races, geographical regions, and different climates. This translates to different skin norms and differences in the epidemiology of dermatological diseases. For instance, the honeycomb pigment pattern is typically associated with people of Fitzpatrick IV–VI and in sun-exposed areas. Testing dermoscopic images from such skin on models trained on types I–III will likely produce poor sensitivities and specificities. Variations in the presentation of the same disease in different skin color types are also well documented. Basal carcinoma is usually pigmented in darker skin phototypes. Furthermore, in skin of color (SoC), squamous cell carcinomas more commonly occur in non-sun-exposed areas such as the lower extremities and anogenital region, where non-UV-related etiologic factors—such as chronic inflammation and scarring—play a significant role. Melanomas are more of the acral lentiginous type, and postinflammatory hyperpigmentation from inflammatory dermatoses like acne is quite common [1].

Various artificial intelligence tools are presently available for use in dermatology, encompassing both ongoing research and commercially available applications. These tools are designed to perform a range of functions, from analyzing

N. A. Enechukwu (✉) · D. E. Malachy
Dermatology Unit, Department of Internal Medicine, Faculty of Medicine, Nnamdi Azikiwe University, Nnewi, Nigeria

E. Karampinis et al. (eds.), *Artificial Intelligence Applications in Dermatology*,
https://doi.org/10.1007/978-3-032-15614-3_22

dermatological images, for example, SkinVision, to assisting in suggesting research topics based on the identified patient as demonstrated by Kim et al. [2]. Current dermatology AI models perform significantly worse on images of darker skin tones and uncommon diseases due to a lack of diversity in training datasets [3]. This is attributable to the limited representation of the unique features of skin diseases in SoC in datasets and concerns about the quality and standardization of the images used [4].

Interestingly, dermatologists, who often provide labels for AI training datasets, also exhibited decreased diagnostic accuracy on images of darker skin tones and uncommon diseases. This suggests that the observed biases are not solely algorithmic but may also reflect broader challenges in clinical practice [4].

Additionally, the Fitzpatrick skin type (FST) classification, which is used by most AI models, is limited in its ability to capture the full range of skin tone variations, even within the narrower spectrum of types IV–VI.

22.1.1 Dermatological Image Analysis and Diagnoses in Cutaneous Malignancies

A substantial portion of AI research in dermatology is concentrated on image classification. In dermatologic malignancies, the primary aim is typically to classify skin lesions based on their potential for malignancy. This mirrors the increasing incidence of cutaneous melanoma in the general population, although the death rate has decreased, partly due to earlier diagnoses facilitated by increased awareness and prompt intervention. The integration of advanced dermatological image analysis techniques significantly improves diagnostic precision and clinical outcomes, particularly in the nuanced evaluation of skin conditions in individuals with skin of color. However, individuals with skin of color continue to be diagnosed at more advanced stages, resulting in lower survival rates and generally poorer outcomes when compared to the overall population.

Diverse training methodologies and classification techniques have been applied. Frequently utilized models include those based on the Squeeze-and-Excitation Network (SENet). These models are considered more sophisticated image processors and are particularly beneficial because they emphasize informative features while suppressing extraneous noise. This characteristic is thought to partially mitigate the issue of varying background skin pigmentation, which might otherwise be interpreted as noise, especially in dermoscopic images. The mechanism is deemed particularly suitable for analyzing dermoscopic images of lesions. Nevertheless, some applications are intended for use by patients, who typically possess phone cameras, not dermoscopes. Using phone cameras introduces additional factors like user proficiency, skin folds, and debris that could potentially distract the model [5]. Another commonly used model is GoogleNet (including Inception 1 and Inception 3). These models offer the advantage of executing multiple convolutions of varying sizes concurrently, thereby reducing the computational time and resources needed. This efficiency makes them well-suited for deployment on mobile applications, which are more accessible to the general public. A notable shared drawback of these models is their training data bias, which heavily favors fairer skin types, potentially leading to overgeneralization when applied to skin of color. Other significant challenges to their application in skin of color include insufficient representation of colored skin in validation research and accessibility issues. Currently, the issue of underrepresentation is receiving increased attention. Inclusion of Fitzpatrick skin types IV–VI in studies has gradually improved, with some recent research including approximately 10% of these skin types. Many researchers now stipulate specific proportions of skin types required for validating a tool. Despite this, even in studies that included skin of color, the representation of darker phototypes (Fitzpatrick V and VI) remained limited. There is also a problem with regional bias [4, 5].

It is important to note that AI models have not yet been widely explored for diagnosing many dermatological conditions commonly seen in individuals with skin of color. However, foot ulcers are an exception, having received comparatively more attention in AI-based diagnostic studies. While these developments are promising in theory, their performance might be suboptimal in real clinical environments. A field study in dermatology found that AI systems demonstrated poor performance when diagnosing skin lesions in clinical settings that involve the presence of "artifacts." Specifically in skin of color, inflammatory conditions frequently exhibit pigment incontinence and reactive sclerotic changes, which can introduce these artifacts and impede accurate diagnosis.

22.1.2 Generative AI and Skin of Color

AI models have also been employed to create images of various skin lesions. These generated images are typically used for educational purposes, such as illustrating disease characteristics for students or training diagnostic AI models. A study of these generative models indicated that skin of color was underrepresented in the images produced [6]. This is thought to be linked to the unequal representation of skin of color in the training datasets used. Figure 22.1 provides an example illustrating these challenges.

22.1.3 Colorimetric Diagnosis in Skin of Color

There are now applications that attempt to perform colorimetric diagnoses using smartphone cameras, such as counting pulse rates or detecting cutaneous signs like cyanosis and jaundice based on skin color changes. These applications face numerous obstacles, including the status of the phone's flash, automatic camera settings (like ISO, aperture, shutter speed), ambient lighting conditions, and crucially, the skin tone of the individual.

Despite these challenges, research is underway to address them. Chen et al. developed a robust Correction System for Oximeter Accuracy designed to manage variations in skin color [7]. By deriving a parameter that strongly correlates for sample quantification, they enabled real-time imaging, which takes the initial steps toward transforming a mobile phone camera into an analytical instrument,

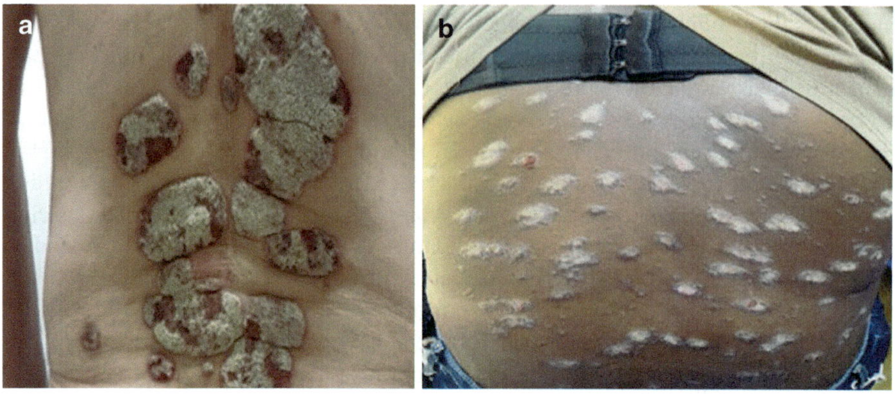

Fig. 22.1 Images (**a**) and (**b**) provide real-world cases between white and dark-skinned individuals with psoriasis

regardless of the phone model, software, or operating system. They showed its clinical utility by imaging patient skin, facilitating quick and convenient diagnosis of cyanosis and measurement of local oxygen concentration with sufficient accuracy for clinical decision-making regarding cardiovascular disease and anemia. Importantly, they demonstrated that their solution accounts for differences in individual skin tones across the Fitzpatrick scale, thereby overcoming potential clinically significant errors in current optical oximetry.

Another study proposed a novel approach utilizing 1D convolutional neural networks (1D-CNN) to estimate bilirubin levels using photos from children, with particular interest at those with early jaundice [8]. This method involves extracting color channel data (RGB, HSV, LAB, and YCbCr) from infant images. Initially, each channel was treated as a time-series input for a 1D-CNN model to predict bilirubin levels via regression. Subsequently, RGB feature maps were combined with those derived from HSV, LAB, and YCbCr channels to enhance prediction performance. The effectiveness was evaluated using RMSE, R-squared, and MAE. The best-performing model was also adapted for classifying jaundice status. The results indicated that the integration of RGB and HSV color spaces yielded the best performance, with an RMSE of 1.13 and an R-squared score of 0.91. This is just a few approaches to this problem [7, 8]. Such approaches, when refined and skin of color accounted for, can have a significant impact on the neonatal outcome of jaundiced children in resource-limited areas like Africa.

22.2 Current Limitations in the Application of AI Dermatology Models to Skin of Color

A primary obstacle identified is the underrepresentation of diverse skin types within the datasets used to train artificial intelligence models. AI relies on recognizing and predicting based on observed patterns; therefore, training datasets need to be substantially inclusive of various skin types for accurate performance across the population. A recent review of 70 studies focusing on image-based AI algorithms for classifying skin conditions found that only a small proportion, specifically 14 (20%), provided details about the race of participants, and an even smaller number, just seven (10%), detailed the skin color. Furthermore, only three of these studies included populations falling under Fitzpatrick skin types IV–VI, and even then, only partially. This lack of diversity in studies is believed to stem from a shortage of publicly accessible datasets that are sufficiently diverse [9]. A systematic review of 39 open-access datasets and skin atlases reported that out of the 14 datasets that mentioned the country of origin, 12 were from countries where the population is predominantly of European ancestry. Given that AI tools are being deployed globally, there is a clear requirement for the creation of more inclusive, open-access datasets specifically targeted to encompass colored skin [5].

Another critical issue pertains to validation bias and the problem of overfitting. The validation research used to test these AI applications often suffers from bias, as most validations, including some showcased on application websites, are conducted on nonpigmented skin. A significant concern arises because most AI algorithms have only been tested using internal datasets—meaning data sampled from the same or very similar populations they were trained on. AI algorithms are susceptible to overfitting, which means they become very good at interpreting the specific data they were trained on but perform poorly when presented with new data from a different source. Overfitting can lead to inflated accuracy measurements when tested only on internal datasets, followed by a substantial drop in performance when exposed to images from a different source. The absence of a standardized model for measuring performance, a lack of publicly available diverse datasets for testing, inconsistent test interfaces, and limited reader studies collectively create barriers to comparing and reproducing the results of AI algorithms effectively. A suggested alternative solution is to evaluate algorithms on standardized public test datasets, maintaining transparency about the algorithm's performance. Testing models on external datasets or images that are "out-of-distribution" (different from the training data) provides a better indication of how the AI model will perform in a real-world clinical setting. Given that public dermoscopic datasets containing diverse skin colors are now becoming available, future algorithms should adopt external testing as the gold standard for evaluation [10].

Beyond the technical data challenges, there are also cost and infrastructure issues. While cost and ease of use are recognized barriers, authors highlight other important considerations for developing mobile health apps for skin cancer screening that may not have been fully anticipated by researchers or dermatologists. A study suggests that people in the Netherlands might be more likely to use mobile health apps for skin cancer screening if the development process is transparent, the developers are seen as trustworthy, and health professionals and regulatory bodies endorse the apps [11]. These insights are particularly vital considering that melanoma incidences remain high and are increasing across Europe, even with existing prevention strategies at both public and policy levels.

Poor image quality and acquisition challenges also significantly impact the performance of AI models. The quality of the images used for both training and testing AI models is crucial, as it is determined by factors like the camera quality and the skill level of the person taking the picture, which directly affects how the model performs in the field. Low image quality includes issues such as low resolution, the presence of noise, or a small dynamic range where details in very dark or very bright areas are lost. Studies have shown that iPhones performed better than Android devices. It is also important to investigate performance variations within the Android ecosystem, especially because recent high-end Android phone processors are specifically designed to run AI models more effectively. Exploring this aspect would allow companies developing these tools to recommend minimum technical specifications. This is particularly important for regions with colored skin where the market share of iPhones is not as high [11].

Finally, ethical and regulatory concerns present a significant limitation. There is growing worry about the emergence of fake applications that make misleading claims. Some apps, such as MelApp and Mole Detective, which claimed to diagnose skin cancers, were found to be largely inaccurate and were compelled by the U.S. Federal Trade Commission to stop making these claims. Individuals from poor socioeconomic backgrounds, including many people of color, particularly in Africa, are especially vulnerable to being targeted by such predatory applications. In response to these issues, the Medicines and Healthcare Products Regulatory Agency (MHRA) in 2024 ruled that any application asserting that it helps diagnose a medical condition must be classified as a medical device [11]. As a medical device, it is required to comply with EU safety and performance standards. This means that the CE mark, which indicates compliance with these EU safety standards, must be clearly displayed either on the app itself or on the developer's website. The presence of largely inaccurate apps poses serious risks, potentially leading to misdiagnoses and delays in individuals seeking necessary healthcare.

22.3 Future Directions

There is a clear need to collect more accurate metadata alongside images. Ultimately, the sources conclude that while efforts like dataset diversification, improved model validation protocols, and advanced data augmentation are underway, the underrepresentation of Fitzpatrick skin types IV–VI, lack of regional data diversity, and validation biases collectively hinder AI tool reliability for these populations, risking the exacerbation of existing health disparities if biased tools are globally deployed. Therefore, there is a pressing need for intentional, community-driven collaborations such as targeted campaigns for hard-to-reach groups and continuous professional development (CPD) for GPs to create a better understanding of unintentional biases and awareness of skin lesions among POC. Priorities must include inclusive research designs, ethical app development practices, robust regulatory oversight, and ensuring representation of skin of color in both the datasets used and the personnel developing these tools. Only through such dedicated and sustained efforts can AI in dermatology truly evolve into an inclusive and globally applicable solution that genuinely enhances care for all skin types. An increased database of expert-confirmed diagnoses across a variety of skin tones.

References

1. Kundu RV, Patterson S. Dermatologic conditions in skin of color: part I. Special considerations for common skin disorders. Am Fam Physician. 2013;87:850–6.
2. Kim J, Chen ML, Rezaei SJ, Ramirez-Posada M, Caswell-Jin JL, Kurian AW, et al. Patient-centered research through artificial intelligence to identify priorities in cancer care. JAMA Oncol. 2025; https://doi.org/10.1001/jamaoncol.2025.0694.
3. Daneshjou R, Vodrahalli K, Novoa RA, Jenkins M, Liang W, Rotemberg V, et al. Disparities in dermatology AI performance on a diverse, curated clinical image set. Sci Adv. 2022;8 https://doi.org/10.1126/sciadv.abq6147.
4. Fliorent R, Fardman B, Podwojniak A, Javaid K, Tan IJ, Ghani H, et al. Artificial intelligence in dermatology: advancements and challenges in skin of color. Int J Dermatol. 2024;63:455–61. https://doi.org/10.1111/ijd.17076.
5. Wen D, Khan SM, Ji Xu A, Ibrahim H, Smith L, Caballero J, et al. Characteristics of publicly available skin cancer image datasets: a systematic review. Lancet Digit Health. 2022;4:e64–74. https://doi.org/10.1016/S2589-7500(21)00252-1.
6. Sakunchotpanit G, Nayudu K, Chen R, Milosavljevic S, Rohan TZ, Ortiz-López L, et al. Representations of skin tone and sex in dermatology by generative artificial intelligence: a comparative study. Clin Exp Dermatol. 2025; https://doi.org/10.1093/ced/llaf126.
7. Chen J, Zhao D, Shi H-W, Duan Q, Jajesniak P, Li Y, et al. Inclusive and accurate clinical diagnostics using intelligent computation and smartphone imaging. ACS Sens. 2024;9:5342–53. https://doi.org/10.1021/acssensors.4c01588.
8. Salami FO, Muzammel M, Mourchid Y, Othmani A. Artificial intelligence non-invasive methods for neonatal jaundice detection: a review. Artif Intell Med. 2025;162:103088. https://doi.org/10.1016/j.artmed.2025.103088.
9. Liu Y, Primiero CA, Kulkarni V, Soyer HP, Betz-Stablein B. Artificial intelligence for the classification of pigmented skin lesions in populations with skin of color: a systematic review. Dermatology. 2023;239:499–513. https://doi.org/10.1159/000530225.
10. Chlap P, Min H, Vandenberg N, Dowling J, Holloway L, Haworth A. A review of medical image data augmentation techniques for deep learning applications. J Med Imaging Radiat Oncol. 2021;65:545–63. https://doi.org/10.1111/1754-9485.13261.
11. Sangers TE, Wakkee M, Kramer-Noels EC, Nijsten T, Lugtenberg M. Views on mobile health apps for skin cancer screening in the general population: an in-depth qualitative exploration of perceived barriers and facilitators*. Br J Dermatol. 2021;185:961–9. https://doi.org/10.1111/bjd.20441.

Can Artificial Intelligence Replace Dermatologists?

23

Emmanouil Karampinis, Dimitrios Mantzaris, and Anna Mavrophorou

23.1 Can AI Replace Dermatologists? Dermatologists' Point of View

It is challenging for a dermatologist to be asked whether the profession that they love so much can be replaced by artificial intelligence (AI) technology. Also, it is known that we worked really hard to gain, with many sacrifices made and significant investments in time and money. We surely are concerned about the increasing use of more and more effective and capable AI technology tools and apps that are advertised and can outperform our experience by analyzing an image in just a few seconds. However, the experience gained by the cases and patients we have encountered, as well as the unique characteristics of the patient we have in front of us, gives us an advantage that AI cannot possess—the real-time and personal interaction between a dermatologist and a patient.

If you had asked me 5 years ago (2020), I would have answered this question as definitely no, considering that AI would never achieve such diagnostic capabilities. If you ask me now, I will answer as perhaps yes or it is possible due to the studies that occur based mainly on CNN programs performing better than experienced

E. Karampinis (✉)
Second Dermatology Department, School of Health Sciences, Aristotle University of Thessaloniki, Thessaloniki, Greece

Department of Dermatology, Faculty of Medicine, School of Health Sciences, University General Hospital of Larissa, University of Thessaly, Larissa, Greece

D. Mantzaris
Computational Intelligence and Health Informatics Lab, Nursing Department, School of Health Sciences, University of Thessaly, Larissa, Greece
e-mail: dmantzar@uth.gr

A. Mavrophorou
Deontology and Bioethics Laboratory, Faculty of Nursing, School of Health Sciences, University of Thessaly, Larissa, Greece

E. Karampinis et al. (eds.), *Artificial Intelligence Applications in Dermatology*,
https://doi.org/10.1007/978-3-032-15614-3_23

dermatologists based on dermoscopy images. Clinical practice, however, is not a study reality. We need to encounter complex studies in a limited time period and not in controlled conditions such as those based on an experiment protocol or a research setting. The dermatologist may also feel certain times as every human being, may be angry or stressed, and those feelings may affect his or her judgment ability to recognize a lesion or dermatosis. Also, the clinician is more likely to make rushed decisions and not conduct a thorough assessment. AI is not affected by those parameters—and this is its greatest advantage—not being human, serving a task without feelings based only on calculations, but this is also its greatest disadvantage—as the empathy and patient need of a human-to-human reassurance is an important part of the treatment approach. We can see doctors who create trust in patients and others who do not—imagine having this concept with AI. Maybe in the future we will see different companies' chatbots to be more persuasive than dermatologists on what treatment plan they suggest.

The last prediction is just an example of how AI application use without restrictions may get beyond control not only for our patients' health protection but also for our specialty preservation. AI systems should be evaluated regularly as continuous adjustments and updates, or new versions may diminish their performance. A committee comprising expert dermatologists can identify possible deviations and alert the responsible company so that the best performance level is maintained. Also, ethical oversight is important in this new AI reality. We upload many images daily—being dermoscopic or macroscopic—to AI assessment software, but we do not know where and to whom those images end up. Would you upload an image of your face on a website when it is not known how it will be use to produce a result? Possibly not. Knowledge of AI technology and understanding of the relationship between inputs and outputs in dermatology are crucial. Therefore, a certificate of AI dermatology based on a booklet of regulatory framework for the use of different AI forms in our specialty would be a great idea and suggestion for the future. Therefore, there are many undefined parameters that need to be addressed to control the AI integration of daily dermatology practice.

Would AI dermatology technology be allowed to be used by nondermatologists? The triage and early recognition of suspicious lesions from general practitioners or doctors without expertise and the following referral to dermatologists when needed can indeed be beneficial for patients. However, the uncontrolled and unsupervised use of AI programs by businesses can have social and financial parameters and create concern. Companies can advertise skin assessments that are performed by an AI system being handled by a technician and not a skin specialist, and this is unethical. Additionally, hospitals do not hire dermatologists based on the fact that the salary given to a dermatologist may be better invested in the purchase and maintenance of an expensive AI system, avoiding the danger of the doctor resigning or complaining due to scheduling conflicts.

Should we ask the patient in case an AI program is used during his or her assessment? I believe yes, especially if the examination contains images and AI-driven diagnosis. The patients should know every detail about how their data are being used and, therefore, may sign a consent form regarding this kind of program in the future.

In conclusion, regarding the hot question of whether AI can replace dermatologists, a subquestion may arise: Replace them in what aspect exactly? These aspects can be diagnostic accuracy, communication, or taking responsibility for medical decisions as dermatology is more than observation. However, the support of dermatologists by AI use is indeed the future of our specialty, and I strongly believe that, although dermatologists may not be replaced by AI, dermatologists who do not use AI would certainly be replaced by dermatologists who have this knowledge.

23.2 Can AI Replace Dermatologists? Bioengineers' Point of View

The rapid advancement of artificial intelligence (AI) has sparked significant interest and debate across various fields, including healthcare. One of the most intriguing questions in this domain is whether AI can replace dermatologists. Dermatology, a specialized field of medicine focused on the diagnosis and treatment of skin conditions, is particularly ripe for AI integration due to the visual nature of many skin diseases. From a bioengineer's perspective, this question involves a multifaceted analysis of technological capabilities, ethical considerations, and the unique human elements that AI may or may not replicate.

From a bioengineering standpoint, the integration of AI into dermatology represents a significant advancement in the field. AI, particularly ML and DP, has shown remarkable potential in dermatology. These technologies can analyze large datasets of skin images to identify patterns and make predictions. For instance, CNNs, a type of deep learning algorithm, have been trained to recognize various skin lesions, with accuracy comparable to that of experienced dermatologists. Studies have demonstrated that AI models can diagnose conditions such as melanoma, basal cell carcinoma, and other skin cancers with a high sensitivity and specificity.

One of the key advantages of AI in dermatology is its ability to process and analyze vast amounts of data quickly and consistently. This can lead to more efficient and accurate diagnoses, potentially reducing the workload on dermatologists and improving patient outcomes. Additionally, AI can assist in triaging patients, prioritizing those who require immediate attention and reducing the time to diagnosis.

Beyond visual diagnosis, AI can also contribute to other areas of dermatology. It can assist in teledermatology, providing remote consultations and triaging patients based on image analysis. This can be particularly beneficial in underserved areas with limited access to dermatologists. Furthermore, AI can be used to personalize treatment plans, analyzing patient data to predict treatment outcomes and optimizing therapeutic strategies. Bioengineers can develop algorithms that integrate genetic information, environmental factors, and clinical data to create personalized treatment recommendations. Moreover, AI-powered smartphone apps could enable patients to perform initial skin checks at home, reducing the burden on clinics and improving access to care in underserved regions.

Additionally, AI systems can act as decision-support tools for dermatologists, helping them analyze complex cases and reducing the likelihood of diagnostic errors. Despite the impressive progress, significant limitations prevent AI from fully replacing dermatologists. One major hurdle of AI in dermatology is its reliance on high-quality training data. AI systems are only as good as the datasets they are trained on, and biases in these datasets can lead to inaccurate or unreliable results. While AI excels in analyzing images with well-defined labels, real-world clinical scenarios are often more ambiguous. Lesions can present with atypical features, and diagnostic uncertainties are common. Dermatologists rely not only on visual assessment but also on patient history, physical examination, and even intuition gained from years of experience. This "art of diagnosis," involving subjective interpretation and contextual understanding, is currently beyond the capabilities of AI systems.

From a bioengineering perspective, while AI holds transformative potential for enhancing dermatology practice, it primarily functions as a tool that complements human expertise rather than as a complete substitute. Dermatologists possess invaluable skills that extend beyond image analysis. Their clinical experience, empathy, communication abilities, and familiarity with treatment regimens play a critical role in patient care. The ability to conduct physical examinations, assess patient histories, and address psychosocial factors remains crucial to effective dermatological practice.

Furthermore, dermatology often involves complex decision-making that integrates patient preferences, systemic considerations, and evolving treatment modalities—an area where human dermatologists thrive. AI systems currently lack the comprehensive understanding required to consider these multifaceted aspects of patient care.

In conclusion, I would answer no. Rather than viewing AI as a potential replacement for the dermatologist, it is more productive to consider its role as an augmentative tool within dermatology. By integrating AI into the diagnostic process, dermatologists can leverage the strengths of both humans and machines. AI can enhance diagnostic assessments by processing large volumes of data quickly, supporting clinicians in making more informed decisions. For instance, AI can aid in screening processes, allowing dermatologists to focus on complex cases requiring their expertise and patient interactions. The collaboration between dermatologists and AI systems could lead to more accurate diagnoses, improved patient outcomes, and a more efficient healthcare system.

23.3 Can AI Replace Dermatologists? Law Specialists' Point of View

AI is a technology that has been evolving and integrating in medical practice very fast over the last decade, providing several advantages in screening, diagnosis, and treatment of patients. Dermatology is one of the specialties in which AI has offered clear benefits by analyzing images of skin conditions, detecting patterns, and even diagnosing certain skin diseases with a high level of accuracy. Conditions like melanoma, acne, and other skin disorders may be detected by analyzing images from dermatological exams. Additionally, in combination with telemedicine, it can provide important healthcare impact in the rural and underserved areas where a shortage of dermatologists may exist.

Because of these capabilities of AI, there has been a concern that it may fully replace physicians in dermatology practice. It is inevitable that with the introduction of AI in general, several medical, legal, and theological concerns have been raised, especially when considering its potential to influence the role of human dermatologists. Nevertheless, besides its potential to play an important role, this idea is more complex and very unlikely to happen in the near future for several reasons that are elaborated below.

Regarding accuracy, reliability, and tailored treatment plans, AI is not infallible and thus may not be fully accounted for by diagnosing rare skin conditions or conditions with overlapping symptoms that require seasoned experience and deep knowledge of a dermatologist. Misdiagnosis due to such errors may lead to inappropriate treatments and patient harm, while dermatologists' reliance on AI outputs will stop them from questioning, leading to complacency or overconfidence and loss of clinical judgment. Also, it may lead to physicians' deskilling, diminishing the need for continuing education and clinical skill improvement from the physicians. Furthermore, personalized treatment plans require a more integrated approach, and it can be made by considering individual preferences, potential side effects, underlying health conditions, and psychosocial factors.

The ethical concern is an issue that cannot easily be surpassed. The cornerstone moral issue in clinical practice is the patient–doctor relationship. It is fundamental in building trust between physicians and patients, ensuring adherence to treatments, and improving outcomes. AI cannot replace this relationship as it does not have the capability to communicate effectively with patients, listen to their worries, assess their views and values, and provide them with education about their conditions and treatment options. Too much reliance on AI may erode trust, making patients feel that the human aspect of care is diminished in the healthcare system.

The legal concerns include accountability in case of malpractice. If AI makes a mistake in diagnosing skin conditions, who is liable? The dermatologist, the developers of the AI tool, or the healthcare institution that used the tool? Additionally, informed consent is fundamental in all jurisdictions. Failure to fully disclose the tools and technologies being used in the patients' care and to ensure that patients understand the limitations and capabilities of the AI system might potentially lead to legal ramifications if patients are dissatisfied with their care. The role of the physician-dermatologist in this process is of paramount importance. Finally, data privacy and security as AI systems in dermatology rely heavily on large datasets, often including sensitive patient information (such as images of skin conditions). Ensuring these datasets are securely stored and protected from breaches and unauthorized access or misuse of personal health data remains a major legal concern. Physicians hold a critical role in ensuring that their patients' datasets remain safe and, if processed, it will be in as much as possible an anonymized way. This can protect healthcare institutions from lawsuits, regulatory penalties, and damage to their trust. As there is currently a lack of uniform global standards regulating the use of AI in healthcare, governments and regulatory bodies need to create clear guidelines for its use to address safety standards, efficacy, and ethical considerations to prevent misuse or harm.

According to these, I would answer no, the ethical and legal boundaries and concerns would not allow AI technology to gain independence from medical science, including dermatology, that makes the presence of a human expert-dermatologist irreplaceable.

23.4 Can AI Replace Dermatologists? AI'S Point of View

Asking chatbots and large language models is becoming an increasingly everyday practice as it is considered more time-saving and practical to ask a specific question to a chatbot rather than searching on websites using keywords in search engines. Therefore, we asked two chatbots the same question, so the AI-created answer is reported and compared with other ones expressed by specialists (Fig. 23.1). Worth mentioning are the different arguments that each responder outlines to defend their thesis. All agree that AI cannot replace dermatologists at present. Dermatologists emphasized not only the practical difficulties but also the economic aspects that AI integration would have. Legal specialists highlighted mainly the ethical parameters and the legal responsibilities in case of medical malpractice, while AI responses provided by chatbots are based mainly on the inherent limitations of the AI technology that would never match a human doctor. All responders agree that the collaboration of AI and dermatologists would form the future of dermatologists, with the need for regulations proposed strongly by the dermatologist and law specialist.

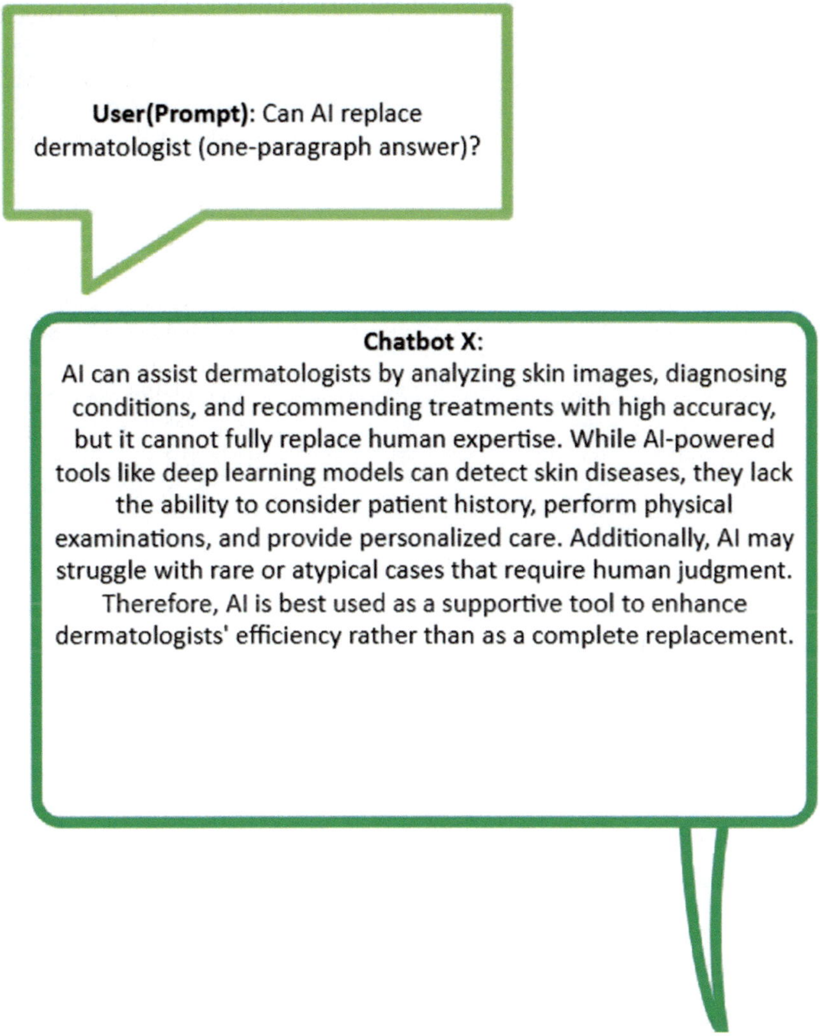

Fig. 23.1 Image displaying the answer to whether AI can replace dermatologists by a chatbot. The input containing the one-paragraph request is made to control the length of the answers. The chatbot concludes that AI would assist but not replace dermatologists based mainly on its limitations in dermatology

GPSR Compliance

The European Union's (EU) General Product Safety Regulation (GPSR) is a set of rules that requires consumer products to be safe and our obligations to ensure this.

If you have any concerns about our products, you can contact us on ProductSafety@springernature.com

In case Publisher is established outside the EU, the EU authorized representative is:

Springer Nature Customer Service Center GmbH
Europaplatz 3
69115 Heidelberg, Germany

Batch number: 10726058

Printed by Printforce, the Netherlands